Cleansing the Fatherland

Cleansing the Fatherland

NAZI MEDICINE AND RACIAL HYGIENE

By Götz Aly, Peter Chroust, and
Christian Pross

Translated by Belinda Cooper

Foreword by Michael H. Kater

The Johns Hopkins University Press
Baltimore and London

The Johns Hopkins University Press
2715 North Charles Street
Baltimore, Maryland 21218-4319
The Johns Hopkins University Press Ltd., London

ISBN 0-8018-4775-3
ISBN 0-8018-4824-5 (pbk.)

Library of Congress Cataloging-in-Publication Data will be found at the end of
this book.

A catalog record of this book is available from the British Library.

Contents

Foreword

by Michael H. Kater

In the decades after World War II, the Nuremberg Code, the Declaration of Helsinki, and the Tokyo Convention were passed, all meant to safeguard ethical standards in medicine following the hideous medical abuses perpetrated by the Nazis and the Japanese during the war. But in recent times, news about medical practices from around the world has not been good—it is as if those codes had never been passed. Newspapers and magazines have published accounts of boys not even in their teens being taken away from their homes to become bonded laborers in the Indian carpet industry, with the help of birth certificates expertly forged by village doctors. They reported that in the Canadian province of Ontario, the College of Physicians and Surgeons had been considering tough new professional ethics laws because of the many doctors who were found to have sexually molested young women and children in their care. According to these news media, physicians allegedly assisted in the post-torture care of German hostages Heinrich Strübig and Thomas Kempter in Lebanon to ensure that, despite all the ill treatment, they would not die. And apparently in Germany itself not everything is well. In the former Stasi penitentiary of Bautzen in the territory of the one-time German Democratic Republic, a prison physician allegedly remained employed even after having purposely neglected his duties in the old regime, causing physical disabilities and even death for political and other inmates. In western Germany, too, dubious medical practices seemed to prevail, locally and regionally. Hence in the psychiatric ward of Straubing Penitentiary in Bavaria, inmates were said to have been treated forcibly with drugs, a situation that Amnesty International has been investigating.

The chapters in this book painfully drive home the point that certainly as far as Germany is concerned, the lessons of the Third Reich may not yet have been learned with any degree of thoroughness. Thus, in his introductory chapter, Christian Pross mentions the emergence to prominence in post-1945 Germany of all stripes of physicians who had compromised themselves during the Nazi regime. In Chapter 3, Götz Aly tells of anatomy professor Hermann Voss, who despised Jews, Poles, and other non-"Aryans" with great fervor. In 1937 Voss tried, unsuccessfully, to advance his career at the expense of a Jewish colleague, a victim of Nazi purges. In 1941, Voss became director of the Anatomical Institute at the Nazi model university of Posen (in territory wrongfully annexed from Poland). There he rejoiced that the Gestapo had use of the institute's crematorium to incinerate the bodies of "impudent" Poles executed by the Nazis. ("Why aren't a hundred Poles . . . executed for each murdered German?") He found looking into "our ovens" to be "very comforting." According to Aly, between 1952 and 1962 Voss was a respected anatomist at the East German University of Jena and thereafter retired peacefully in Hamburg, in the West.

In chapters 2 and 4 as well, Aly writes about the Nazi murder of the handicapped, mental patients, and others deemed to represent, by Nazi standards, "useless life." His sad tale serves as background for disconcerting information that Ernst Klee, another critical German writer, has recently divulged, namely that sufferers from Nazi euthanasia to this day have not been formally recognized by the Bonn government as victims of Nazi terror. Neither have Gypsies—Sinti and Roma—regarding whose fate at Nazi hands Aly has written much in his previous publications.

Götz Aly, Ernst Klee, Christian Pross, and Peter Chroust belong to a new generation of German scholars whose declared aim is not only to uncover Nazi medical irregularities and crimes but also to identify the lack of redress of such crimes after 1945. Yet while their publications have already met with widespread acceptance among younger health-care workers, physicians, and a more enlightened reading public, they are still largely ignored by the German medical establishment. The ban applies particularly to Aly and Pross. Their courageous endeavor some years ago of founding a critical medical-history group, Verein zur Erforschung der nationalsozialistischen Gesundheits- und Sozialpolitik, was anything but hailed by the publicity organs of the medical powers that be, and it remains an idealistic rather than a commercial venture. When the two authors organized an international symposium on the occasion of the critical exhibition *Der Wert des Menschen* (The value of the human being) in West

Berlin in 1989, the event was supported only by the left-leaning Berlin chapter of the Federal Chamber of Physicians; the Cologne-based federal organization turned its back on the event. The national organization subsequently refused to assist Aly and Pross in taking the exhibition to selected West German medical schools—but could not prevent its international success a few years later in Canada, the United States, and Japan. Recognition of any kind for Aly and Pross's work will not sit well with the medical establishment's constituents, who might insist that the authors' interpretations are exaggerated or twisted out of all proportion. It is true that some of Pross and Aly's writings have been controversial in the past and will probably continue to be so for some time—partly due to emphases they place on other than the conventionally treated trouble spots, such as issues directly related to the Holocaust. But it is equally true that they have forced us to accept the existence of new problems, the formulation of new questions about them, and, in some cases, even new and plausible explanations.

Precisely because in Germany and elsewhere ignorance and abuse linger as if the Third Reich had never happened, these significant attempts by younger recruits to the larger medical establishment to change things through eye-opening reflection and analysis, however uncomfortable, deserve support. Such support should be international in scope. Hence the essays by Aly, Chroust, and Pross presented in this volume, some after translation and adaptation from the German *Beiträge zur nationalsozialistischen Gesundheits- und Sozialpolitik* originals, even if controversial, are bound to be of great interest to empathetic English-language readers, certainly to those who are capable of recognizing not only the historic German crimes but also the potential for similar or parallel occurrences in their own countries.

Peter Chroust has produced an annotated English-language version of neurologist Friedrich Mennecke's letters to his wife, Eva, written while he was a punctilious, patriotic euthanasia killer during World War II. As in the case of anatomy professor Hermann Voss, Mennecke turns out to have been a virulent hater of Jews, Communists, and racial "inferiors": "He who fights Judas saves our people and our Reich!" is Mennecke's message to his wife. When stationed in Russia, he wrote of the poverty-stricken peasants that they had been molded by "Jewish Bolshevism" and that "a single human life means as little here as in any lower order of animals." This from a man who was condemned to death at Nuremberg for the murder of at least 2,500 people in psychiatric hospitals and concentration camps. As I was reading about these men I was once again reminded that in Nazi Germany, from 1933 to 1945, a physician did not have to be dressed in an SS uniform or to perform liquidation functions in an eastern extermination camp to be recognizable as a hater of Jews and other "inferiors." In retrospect, this underscores what I found to hold true during the research for my own book on medical doctors in the Nazi regime a few years ago, namely that exactly half of the men in the profession were members of the Nazi party, and that 26 percent of them were storm troopers and over 7 percent in the SS—much higher rates than those for any other academic profession.

In contrast, the history of Jewish physicians in Germany is instructive. It is well to remember the tradition of excellent medical practice which Jewish physicians founded in Germany before the Holocaust was initiated in 1939. Not that this pre-Nazi era was one entirely free of Judeophobia, one in which Jewish physicians could do nothing but thrive. Just as the Nazi Holocaust in its wider setting had precursors, so, too, did Jewish doctors suffer from early bouts of envy, greed, and malice on the part of their Gentile colleagues.

At the end of the nineteenth century, Jewish physicians in Germany were professionalized—a process contingent on the professionalization of all German doctors as an academically educated group. This process also interacted with the final stages of the emancipation of German Jews, ultimately as a consequence of the French Revolution and Napoleon's influence on the country. Yet, ironically, in its final stages at the turn of the nineteenth century, this process evoked a new kind of anti-Semitism. Typically, in the last few decades before World War I, Jewish physicians in the Wilhelmine Empire were hated by their Gentile colleagues, both for their earning power and for their skill and their subsequent successes in treating patients. Added to this economically based envy, the pseudoscientific, racist mold of German anti-Semitism, new since the 1880s, which has rightly been associated with Social Darwinism, claimed, among other monstrosities, that Jews were bent on poisoning the blood of Gentiles through an infusion of their own. Thus, Jewish male doctors were viciously charged with sexual predation against non-Jewish female patients.

Other charges were leveled in those decades before World War I. At that time there existed an oversupply of physicians, for which the Jews were blamed. Quackery, too, was said to be caused by Jews. Gentile doctors alleged to have uncovered plots by Jewish colleagues to boycott non-Jewish physicians, and yet it was the Gentiles who were guilty of conspiracy. If possible, Jews were even to be kept out of the professional organizations. Virulently anti-Semitic deputies of the Reichstag, the national parliament, were eager to restrict the number of Jewish physicians to be licensed, if to no avail.

In the context of such forms of discrimination, it comes as no surprise that Jews were also hampered in the medical faculties. At the professorial level, despite all other manifestations of emancipation, Jewish medical scholars were kept from occupying full chairs, unless they converted. Few Jews were associate professors; most remained at the level of an economically insecure lecturer. At the University of Kiel, not even scholars with one Jewish parent could then be promoted to full professor, and in all German medical faculties, disciplines with sexual connotations or implications, such as gynecology and even surgery, were reserved for the Gentile professors.

Jewish medical students fared accordingly. In 1891, Dr. Gustav Stille, one of the more vituperative anti-Semitic physicians, lamented that one of every five medical students in Prussia—encompassing two-thirds of Germany—was a Jew and that Jewish medical students were hampering their Gentile fellows. Conflict deepened when in the decade immediately before World War I, after the aborted Russian Revolution of 1905, many young Russian Jews arrived at German universities to pursue medical studies there. By that time, every second Jewish student in the Reich was enrolled in medicine. Now efforts were renewed at governmental levels to apply quotas to Jewish students, efforts that were defeated only after Social Democratic deputies intervened.

When war broke out in August 1914, both Jewish physicians and Jewish students of medicine, thinking of themselves as the good Germans that they were, volunteered for the colors like everyone else. Without a doubt they were hoping that the war would remove the still existing injustices in society engendered by Judeophobia; however, the prejudice that held that no Jew could fit the Prussian ideal of martial masculinity was difficult to dispel.

After the defeat of the Wilhelmine Empire by 1918, the new Weimar Republic buoyed the hopes of progressive citizens that the lot of all German Jews would be improved from then on. Jewish physicians expected this to happen within their specific professional situation, for they correctly believed that the new democratic constitution supported them. On the one side, conditions did indeed get better: throughout the Weimar period, German Jewish physicians made great strides as researchers, teachers, specialists, and in general practice, and they contributed significantly to the fledgling discipline of social medicine. Yet the beginning of the republic also saw the rise of reactionary forces, who at first clamored for the return of the Wilhelmine Empire and then, by about 1923, decidedly opted for a fascist type of leadership. Their vanguard were the rabidly militaristic and increasingly illegal freecorps, and their antidemocratic tenets were determined, above all, by virulent anti-Semitism. Jew-hating physicians played key roles: they were in the front ranks of the freecorps, they helped Adolf Hitler and his National Socialists in the formulation of early party dogma, and, as Nazis at the end of the 1920s, they initiated the National Socialist German Physicians' League.

If throughout the 1920s the racial brand of anti-Semitism that had been sired by Social Darwinism, coupled with the more firmly entrenched stereotypical economic arguments, came to supplant the ancient, religious type of Judeophobia almost completely, this was to no small degree the work of these and other Nazi-beholden, racist physicians. In the forefront of them was Dr. Gerhard Wagner, a former post–World War I freecorps fighter who in 1933 institutionalized the Nazi Physicians' League within the Third Reich. When Wagner died in the spring of 1939, he was succeeded by Dr. Leonardo Conti, also with a freecorps past, who survived World War II only to be captured by the Allies and put in an isolation cell at Nuremberg to await his trial for crimes aginst humanity.

Both Wagner and Conti were personally responsible for most of the measures enacted against their Jewish colleagues between 1933 and 1945. Twenty-six hundred Jewish physicians were removed from the German medical establishment by early 1934; this translated into a reduction of the former Jewish percentage of approximately 16 percent to about 11 percent. The ousted physicians were quickly succeeded by young "Aryan" doctors. Repeated dragnets by SS and Gestapo and all manner of daily harassment forced many Jewish doctors to emigrate by 1935. Three years later, all German Jewish physicians were professionally decertified; only a small number were left to practice medicine among the remaining Jews in the Reich. After the beginning of World War II, in September 1939, the Jewish doctors still in the country fell victim to the lethal deportations to the eastern ghettos and camps, where, after brave attempts to continue their professional practice of medicine, most of them died.

In the final analysis, a demographic reckoning concerning the fate of German Jewish physicians from 1933 to 1945 is difficult because of uncertain Holocaust statistics and the relative absence of records in foreign countries. Between 1932 and 1945, anywhere from 4,500 to 6,000 Jewish physicians were expelled from Germany, which would amount to some two-thirds of all non-"Aryan" doctors. Five percent, or several hundred of all the Jewish physicians in Germany, probably committed suicide. In the end, it is safe to say that close to 2,000 Jewish doctors, meaning no fewer than one-quarter of the entire professional group, perished in the Nazi Holocaust.

The Jews are the best-known, and were the most systematically persecuted, group that fell victim to the Nazis in Germany. As Christian Pross notes in his introductory chapter, a combination of pseudoscientific racism, socioeconomic crisis, and abandonment of the ideal of physician as healer produced doctors who sterilized or killed so-called inferiors and social deviants in the name of science. And surely it does not diminish the acknowledged horrors of the Holocaust or dishonor the memory of its victims to point out, as Pross, Aly, and Chroust do, that many of these expendable individuals were non-Jewish Germans: tuberculous or handicapped children; mentally ill or retarded adults; the institutionalized elderly; the unemployed poor; prostitutes; alcoholics. Their extermination meant fewer "useless mouths" to feed, hospital beds freed for wounded German soldiers, "active" psychiatric treatment of mental patients deemed curable, and—it was hoped—greater scientific understanding of mental illness and retardation.

Who committed these crimes? As Pross states, it was not only "the tiny number of 350 black sheep among the German medical profession who were involved in medical crimes, but . . . many more were involved directly or indirectly, among them the cream of German medicine, university professors, outstanding scientists and researchers." He cites Richard Toellner, medical historian at the University of Münster, as stating in 1989: "The whole range of normal representatives of the medical profession was involved and they all knew what they were doing. . . . A medical profession that accepts mass murder of sick people as normal, and to a large degree explicitly approves of it as a necessary, justified act for the sake of the community, has failed and betrayed its mission."

It is appropriate that the memory of victims of a German medicine gone astray be honored by contributions of the kind to follow. And it fills us with hope that these essays should have been authored by a younger and infinitely more sensitive generation of medical-historical scholars than would have existed in Germany as recently as twenty years ago.

Translated Terms

Adviser, consultant: Gutachter

Alien to the community: gemeinschaftsfremd

Association of German Children's Hospitals: Verein "Deutsches Kinderkrankenhaus e.V."

Central Clearinghouse for Mental Hospitals: Zentralverrechnungsstelle Heil- und Pflegeanstalten

Central Office T-4: Zentraldienststelle T-4

Federal Chamber of Physicians: Deutscher Ärztekammer

Führer's Office: Kanzlei des Führers

German Institute for Psychiatric Research: Deutscher Forschungsanstalt für Psychiatrie

Law for the Prevention of Genetically Diseased Offspring: Gesetz zur Verhütung erbkranken Nachwuchses

Law on Euthanasia for the Incurably Ill and Aliens to the Community: Gesetz über die Sterbehilfe für Lebensunfähige und Gemeinschaftsfremde

Lecturers' Association: Dozentenbund

Main Department: Hauptabteilung

Main Reich Security Office: Reichssicherheitshauptamt, also known as RSHA

National community: Volksgemeinschaft

Nazi seizure of power: Machtergreifung

Pediatrics department, pediatrics ward: Kinderfachabteilung

Public Ambulance Service, Ltd.: Gemeinnützige Kranken-Transport GmbH (GEKRAT)

Public Foundation for the Maintenance of Asylums: Gemeinnützige Stiftung für Anstaltspflege

Reich Association of Mental Hospitals: Reichsarbeitsgemeinschaft Heil- und Pflegeanstalten

Reich Commissioner for Mental Hospitals: Der Reichsbeauftragte für die Heil- und Pflegeanstalten

Reich Committee for the Scientific Processing of Serious Genetic Diseases: Reichsausschuß zur wissenschaftlichen Erfassung erb- und anlagebedingter schwerer Leiden

Reich Health Office: Reichsgesundheitsamt

State Security Service: SD (Staatssicherheitsdienst)

CHAPTER ONE

Introduction

by Christian Pross

The Topicality of Nazi Medicine

Fear of breathtaking advances in medical technology, the uncertainty of how to handle them, and the perceived erosion of traditional ethical standards lead people to look for lessons in the Nazi experience. Yet it has never been easy to find answers to present-day problems by exploring historical analogies. Long before 1933, some physicians and anthropologists had tried to prove that certain human beings' lives were less valuable than others'.

In the nineteenth century, the theory that there were different human races, which could be differentiated as "superior" and "inferior," served as the basis for the attack by the declining European gentry on the demand for "liberty, equality, and fraternity" and the declaration of the rights of man posited by the French Revolution. This theory provided *ideological tools* for a *biological solution* to a *social problem*. Despite the notable spread of venereal disease, tuberculosis, and alcoholism in urban slums during the period of industrialization, the social causes of these ills were denied, and the individual was blamed for being poor and being sick. Poverty was seen as a sign of "degeneration" and "hereditary inferiority." Leading psychiatrists and anthropologists translated these ideological slogans into scientific categories and applied them as apparently objective medical diagnoses.[1] The new science that embraced these categories was called *racial hygiene*.

The Nazis' seizure of power in 1933 provided the long-desired opportunity for the theory of racial hygiene to be applied in practice. The

Nazis proposed to solve the economic and social crisis of German society with a radical biological cure. Yet racism was not the only source of the disaster. Alexander Mitscherlich, the official delegate of the West German Chamber of Physicians at the Nuremberg doctors' trial, in 1947 gave his first-hand impressions: "Before such monstrous deeds and thoughts could shape everyday routine and real life, the disaster must have originated from many sources. Only in the crossing of two currents could the doctor turn into a licensed killer and publicly employed torturer: at the point where his aggressive search for the truth met with the ideology of the dictatorship. It is almost the same thing to see a human being as a 'case' or as a number tattooed on his arm. This is the double facelessness of a merciless epoch."[2]

Indeed, the search for truth, for new ideas, has motivated scientists and doctors for centuries. Without it there would be no progress, no modern diagnostic and therapeutic knowledge or techniques. In the nineteenth century, however, this search became, for science, more and more a search for objective truths. The search for truth in medicine turned into destruction when medicine abandoned both the Hippocratic *nil nocere* and its true purpose of healing the sick individual, of alleviating suffering—and when this was done for science's own "superior" aims.

What physician is not tempted by the enormous range of invasive diagnostic measures and fascinated by the chance to look into the most remote parts of the human organism? Today sheer curiosity, competition, and careerism among doctors, protective medicine, the corporatization of medicine, and the disappearance of such classic elements of medicine as the art of listening to the patient and using one's senses in diagnosing him or her have led to a burgeoning application of technology. Technology seduces the physician, who is continually confronted with the imperfect, unpredictable human being, to escape into the apparently safe world of laboratory parameters and computer scans. In the Weimar Republic, numerous physicians complained about the decay of medicine into purely diagnostic science.[3] Under the Nazis, it was as if an already weak dam had broken. The abundant availability of human guinea pigs among people labeled as inferior or subhuman was exploited by doctors as a unique opportunity for scientific research. The chief managers of "euthanasia" did not simply kill their victims, as Götz Aly shows in this book, but they thoroughly investigated them before and after and hoped eventually to find the clue to the nature of mental disease.

Another source of the disaster was the tension between the physicians' fantasies of omnipotence and their actual impotence. Medicine is often a labor of Sisyphus, because it alone can do little to overcome the misery of many patients, nor can it change human nature, which is often puzzling and stubborn. When young physicians graduate from medical school and enter the rough reality of medical practice, they quickly feel the limitations of their professional skills and their own helplessness. They can change neither individuals nor society. The idealism of the helpless helper can turn into an aggressive attitude toward the sick and a search for radical and final prescriptions. The relapsing, chronically ill, even incurable patient mobilizes the helper's hidden fears of disease and death. If these emotions coincide with a loss of job security, a financial crisis in the health care system, and a fear of the future, ethical standards tend to erode very quickly. The propaganda promoting the sterilization of the "inferior" and the elimination of "unnecessary eaters" in Weimar Germany only gained broad support when the Great Depression of 1929 caused an acute shortage of funds in the health service. Growing unemployment by 1929 drove thousands of doctors into the ranks of the newly formed Nazi Physicians' League.

In contemporary Germany, dramatic official rhetoric about the "cost explosion" in health care and continuous cuts in spending have produced new prophets of euthanasia. In a video made in 1981 and later aired on German television, the surgeon Julius Hackethal handed a cancer patient potassium cyanide and advocated active euthanasia.[4] A growing number of court cases are reported in which nurses have intentionally killed old and chronically ill patients in nursing homes and intensive care units.[5] The *Journal of the American Medical Association* in 1988 published the anonymous report of a young physician on duty who gave a young cancer patient, whom he did not know but whom he had just come across during his night shift, a fatal injection.[6] What did the editors have in mind when they published the report? Neither America nor West Germany of the late 1980s was pre-Nazi Germany, certainly, and yet in both countries there was an economic crisis, there was unemployment, there were serious cuts in health care spending, and there was new talk about certain people being less deserving of full medical care than others. Daniel Callahan, a leading American ethicist, has called for a discontinuation of sophisticated medical care and life-prolonging measures for anyone beyond the age of 75; has this been the catalyst for an attack on the life of the elderly,[7] in the same way that Binding and Hoche's call for "the destruction of worthless life" was an attack against the mentally ill and the handicapped in 1920s

Germany?[8] Probably not, since contemporary Germany and the United States are very different from Nazi Germany. And yet, we must be alert, and we must proceed with extreme caution.

An example of how much the life of the elderly is jeopardized by false prophets of an easy death is the current scandal over the German Society for Humane Dying. The society, founded in 1980, gained more than 50,000 members in 12 years by proposing to provide death for terminally ill patients and elderly people. Members could file written statements asking for passive euthanasia in case of a terminal illness; potassium cyanide and instructions for suicide were also made available to them. Last but not least, the society petitioned to change the law in order to allow active euthanasia and assistance for those wishing to commit suicide. The society presented itself as "a civil rights movement, which wants to realize human self-determination even for the dying."[9] The society was supported by celebrities such as the popular actress Inge Meysel and the surgeon and media star Julius Hackethal. On several occasions the society organized media events, such as handing out potassium cyanide to cancer patients in front of TV cameras, which produced an immediate rise in applications for membership.

The reason for the German Society for Humane Dying's success is the widespread fear of endless suffering in the process of dying and the fear of medicine as a soulless machine that allows alienated, inhumane life-prolonging measures. One must question the practice of prolonging life by all means possible in intensive care units. The recently revealed secret practices of the society, however, made clear that it exploited those fears under the cover of charity by criminal means. In January 1993, the president of the society, Hans Henning Atrott, was arrested after the police had obtained proof that Atrott and his followers were a ruthless Mafia of potassium cyanide dealers who had sold the drug to the society's members and clients at an extremely high profit—and with no regard for the plight of the individual recipient. There was no pretense of providing counseling for the dying; instead, people were given the drug by medically and psychologically unskilled minions who were simply motivated to sell as much of the death medicine as they could as quickly as possible, and at a price of at least 3,000 DM ($1,875) apiece. They did not bother to ascertain the personal situation of the patient, nor did they communicate with relatives. Caring relatives in a number of cases reported to the police that those who were given the death drug were not terminally ill but instead had suffered from a temporary depression or a stroke from which they might have recovered physically and mentally, perhaps eventually regaining the will to live.

Atrott threatened dissidents within his own ranks who left the organization because of scruples about its methods. The prosecutors were amazed by the criminal energy and the ruthlessness of its perpetrators.[10]

Historiography and Politics

It is by now well known that it was not only the tiny number of 350 black sheep among the German medical profession who were involved in medical crimes, but that many more were involved directly or indirectly, among them the cream of German medicine—university professors and outstanding scientists and researchers. As Alexander Mitscherlich and Fred Mielke noted in 1947, "Only the secret consent of the professions of science and politics can explain why the names of high-ranking scientists are constantly dropped during this trial, of men who perhaps did not right off commit any crime but took advantage of the cruel fate of defenseless individuals."[11] Mitscherlich and Mielke had the courage to break the esprit de corps of their profession by publishing trial documents that charged Germany's premier surgeon, Ferdinand Sauerbruch, and Wolfgang Heubner, director of the Pharmacological Institute of Berlin University, with being accessories to medical crimes for knowing of, but failing to prevent, the extremely cruel and sometimes fatal sulfonamide experiments at Ravensbrück.[12] Mitscherlich paid a high price for this disclosure: Sauerbruch and Heubner sued him and forced him to remove this paragraph from the trial report. At the same time, the leading Göttingen physiologist and specialist in aviation medicine, Friedrich Rein, accused Mitscherlich of irresponsibly attacking the foundation of scientific research and tarnishing the honor of the German medical profession.[13]

Ten thousand copies of the final version of Mitscherlich's documentation of the Nuremberg doctors' trial were printed in 1949 exclusively for the members of the West German Chamber of Physicians.[14] Yet the book did not become known to the public: there were no reviews, no letters to the editor. "It was as if the book had never been written," Mitscherlich recalled. One must assume that 10,000 copies disappeared in the basement of the West German Chamber of Physicians without a single German doctor ever having read the book. The World Medical Association received a copy, however, and took it as proof that the German medical profession had distanced itself from the medical crimes committed under the Nazis and thus was qualified for renewed membership.[15] In return Mitscherlich, who had helped save the international reputation of the German medical profession, faced a campaign of slander by his colleagues, who labeled him a traitor to his country and were successful in damaging his career. In 1956, the medical faculty of Frankfurt University refused to let him become the director of the new Institute of Psychoanalysis and Psychosomatic Medicine, which the state government had offered him. In his autobiography, Mitscherlich bitterly notes that he had virtually rescued the reputation of his profession but had been stabbed in the back for it.[16]

In the three decades following the repression of Mitscherlich's documentation, there was virtual silence. Little was published, and what was published got little public attention.[17] In 1960, there was some news coverage of the leading protagonist in the killing of handicapped children in the Third Reich, Werner Catel, who was forced to resign as director of the pediatric hospital of Kiel University.[18] In 1959, Werner Heyde, former professor of psychiatry at Würzburg University and chief manager of euthanasia, was arrested. For fifteen years he had been practicing medicine in a small town in northern Germany under a false name, protected by the local medical establishment, who knew his identity. Heyde committed suicide in prison and thus evaded trial.[19] The East German lawyer Friedrich Karl Kaul, who was an observer in many trials against Nazi criminals in West Germany, published a book on the cover-up of Heyde as well as one on physicians at Auschwitz, some of whom stood trial in Frankfurt in the mid-1960s.[20] But in the days when the cold war was raging, anything from an East German source was considered suspect. As a result of those events, at least, Mitscherlich's documentation was republished.[21] During the student rebellion in the late sixties, facts were revealed about the Nazi past of prominent faculty members of medical schools. In 1968 the director of the National Cancer Institute in Heidelberg, Karl Heinrich Bauer, faced a sit-in by medical students confronting him with his involvement in compulsory sterilization during the Third Reich. Documentation was published but did not become known beyond the Heidelberg academic community. The whole medical faculty backed Bauer, and the document's author was expelled from Heidelberg University.[22]

With few exceptions, historians of medicine at German medical schools produced the literature on the profession's past that its leaders were asking for. Hans Schadewaldt, the late director of the Institute of the History of Medicine in Düsseldorf, in a 1969 essay on the 75-year history of the largest of the physicians' lobbying organizations, Hartmannbund, denied that its pre-1933 leaders had actively participated in the Nazi seizure of power.[23] Until recently, Schadewaldt was the official historian of the German Federal Chamber of Physicians. Another influential figure in the postwar German history of medicine was Paul Diepgen, who as director of the prestigious Berlin Institute during the Third Reich had created a list of Jewish authors who were no longer to be cited.[24] In the 1947 and 1953 editions of his popular textbook *Die Heilkunde und der ärztliche Beruf*, he cleaned out all Nazi phraseology that the 1938 edition had included.[25] Another example of this *Zeitgeist* is the 1972 festschrift marking the 100th anniversary of the renowned Moabit Hospital in Berlin, in which Berlin medical historian Manfred Stürzbecher gave a thorough and detailed account of patient admissions, hospital budgets, the construction of new buildings, and the changing patient menus of the past hundred years, while almost entirely skipping the events between 1933 and 1945, when the hospital's predominantly Jewish physicians were persecuted and an underground resistance group of physicians was arrested and some of its members killed.[26] Here is the blank spot that one typically finds in postwar German festschriften and biographies.

Another factor interfered with an open examination of the profession's past: up until the end of the 1970s, many university chairs and leading positions in professional organizations were held by physicians who had been active members of the Nazi party or its affiliated organizations, the SA and the SS. As recently as 1983, the president of the West Berlin Chamber of Physicians was the surgeon Wilhelm Heim, who had been a member of the SA squad that was involved in a purge of Jewish physicians at the Urbankrankenhaus in Berlin in 1933.[27] Important data on these physicians can be found in the archives of the U.S.-administered Berlin Document Center, which until recently was rarely accessible to German researchers. Equally significant are the files of the Kassenärztliche Vereinigung Deutschlands, the federation of national health insurance physicians, which revoked the licenses of Jewish doctors after 1933. These files were discovered in the late 1970s in the archives of the Berlin office of the Kassenärztliche Bundesvereinigung, the West German national health insurance physicians' federation, by the Canadian historian Michael H. Kater. Kater was farsighted enough to copy most of the material and move it to the archives of York University in Ontario, Canada—because by the time researchers asked for the files, a couple of years later, the files had mysteriously disappeared. After repeated requests for information, Kater in 1986 received an official letter from the Kassenärztliche Bundesvereinigung headquarters in Cologne informing him that "unfortunately" the papers had now been "destroyed."[28]

By the late 1970s and early 1980s, partly as a result of the influential American television series "Holocaust," the political climate had changed. The old Nazi generation had begun to retire, and some Nazis had died. As a result, archives that had never been accessible were suddenly flung open. Grass-roots historians feverishly sought out reminiscences, their activities reaching a crescendo in the commemoration of the fiftieth anniversary of the *Machtergreifung,* the Nazi seizure of power, in 1983, and the fiftieth anniversary of the Kristallnacht pogrom, in 1988. Political and professional organizations, village and city governments, suddenly discovered their Jewish "fellow citizens" and invited and honored the survivors on a grand scale. As Raoul Hilberg had noted in 1962, in a sarcastic commentary on the reception of Anne Frank's diary in Germany, the Germans tend to praise and deify their former victims with an ardor that seems uncanny.[29] Quite apart from all the official memorial ceremonies, however, grass-roots historians began to unearth document after document describing what happened between 1933 and 1945. They continued where the Nuremberg trials and the postwar German trials against perpetrators had left off. The evidence they provided about the involvement of almost every public institution and professional organization, and about the forgotten victims—Gypsies, Communists, homosexuals, sterilization victims, deserters, and conscientious objectors—who were never compensated, pervaded the consciousness of a broader public and has to a certain extent influenced official rhetoric ever since. It is this new consciousness that so far has prevented conservative historians like Ernst Nolte from quietly implanting their revisionist version of history—without any public debate— into the concept of a planned National Museum of History in Berlin.

In the historiography of Nazi medicine, the tide turned during the Gesundheitstag, a national conference of physicians and health workers convened in West Berlin in May 1980. This was deliberately held as a counter-conference to the simultaneously occurring annual meeting of the Deutsche Ärztetag, the physicians' congress, hosted by the above-mentioned former SA member Wilhelm Heim. In an attempt to recapture destroyed alternative models of health care from the Weimar period, the organizers of the Gesundheitstag invited five Jewish refugee physicians from abroad, most of them former members of the Socialist Doctors Association (Verein Sozialistischer Ärzte). "Medicine under National Socialism: Repressed Past or Unbroken Tradition?" was the title of the conference, which for the first time presented the work of a small group of outsiders.[30] Among them were the investigative reporter Günther Schwarberg, who had written a book on fatal experiments with tuberculous children in Hamburg;[31] the Bremen law professor Stephan Leibfried and the Kassel sociologist Florian Tennstedt, who had documented the purge of Jewish and socialist doctors from the health insurance panels;[32] the historian Walter Wuttke-Groneberg, who had published a voluminous collection of documents on Nazi health policy;[33] and the Hamburg family physician Karl Heinz Roth, who had studied family planning and population control in the Third Reich.[34] From the institutes of the history of medicine, two nonconformists had the courage to attend the conference: Fridolf Kudlien from Kiel University, who gave a paper on anti-Nazi resistance among physicians, and Gerhard Baader, who spoke about the history of Social Darwinism.[35]

The conference had far-reaching repercussions and inspired further research. A social worker for the handicapped, Ernst Klee, came out with a major study of euthanasia based on material from the archives of mental hospitals run by the Innere Mission, the charitable organization of the Lutheran church.[36] Walter-Wuttke Groneberg and associates created an exhibit, shown all over West Germany, which focused on the role of psychiatrists, occupational health care, and the preference of early Nazi health policy for holistic medicine and natural healing over decadent "Jewish" scientific medicine.[37] Benno Müller-Hill, a geneticist from Cologne University, revealed the involvement of leading German geneticists and anthropologists in the selection of Jews, Gypsies, and the mentally ill and retarded for sterilization and genocide. Among these professionals he focused on Otmar von Verschuer, the director of the prestigious Kaiser Wilhelm Institute for Anthropology, Human Genetics, and Eugenics (Kaiser-Wilhelm-Institut für Anthropologie, menschliche Erblehre, und Eugenik), who directed Josef Mengele's research on twins in Auschwitz.[38] To this day, Verschuer's studies are honored and cited by many of the world's leading geneticists.[39] The Berlin historian Gisela Bock published an important study of compulsory sterilization in which she suggested that sterilization was mainly directed against women, who were considered an inferior species.[40] Other classics that came out after the Gesundheitstag are Götz Aly and Karl Heinz Roth's analysis of compulsory registration of the German population (implemented in 1938, this registration provided the technical foundation for the selection of racially and hereditarily based superiors and inferiors);[41] Michael H. Kater's studies of the Nazi Physicians' League, the high percentage of physicians in Nazi organizations, and the power struggle within the Nazi health administration;[42] Georg

Lilienthal's study of the Lebensborn, an SS-run foundation that established maternity homes for unmarried mothers and orphanages to raise racially selected children;[43] Geoffrey Cocks and Regine Lockot's history of psychoanalysis and psychotherapy in Nazi Germany;[44] Angelika Ebbinghaus and her associates' study of the Nazi model for a "modernized" health care system in the city of Hamburg;[45] and many other local studies.[46]

To coordinate and fund this new wave of research, which in general was not welcomed and sometimes even obstructed by the academic community, Karl Heinz Roth, Götz Aly, and others in 1983 founded the Association for Research on Nazi Health and Social Policy (Verein zur Erforschung der nationalsozialistischen Gesundheits- und Sozialpolitik). The association received private contributions, and some of its members were sponsored by the foundation Hamburger Institut für Sozialforschung. In 1985 the association began issuing the journal *Beiträge zur nationalsozialistischen Gesundheits- und Sozialpolitik,* of which ten volumes have appeared.[47] Translations of selected essays from volumes 1, 2, and 4 are published in this book.

The impact of these numerous publications has been powerful enough to force the German Federal Chamber of Physicians to change its attitude. On the fiftieth anniversary of the Nazi seizure of power, however, the *Deutsches Ärzteblatt* (the German equivalent of *JAMA*) still maintained in an editorial that "the new masters had appeared overnight" and had seized control of the reluctant professional organizations, simultaneously denying the fact that the leaders of these same organizations had enthusiastically supported the new regime.[48] When the German pediatrician and peace activist Hartmut Hanauske-Abel published an article in the *Lancet* in 1986 about the medical profession's continuing denial of the truth,[49] the chairman of the Federal Chamber of Physicians, Karsten Vilmar, angrily accused him of distorting facts and collectively slandering the profession.[50] Hanauske-Abel subsequently lost his position as emergency physician with the panel doctors' association (i.e., the association of doctors working under contract with the health insurance association) in Mainz. Hanauske-Abel's politically based firing and Vilmar's retrograde attitude were depicted by the leading German newspapers as a scandal.

In May of 1989, the Berlin Chamber of Physicians, which was by this time controlled by the organizers of the 1980 Gesundheitstag, used the opportunity of hosting the 1989 annual meeting of the Deutsche Ärztetag to force Karsten Vilmar to place the topic of medicine under the Nazis on the agenda. Against considerable resistance from some state physicians' chambers, an exhibit of photos and documents was created and officially opened at this annual meeting.[51] Simultaneously, an international scientific symposium under the aegis of the Federal Chamber of Physicians was organized and a series of articles was published on medicine under the Nazis in the *Deutsches Ärzteblatt*.[52] At the opening of the exhibit Richard Toellner, medical historian at the University of Münster, stated in a widely noted speech that the German medical profession had to acknowledge that the majority of physicians had actively or passively participated in medical crimes and that the burden of the past had to be faced and no longer repressed: "The whole range of normal representatives of the medical profession was involved and they all knew what they were doing. . . . A medical profession that accepts mass murder of sick people as normal, and to a large degree explicitly approves of it as a necessary, justified act for the sake of the community, has failed and betrayed its mission. Such a medical profession as a whole has become morally culpable, no matter how many members of the profession directly or indirectly participated in the killings of sick people in a legal sense." Toellner's unequivocal statement was printed in the *Deutsches Ärzteblatt* and must be taken as the new official attitude of the Federal Chamber of Physicians toward the past.[53] Does this mean that in 1989 the German medical profession finally expressed the remorse that Mitscherlich had asked for in vain 42 years earlier? The attitude of the official representatives of the profession has remained contradictory.

The 1989 Deutsche Ärztetag in Berlin certainly triggered a debate within the profession that was unthinkable before, and the articles in the *Deutsches Ärzteblatt* caused angry reactions among a number of readers. Some letters to the editor were full of anti-Semitic and German chauvinist sentiments.[54] Karsten Vilmar revised Toellner's ideas during a 1989 memorial rally for the victims of Nazism in Bremen by saying that the majority of German physicians had altruistically worked for their patients and had never been involved in or approved of any atrocities.[55] Another illustration of how seriously the official representatives of the Federal Chamber of Physicians have confronted the past is the election of former SS member Hans Joachim Sewering as president of the World Medical Association. Sewering, whose election was backed by the association, finally had to resign after strong protests from American, Canadian, Israeli, and German physicians.[56] The system of silence, lies, half-truths, excuses, and angry denials of the last four and one half decades is on the retreat, however. The open debate about the Nazi past has raised the consciousness of many German doctors and parts of the German public about contemporary medical abuses. It has shaken the German doctor's self-image of infallibility, of belonging to a profession that stands neutrally above political and social forces and that presumably has always had a clean record and acted out of noble, altruistic motives.

The Trivialization of the Holocaust

Anti-Nazism and *Vergangenheitsbewältigung* (overcoming the past) have turned into an integral part of the official state ideology in Germany. We witness a simultaneous commercialization and trivialization of the Holocaust. The media have discovered that the topic is in vogue, that it sells. Many of the numerous books and articles are derivative; they not only copy original work but also dilute it and offer easy, even revisionist explanations of what the Holocaust presumably was all about.

In addition, it has become fashionable to use oral history in researching the Third Reich. Undoubtedly a valuable method in areas where little documentation is available (for example, in the history of resistance or emigration), oral history is extremely unreliable when applied to former perpetrators, as Robert J. Lifton has done in *The Nazi Doctors*.[57] The fundamental message of Lifton's book, which is the first major publication on medicine under the Nazis in the Anglo-Saxon world, is misleading. From personal interviews with former Nazi doctors he develops a model that explains how doctors were able to torture and kill through a process that he calls the "doubling" of the doctors' personality into the "Auschwitz-Self" of the murderer and the pre-Nazi self of the humane physician healer. Apart from the fact that "doubling" is a neologism for the well-known phenomenon of a personality split, Lifton's model may be valid as a postwar psychopathological study of some of his interviewees, but it certainly cannot be applied to Nazi doctors in general—nor does it provide, as Lifton suggests, the essential clue to the source of medical crimes. The postwar German generation, which grew up in a society ruled by the old Nazi power elite (smoothly converted into "good democrats") experienced this kind of oral history as a history of nothing but silence, excuses, legends, lies, and aggressive denial. Today the perpetrators are old men who have rehearsed the legends about their lives for decades, with the result that they firmly believe them. Even the most skilled psychohistorian will not be able to extract any new insights into the nature of Nazism from them. To shine more light into the darkness it is necessary to identify names, institutions, planning authorities, and brain trusts, and the way in which they were interrelated through personal connections. This can only be achieved through a diligent study of documents and archival material, something that Lifton largely neglected. Instead, he concealed the names of his interviewees and collected a great deal of hearsay information; thus, he did more to obscure than to clarify the issues. As the new magic clue to the origins of genocide, Lifton's neologism "doubling" is widely used as a substitute for the necessary intellectual effort required to study and to understand the nature of Nazism.

The doubling theory psychologizes political phenomena by projecting the contradiction between healing and killing into the psyche of the individual Nazi doctor. Healing and killing, however, were an integral part of selective social policy. "Superior" citizens were to receive the best and most modern medical treatment and social services available, whereas the genetically "inferior," the subproletariat, children in foster homes, prostitutes, the mentally retarded, alcoholics, and the mentally ill, as well as the racially "inferior" Jews, Gypsies, and Slavs, were to be sterilized or killed. Elimination of the inferior provided the funds and facilities for the privileges of the superior. For example, Carl Schneider, professor of psychiatry at Heidelberg, a leading manager of the mass killings of "hereditarily" deficient and incurable patients in German hospitals, was simultaneously an innovative and humanistic liberal reformer of traditional German psychiatry (something Götz Aly points out in Chapter 4). Schneider's double role cannot simply be explained, as Lifton suggests, by his "psychiatric idealism"—there was no doubling into the healer-and-killer-personality. Schneider did what he did as an executor of selective social policy.

The personality split is something that did not exist in most Nazi doctors during the Nazi period but occurred after 1945, when they were accused and tried to deny their involvement and find excuses: "It cannot be me who did that." Lifton's fundamental error was to project something he found in postwar confessions of Nazi doctors onto the reality of 1933–45. The diaries, letters, and publications of Nazi doctors of the time (some of which are published in this volume) contain few elements of idealism or the high ethical standards of the "physician-self," and thus scant evidence of doubling. Dominating these documents, instead, are small-minded greed for money and privileges, careerism, and a mixture of envy, inflated self-esteem, and contempt for the so-called inferior. Lifton, who used neither contemporary personal documents of this kind nor the extremely rich interrogation records from the Nuremberg doctors' trial, set out to analyze the normality of the Nazi perpetrator and to point to the potential Nazi in every human being. The result of his study, however, is an apologia. According to Lifton, the Nazi doctors were blinded idealists who believed in healing the sick body of the Volk—tragically misled scientists, "Faustian" figures, as he labeled them, seduced by the Mephistophelian Hitler to murder for the sake of a higher purpose. Lifton has added a legend of his own to the many legends that already exist about Nazism.

Destruction and Modernization — a New View of the Nature of Nazism

One purpose of the research presented in this book is to overcome German postwar legends about Nazism. The work of the new generation of scholars has contributed to a better and deeper understanding of health policy in Nazi Germany and of the motives and actions of Nazi physicians by uncovering hitherto unknown material and putting old material into a new context. Anti-Semitism and racism can no longer be identified as the only driving forces behind Nazi politics, nor can the Nazi power elite be viewed as a small group of deviant monsters who misled a supposedly passive constituency. What for us today appears to be the contradictory nature of Nazism in fact explains its success: the connection between destruction and modernization. Auschwitz cannot be seen without the Volkswagen plant in Wolfsburg, nor the SS regime of terror without the social security, health, and recreation program provided by the Nazi trade union Deutsche Arbeitsfront. The so-called *Neue deutsche Seelenheilkunde* (New German Psychotherapy) for the superior members of the Volk complemented the mass sterilization of the inferior. The destruction of the latter created social guarantees for the former and thus secured the standard of living of the productive community of a conformist petit bourgeoisie and working class at the expense of excluded minorities.

Along with the homeless, the beggars, the inmates of insane asylums, and the Jews of the Eastern European ghettos, the German authorities eliminated the visible poor, those people who required "unnecessary expenditures" during their lifetime. Their mistreatment and liquidation provided housing, employment, assets, and old age pensions for others. In this sense, the National Socialist *Volksgemeinschaft* (national community) really existed. Health policy in Nazi Germany—scientifically labeled "Hereditary and Racial Hygiene"—was a concept of rule. It unified German policy regarding the population, economics, and society to achieve one goal: the final solution of the social question. On the whole, the functionaries of the Nazi state were extraordinarily young, and they consciously relied on the results of scientific research. Germany has never had a younger or more mentally flexible elite than it had in those years. This elite did away with rusty old structures and started to put their utopian political ideas—such as the concept of a common *Gesundheitspflicht* (obligation of health)—into practice. To cleanse the body of the Volk of everything sick, alien, and disturbing was one of the dreams of the German intelligentsia.

In Chapter 2, Götz Aly deals not only with the euthanasia program Operation T-4 of 1940–41 directed against the incurably mentally ill, the handicapped, and the malformed, but also with a hitherto unknown chapter of mass murder, the ways in which other "useless" members of society were singled out and deported into killing hospitals, where they were starved to death or killed by injections. The "useless" consisted of "antisocials" or *Gemeinschaftsfremde* (aliens to the community), as the Nazis called them, maladjusted adolescents, sick foreign slave laborers, and civilians who had suffered psychic breakdowns and lost their orientation to reality after air raids and were considered to pose a threat to public order and discipline. Aly identifies the planning and executing forces—labor offices, health authorities, mayors—who organized the killings and examines the rationale behind the murders. One goal was providing beds for physically wounded soldiers and civilians during all-out war by emptying mental hospitals, foster homes, and institutions for the handicapped. These issues were only marginally dealt with in the Nuremberg doctors' trial of 1946–47 and the postwar trials of euthanasia doctors, because the prosecutors were interested in finding evidence for the individual guilt of the defendants and not in the overall context and the network in which they had functioned.

Chapters 3 and 5—the Posen diaries of the anatomist Hermann Voss (with commentary by Götz Aly) and the letters of the euthanasia doctor Friedrich Mennecke to his wife (with commentary by Peter Chroust)—provide an unusual insight into the inner life of two rather average perpetrators. These documents were honest and uncensored, written without any excuses and without any idea of the need to construct some kind of postwar identity. To a certain extent, they resemble the autobiography of the commander of Auschwitz, Rudolf Höß, written after his arrest by the Allies. His whining and philistine language bore the stamp of the typical culprit: the German sentimentality of the mass murderer, who claims his own suffering in the face of the mountains of corpses he himself produces.

The autobiography of Rudolf Höß gave proof to Hannah Arendt's notion of the "banality of evil." Remarkably, few other concepts have made as significant a contribution to the dissemination of a sense of threat emanating from the continued presence of these men in Germany. The formula quickly became the common currency of the task of mastering the past, utterly contrary to Hannah Arendt's intent. Intended as a rhetorical spur to focus attention on the inconceivable, the concept merely diminished the power of the inconceivable so that it could be shunted aside. As a consequence, Höß, the common criminal, managed to disappear behind the image of Höß, the evil perpetrator. He was perfectly willing to admit to mass murder, but he did not mention the removal of three carloads of valuables from Auschwitz. This silence concerning the evidence of baser motives was accepted without question. Amazingly, it seemed easier to deal with a profile of the perpetrator which remained unblemished by any trace of sadism or greed.

Voss's diary and Mennecke's letters, on the other hand, reveal such baser motives as envy, greed, careerism, and competitiveness, as well as malicious joy and contempt for the subhumans who are at the perpetrators' disposal. They exhibit a peculiar coexistence of such joys of everyday life as tender feelings for loved ones and such atrocities as selecting and killing other human beings. Even if one expects petit bourgeois intimacy and human destruction to be linked in these private documents, actually seeing the mixture of these two elements in their particularity is a shock. Voss's diary is a combination of whining over his unsatisfactory career, humming with pleasure in nature, and unrestrained expressions of greed for the marginal profits of the great war, for its "special bonuses." The conquest of the East brings him a professorship at the university in Posen. Even if his drive for advancement cannot be satisfied by this position, the anatomical institute of the Reichsuniversität Posen represents one object of his desire: the crematorium in the service of the Gestapo. The oven is his social utopia: "The Poles are quite impudent at the moment, and thus our oven has a great deal to do. How nice it would be if we could drive the whole pack through such ovens!" "Yesterday, two wagons full of Polish ashes were taken away. Outside my office, the robinias are blooming beautifully, just as in Leipzig." These quotes from an average doctor demonstrate to what extent the officially organized murders were supported by the anticipatory consent of the people, including the intelligentsia. The German intelligentsia lent a vocabulary to the hatred felt by ordinary people and rationalized the desire for annihilation to the point where it could become realized. It is, in fact, a singular accomplishment of the German intelligentsia that the crematoriums could be promoted as a solution for social ills. Above all, Voss's diary is important because it shows that it was not only unrestrained desire for knowledge which energized the fury of destruction, but also simple hatred.

In Chapter 4, Götz Aly deals with the connection between murder and modernization in German psychiatry, describing how reforms required the destruction of patients and how the reformers—as advocates of an intensive therapy and rehabilitation program—demanded the destruction of incurable patients. To decrease the size of hospitals, reorganize their internal structure, shorten the duration of inpatient care, simplify the reimbursement of expenses, create a variety of outpatient care facilities, and perform systematic research on the causes of mental disease—all these considerations went into the professional ethos and identity of the doctors who performed mass murder not simply for its own sake. They had been among the leaders of psychiatric reform in the Weimar period, and in 1941/42 they believed they had achieved the goal set out in their plans, which had been massively promoted and accelerated by the euthanasia program. As unfinished as their programs were in 1945, the military defeat of German fascism did not make them disappear.

National Socialism removed barriers that in a democratic system would at least have considerably impeded quick reforms and radical scientific experiments. It offered certain researchers and reformers unusual chances. At the same time, a modern social strategy and science gave National Socialism the chance to rationalize its irrational ideology and rationally to legitimize its crimes as scientifically and economically reasonable. These scientific procedures did not require any *Gleichschaltung* (synchronization). Their inner form, guided by their abstract interest, complied with the logic of Nazi rule.

Can we develop new definitions of the Nazi program and the Nazi perpetrator from the work presented in this book? The answer is no. And it is not even definition that we seek, but illustration of the fact that all definitions have served to obscure the details. Only details can uncover the historical truth.

Notes

1. For the history of the politics of eugenics in Germany, see Hedwig Conrad-Martius, *Utopien der Menschenzüchtung: Der Sozialdarwinismus und seine Folgen* (München, 1955); Gerhard Baader, "Die Medizin im Nationalsozialismus: Ihre Wur-

zeln und die erste Periode ihrer Realisierung 1933–1938," in *nicht mißhandeln,* ed. Christian Pross and Rolf Winau, pp. 61–75 (Berlin, 1984); Anna Bergmann, Gabriele Czarnowski, and Annegret Ehmann, "Menschen als Objekte humangenetischer Forschung und Politik im 20. Jahrhundert: Zur Geschichte des Kaiser Wilhelm Instituts für Anthropologie, menschliche Erblehre, und Eugenik in Berlin-Dahlem (1927–1945)," in *Der Wert des Menschen: Medizin in Deutschland 1928–1945,* ed. Ärztekammer Berlin, in cooperation with the Bundesärztekammer, redacted by Christian Pross und Götz Aly, p. 121ff. (Berlin, 1989); Sheila Faith Weiss, *Race Hygiene and National Efficiency: The Eugenics of Wilhelm Schallmeyer* (Berkeley, 1987).

2. Alexander Mitscherlich and Fred Mielke, eds., *Das Diktat der Menschenverachtung* (Heidelberg, 1947).

3. See Heinz-Peter Schmiedebach, "Zur Standesideologie in der Weimarer Republik am Beispiel Erwin Liek," in *Der Wert des Menschen,* pp. 26–35, and Susanne Hahn, "Revolution der Heilkunst—Ausweg aus der Krise? Julius Moses (1868–1942) zur Rolle der Medizin in der Gesundheitspolitik in der Weimarer Republik," in *Der Wert des Menschen,* pp. 71–85.

4. See Chapter 2, below.

5. The most recent one is the case of the "Vienna death nurses": "Die Mordschwestern von Wien, 'Ruhig, unauffällig, hilfsbereit,'" *Stern,* no. 17, 20 April 1989, pp. 32–39.

6. Anon., "It's Over, Debbie," *JAMA* 259 (1988): 272.

7. Daniel Callahan, *Setting Limits: Medical Goals in an Aging Society* (New York, 1987). See also Amitai Etzioni's critical review of Callahan's book, "Spare the Old, Save the Young," *Nation,* 11 June 1988, pp. 818–22.

8. Karl Binding and Alfred Hoche, *Die Freigabe der Vernichtung lebensunwerten Lebens: Ihr Maß und ihre Form* (Leipzig, 1920).

9. Hans Henning Atrott, *Deutsche Gesellschaft für Humanes Sterben: Ihre rechtspolitischen Forderungen* (pamphlet published by Deutsche Gesellschaft für Humanes Sterben—The German Society for Humane Dying), p. 5.

10. The case of the German Society for Humane Dying is extensively documented in "Sterbehilfe—zur Argumentation der DGHS," *Dr. med. Mabuse,* no. 54, June/July 1988, pp. 18–22; and in "Die Zyankali-Bande, Sterbehilfe gegen Bargeld," *Der Spiegel,* no. 8, 22 February 1993, pp. 90–101.

11. Mitscherlich and Mielke, *Das Diktat der Menschenverachtung.*

12. Ibid., pp. 83–84.

13. Rein, Sauerbruch, and Heubner's campaign against Mitscherlich is documented in the *Göttinger Universitätszeitung,* no. 14 (1947), pp. 3–5; no. 17/18 (1947), pp. 6–8; no. 3 (1948), pp. 4–7; no. 10 (1948), pp. 6–8.

14. Alexander Mitscherlich and Fred Mielke, *Wissenschaft ohne Menschlichkeit* (Heidelberg, 1949).

15. Alexander Mitscherlich and Fred Mielke, *Medizin ohne Menschlichkeit* (Frankfurt, 1978), p. 15.

16. Alexander Mitscherlich, *Ein Leben für die Psychoanalyse* (Frankfurt, 1980), pp. 144–47, 157, 189–92.

17. In 1965, a whitewash of Nazi euthanasia was published by the prominent psychiatrist Helmut Ehrhardt (*Euthanasie und die Vernichtung "lebensunwerten Lebens"* [Stuttgart, 1965]). In his book, Ehrhardt denied the true extent of the euthanasia program, did not name all the physicians involved, and overemphasized the resistance against the killing of patients by some psychiatrists. In the same year, a report about

the killings in the state psychiatric hospital Eglfing Haar (near Munich) was published by its postwar director, Gerhard Schmidt (*Selektion in der Heilanstalt, 1939–1945* [Stuttgart, 1965]).

18. Ulrich Schultz, "Dichtkunst, Heilkunst, Forschung: Der Kinderarzt Werner Catel," in *Beiträge zur nationalsozialistischen Gesundheits- und Sozialpolitik,* vol. 2, *Reform und Gewissen: "Euthanasie" im Dienst des Fortschritts* (Berlin, 1985), p. 122.

19. Ernst Klee, *Was sie taten — Was sie wurden: Ärzte, Juristen, und andere Beteiligte am Kranken- oder Judenmord* (Frankfurt, 1986), pp. 19–29.

20. Friedrich Karl Kaul, *Dr. Sawade macht Karriere: Der Fall des Euthanasie-Arztes Dr. Heyde* (Frankfurt, 1971); Friedrich Karl Kaul, *Ärzte in Auschwitz* (Berlin [GDR], 1968).

21. Of the first new edition under the title *Medizin ohne Menschlichkeit* (see n. 15, above), 50,000 copies were printed in 1960 and another 25,000 in 1962.

22. "Dokumentation des Arbeitskreises Medizin und Verbrechen, Arbeit, Aktionen Analysen zum Thema Zwangssterilisation im 3. Reich, Kritik heutiger Medizin," Kritische Universität Heidelberg (Critical University, Heidelberg), July 1968. Typewritten brochure in author's possession. The main initiator and author of the brochure, Ernst Scheurlen, a young internist, lost his job in the Department of Medicine at the University of Heidelberg. In 1936, Bauer had published the standard textbook on the sterilization of males under the Nazi racial hygiene program concerning the "hereditary inferior" (Karl Heinrich Bauer and Felix von Mikulicz-Radecki, *Die Praxis der Sterilisierungsoperationen* [Leipzig, 1936]). Bauer, who to this day is wrongly regarded as an anti-Nazi, was made the first postwar president of the University of Heidelberg by the American military government.

23. Hans Schadewaldt, *75 Jahre Hartmannbund: Ein Kapitel deutscher Sozialpolitik* (Bonn–Bad Godesberg, 1975), p. 79. A detailed correction of Schadewaldt's defense has been made by Michael Hubenstorf, "Deutsche Landärzte an die Front!—Ärztliche Standespolitik zwischen Liberalismus und Nationalsozialismus," in *Der Wert des Menschen,* pp. 200–223.

24. Werner Leibbrand is reported as saying this in a biographical article written by Fridolf Kudlien, "Werner Leibbrand als Zeitzeuge: Ein ärztlicher Gegner des Nationalsozialismus im Dritten Reich," *Medizinhistorisches Journal* 21 (1986): 344.

25. A summary of the Diepgen story is given by William Coleman in "The Physician in Nazi Germany," *Bull. Hist. Med.* 60 (1986): 238–40.

26. Manfred Stürzbecher, "Aus der Geschichte des Städtischen Krankenhauses Moabit," in *1872–1972 Städtisches Krankenhaus Moabit: Festschrift zum 100 jährigen Bestehen* (Berlin, Bezirksamt Tiergarten von Berlin: Abteilung Gesundheitswesen, 1972), pp. 13–98. For comparison, see Christian Pross, "Das Krankenhaus Moabit, 1920, 1933, 1945," in Pross and Winau, *nicht mißhandeln* (Berlin, 1984), pp. 7–10, 109–261.

27. Michael Kater, "The Burden of the Past: Problems of a Modern Historiography of Physicians and Medicine in Nazi Germany," *German Studies Review* 10 (1987): 31–56.

28. Ibid., p. 40.

29. Raoul Hilberg, *Die Vernichtung der europäischen Juden: Die Gesamtgeschichte des Holocaust* (Berlin, 1982), p. 802.

30. The proceedings of the Gesundheitstag 1980 were published in Gerhard Baader and Ulrich Schultz, eds., *Medizin und Nationalsozialismus, Tabuisierte Vergangenheit — ungebrochene Tradition?* (Berlin, 1980).

31. Günther Schwarberg, *Der SS-Arzt und die Kinder* (Hamburg, 1979).

32. Stephan Leibfried and Florian Tennstedt, *Berufsverbote und Sozialpolitik 1933: Die Auswirkungen der nationalsozialistischen Machtergreifung auf die Krankenkassenverwaltung und die Kassenärzte*, Arbeitspapiere des Forschungsschwerpunktes Reproduktionsrisiken, soziale Bewegungen und Sozialpolitik, no. 2 (Universität Bremen, 1979).

33. Walter Wuttke-Groneberg, *Medizin im Nationalsozialismus: Ein Arbeitsbuch* (Tübingen, 1980).

34. See n. 30.

35. See n. 30.

36. Ernst Klee, *"Euthanasie" im NS-Staat: Die "Vernichtung lebensunwerten Lebens"* (Frankfurt, 1983).

37. Projektgruppe Volk und Gesundheit, *Volk und Gesundheit: Heilen und Vernichten im Nationalsozialismus,* Tübinger Vereinigung für Volkskunde e.V. (Tübingen, 1982); see also Walter Wuttke-Groneberg's paper at the 1980 Gesundheitstag, "Von Heidelberg nach Dachau: 'Vernichtungslehre' und Naturwissenschaftskritik in der nationalsozialistischen Medizin." See n. 30, pp. 113–38.

38. Benno Müller-Hill, *Tödliche Wissenschaft: Die Aussonderung von Juden, Zigeunern und Geisteskranken, 1933–1945* (Reinbek, 1984). The book is now available in English as *Murderous Science: Elimination by Scientific Selection of Jews, Gypsies, and Others in Germany, 1933–1945,* trans. George Fraser (Oxford, 1988).

39. See, for example, Victor McKusick, "Medical Genetics," in A. McGhee Harvey et al., *The Principles and Practice of Medicine,* 21st ed. (Norwalk, Conn., 1984), p. 433.

40. Gisela Bock, *Zwangssterilisation im Nationalsozialismus* (Opladen, 1986).

41. Götz Aly and Karl Heinz Roth, *Die restlose Erfassung, Volkszählen, Identifizieren, Aussondern im Nationalsozialismus* (Berlin, 1984).

42. Michael H. Kater, "Hitlerjugend und Schule im Dritten Reich," *Historische Zeitschrift* 228 (1981): 572–623; *The Nazi Party: A Social Profile of Members and Leaders, 1919–1945* (Cambridge, Mass., 1983), p. 112; "Hitler's Early Doctors: Nazi Physicians in Predepression Germany," *Journal of Modern History* 59 (1987): 25–52; "The Nazi Physicians' League of 1929: Causes and Consequences," in *The Formation of the Nazi Constituency, 1919–1933,* ed. Thomas Childers (London, 1986), pp. 147–81; "Doctor Leonardo Conti and His Nemesis: The Failure of Centralized Medicine in the Third Reich," *Central European History* 18 (1985): 299–325; *Doctors under Hitler* (Chapel Hill, N.C., 1989).

43. Georg Lilienthal, *Der "Lebensborn e.V."* (Stuttgart, 1985).

44. Geoffrey Cocks, *Psychotherapy in the Third Reich: The Göring Institut* (New York, 1935); Regine Lockot, *Erinnern und Durcharbeiten: Zur Geschichte der Psychoanalyse und Psychotherapie im Nationalsozialismus* (Frankfurt, 1985).

45. Angelika Ebbinghaus, Heidrun Kaupen-Haas, and Karl Heinz Roth, *Heilen und Vernichten im Mustergau Hamburg* (Hamburg, 1984).

46. To mention only a few examples: Christian Pross, "Das Krankenhaus Moabit, 1920, 1933, 1945," in Pross and Winau, *nicht mißhandeln;* Arbeitsgruppe zur Erforschung der Karl-Bonhoeffer-Nervenklinik, ed., *Totgeschwiegen 1933–1945: Die Geschichte der Karl-Bonhoeffer Nervenklinik* (Berlin, 1988); Michael Wunder, Ingrid Genkel, and Harald Jenner, *Auf dieser schiefen Ebene gibt es keine Halten mehr — Die Alsterdorfer Anstalten im Nationalsozialismus* (Hamburg, 1987); Matthias Leipert, Rudolf Styrnal, and Winfried Schwarzer, *Verlegt nach unbekannt: Sterilisation und*

Euthanasie in Galkhausen, 1933–1945 (Cologne, 1987); Dagmar Hartung von Doetinchem, *Zerstörte Fortschritte — Zur Geschichte des Jüdischen Krankenhauses zu Berlin, 1756-1861-1914-1989* (Berlin, 1989).

47. *Beiträge zur nationalsozialistischen Gesundheits- und Sozialpolitik* is published by Rotbuch Verlag Berlin. The published volumes are as follows: vol. 1, *Aussonderung und Tod* (1985); vol. 2, *Reform und Gewissen* (1985); vol. 3, *Herrenmensch und Arbeitsvölker* (1986); vol. 4, *Biedermann und Schreibtischtäter* (1987); vol. 5, *Sozialpolitik und Judenvernichtung* (1987); vol. 6, *Feinderklärung und Prävention* (1988); vol. 7, *Internationales Ärztliches Bulletin,* Reprint (1989); vol. 8, *Arbeitsmarkt und Sondererlaß* (1990); vol. 9, *Bevölkerungsstrucktur und Massenmord* (1991); vol. 10, *Modelle für ein deutsches Europa* (1992). Another series of books and a journal are published by the Hamburg branch of the Verein: Schriften der Hamburger Stiftung für Sozialgeschichte des 20. Jahrhunderts. Vol. 1, *Der Griff nach der Bevölkerungspolitik; vol. 6, Die Träume der Genetik,* 1987–; 1999, *Zeitschrift für Sozialgeschichte des 20. und 21. Jahrhunderts,* vol. 1, 1986–.

48. Norbert Jachertz, "Die neuen Herren kamen über Nacht," *Deutsches Ärzteblatt* 80 (1983): 23–26.

49. Hartmut Hanauske-Abel, "From Nazi Holocaust to Nuclear Holocaust: A Lesson to Learn?" *Lancet,* 2 August 1986, pp. 271–73.

50. "Die 'Vergangenheitsbewältigung' darf nicht kollektiv die Ärzte diffamieren," interview with Dr. Karsten Vilmar, *Deutsches Ärzteblatt* 84 (1987): 767–79.

51. *Der Wert des Menschen,* an exhibition catalogue containing an anthology of scientific contributions, was published in 1989 (see n. 1).

52. The series of articles in the *Deutsches Ärzteblatt* was published as an anthology: Johanna Bleker and Norbert Jachertz, eds., *Medizin im Dritten Reich* (Cologne, 1989).

53. Richard Toellner, "Ärzte im Dritten Reich," Lecture delivered at the first plenary session of the 92d German Physicians' Congress in Berlin, *Deutsches Ärzteblatt* 86 (1989): 1427–33.

54. See letters to the editor in *Deutsches Ärzteblatt* 85 (1988).

55. "Rolle der Medizin bleibt umstritten," *Süddeutsche Zeitung,* 13 October 1989.

56. The Sewering case is documented in *Der Spiegel,* no. 4, 1993, p. 195; "Deutsche Ärzte protestieren," *Die Zeit,* 22 January 1993; "Sewering verzichtet auf Ehrenamt," *Süddeutsche Zeitung,* 23 January 1993; "Prof. Sewering Ziel einer Verleumdungsaktion," *Deutsches Ärzteblatt,* no. 4, 29 January 1993; "Sewering—Ende einer Karriere," *Deutsches Ärzteblatt,* no. 5, 5 February 1993, p. C-161; "Nazi Links Force Doctor to Give Up World Health Post," *New York Times,* 25 January 1993.

57. Robert Jay Lifton, *The Nazi Doctors* (New York, 1986).

CHAPTER TWO

Medicine against the Useless

by Götz Aly

Between 1940 and 1945, an inconspicuous office at number 4, Tiergartenstrasse in Berlin organized the murder of more than two hundred thousand psychiatric patients, camp inmates who had fallen ill, people suffering from major depression, and nonconformists. This state-organized killing organization's cover name, "Operation T-4," was derived from the office's street address. The building was an "Aryanized" urban villa with a wing of offices attached. Until their almost complete destruction through bombardment, the villa and an office barracks erected later were located almost exactly where the bus stop in front of the main entrance to the Berlin Philharmonic now stands.

"Processing" of patients in psychiatric institutions "for wartime economic purposes" began on 9 October 1939. The Reich Ministry of the Interior sent questionnaires to various mental institutions in which it asked, among other things, for information on each patient's type of illness, length of stay, and ability to work. Asylum directors were not informed of the purpose of these questionnaires. Later, on the basis of the completed questionnaires, three of the approximately thirty medical advisers at T-4 decided which patients would live and which would die. A few weeks later, the asylums received lists of patients they were to prepare for transfer, supposedly at the behest of the Reich Defense Commissar.

Following problems at the start, transports from the "asylums of origin" were no longer sent directly to the killing centers; instead, they took a detour through "interim asylums." This detour made it possible to correct errors. Above all, it was intended to erase all trace of the patients, while at the same time making it possible to release transferred patients whose relatives intervened quickly and firmly. Asylum directors soon became aware of the transfer routes, as well as the planned goal of exterminating these patients; however, they generally kept this information from the relatives.

On the same date that processing began, 9 October 1939, the organizers also established a figure of sixty-five thousand to seventy thousand people to be killed in Operation T-4. This target figure had been exceeded by 273 persons before the program was suspended, as it was termed, in August 1941. This "suspension" might more accurately be called a pause for reorganization. The period of reorientation that followed resulted in an ever-increasing number of groups being included among those slated for selection and possible extermination—tuberculous patients, the elderly, the homeless, and people deemed unwilling to work.

A parallel killing program in concentration camps, disguised as a file number—Operation 14 f 13—had already gotten under way by April 1941. Its aim was to gas, by the winter of 1944–45, all concentration camp prisoners who were unable to work, disruptive, or simply exhausted. Selection, deportation, and execution were placed in the hands of what concentration camp personnel called "the famous Berlin organization," T-4. The practical work of this extermination program combined medical and social criteria, treating them as interchangeable. The program was one of the links that made it possible for the crime against German patients known as *euthanasia* to become a model for far more extensive mass murders. Thus, in 1941 and 1942, Tiergartenstrasse 4 donated one hundred of its experts to the "final solution of the Jewish question in the east." The original commandants of Belzec, Sobibor, and Treblinka came from T-4 and were on its payroll.

Patients in mental institutions were killed because it was cheaper than caring for them. The most important criterion for allowing them to live was their ability to work. On the other hand, patients legally committed to preventive detention and those of Jewish origin were murdered simply because of their social or racial classification. No medical recommendation whatsoever was necessary.

The basis for Operation T-4 was neither an order nor a law, but an informal secret letter from Hitler "authorizing" the killing. In response to pressure from the Minister of Justice and the doctors involved, however, the Law on Euthanasia for the Incurably Ill was drafted in 1940.

Most likely in October 1940, a commission of some thirty experts met to discuss a euthanasia law. The Expert Council on Population and Racial Policies was represented by eugenics expert Fritz Lenz; the Main Reich Security Office sent Reinhard Heydrich. State health authorities were also present; T-4 advisers and professors clearly outnumbered other participants. This conference precisely defined the authority to kill. "Arbitrary measures" involving, for example, handicapped persons who still retained their faculties (though only those over two years old!) or senile patients were prohibited; an observation and recommendation period of two years in an asylum, accompanied by "active" therapy, became mandatory. The discussion on implementation, in particular, indicated that this legal project was, in fact, part of a long-term strategic plan to turn the ad hoc extermination practiced by T-4 into a professional system to exterminate the incurably ill. The minimum age for "euthanasia on demand" would be 21 or 25 (§1); on the other hand, there was no talk of such an age limit in the case of §2 (state-ordered extermination against the will of the victim). In this case, "substantial mental infirmity" referred to people of all ages. And in order to prevent any misunderstanding, "Easing death throes once they have begun [was] not the object of this law."

These guidelines remained largely unimplemented, mainly for fear of objections from abroad or from the church. Those responsible also hoped to avoid provoking popular opposition or disturbing the consciences of patients' relatives. Although they often accepted murder of the chronically ill with suspicious—and therefore suppressed—indifference, the overwhelming majority of Germans were not so lacking in conscience as to agree consciously to legally authorized euthanasia of their relatives.

In contrast, the politicians, physicians, and professors who discussed the euthanasia law were quite serious about establishing precise criteria for scientific killing. In addition to advocating anonymous, assembly line murder of patients classified as incurable, their notion of progress included the conviction that, after the era of mass killings, the number of chronically ill patients could be reduced still further through continuing reform of "active therapy." The doctors involved in T-4 saw themselves as reformers; they were the ones, they felt, who would deal a death blow to the gloomy institutional milieu. They planned to reduce the number of chronically ill patients, not only through their particular brand of clinical execution, but also through the earliest and most intensive possible therapy.

In this context, it is understandable that T-4 opened two departments of its own for basic psychiatric and neurological research in 1942, and even planned to establish its own scientific journal to publish the results of this broad-based research. These plans soon had to be shelved due to the military defeats that began in 1942. The course of the war favored T-4's tendency to include more and more people in the category of possible victims, while involving more and more asylums and physicians in the killing.

In the end, increasing numbers of people who were considered useless in some form or other fell into T-4's deadly clutches. They extended far beyond simply the mentally ill. While within Germany the Nazis expanded and varied the criteria for clinical executions, in the Soviet Union all inmates of psychiatric hospitals, without exception, were killed by the Nazis immediately after the invasion. Reliability and ability to perform productive work increasingly determined the worth of human lives.

In July 1943, the T-4 professors and advisers decided to kill psychiatric patients in order to make beds available for victims of Allied bombing raids. When local authorities needed blankets, medical equipment, and beds for the wounded, the mentally ill and infirm were transferred to public asylums, where they were killed in great numbers through overdoses of tranquilizers. Among the victims of this type of emergency medical care were people who became distraught in Germany's burning cities; they were committed to mental hospitals as "disturbed air-raid victims."

Starting in 1943, slave laborers who were no longer capable of working were also systematically killed. These included people who were psychologically ill (or were thought to be), as well as tuberculosis patients. (In addition, "racially undesirable" children of female slave laborers were either killed outright or allowed to die from miserable conditions and undernourishment. The scenes of these crimes were called "infant homes" or "infant concentration camps"; they were the responsibility of the labor offices, and sometimes of local insurance companies.)

The interruption in August 1941 that ended the first phase of the asylum murders was also the point at which T-4 abandoned its informal, extrainstitutional character. From this point on, the Reich Ministry of the Interior took the lead in exterminating "unusable" Germans; it did so on the basis not of a vague authorization from the Führer, but of a published law. While the Ministry of the Interior had previously acted as an auxiliary to the Reich Association of Mental Hospitals and to the Führer's Office, which supported it, the reverse was now the case. But this did not yet complete T-4's transformation into a normal government office. At the beginning of 1944, the director of T-4 suggested that the "entire body of mental health law be standardized" and that "the incredibly large number" of individual regulations be nullified. Plans called for a Central Office for Care of the Mentally Ill, which would fully institutionalize T-4. In the draft, it was referred to as the Reich Office for Mental Hospitals. Two self-contained subsections would take care of so-called practical work. One would be responsible for finances, the other for "evaluation of question-naires and execution of measures arising from them."

Those involved hoped Operation T-4 would increasingly become part of the legally regulated routine of state administration. Clinical execution of defenseless, chronically ill people was to become a normal part of medical routine and community life.

"Worthless Life"

Hitler's authorization of murder in asylums, dated 1 September 1939, took into consideration the value of a precise, well-defined procedure. Following a "most careful evaluation of their condition," patients "who [were] most likely incurable [were] to be granted a merciful death." In 1940, to make the procedure still more objective, a draft law designed to reassure the protagonists was announced and distributed. In its final known version, called the Law on Euthanasia for the Incurably Ill, it included a preamble, six paragraphs, and provisions for implementation.

> Preamble
> Preservation of the life of persons who desire an end to their suffering due to incurable illness, or who are incapable of productive existence as a result of incurable chronic ailment, . . . [remainder of text unavailable; probably something like "is incompatible with the moral norms of the national community"].
>
> §1
> Persons suffering from an incurable illness burdensome to themselves or others or certain to be fatal can, at their express request and with the permission of an authorized physician, receive euthanasia from a doctor.
>
> §2
> The life of a patient otherwise requiring lifelong care as a result of incurable mental illness can be ended by medical means imperceptible to him.[1]

Extension of what was allowable under the penal code was the subject of the film *I Accuse* (September 1941). In its final scene, the film blames human suffering on supposedly inhuman, rigid laws.* This continues to be the issue for those in Germany—and elsewhere—who are once again discussing "humane death." At the heart of the matter lies the idea of one's own death, and the desire for a quick, painless death—through suicide, if necessary, with the required assistance.

In 1981, a prominent German doctor, Julius Hackethal, made the death of a woman with facial cancer the subject of a video that was later broadcast on television. He provided his patient, more or less officially—and at her own request—with cyanide. Over 60 years earlier, it had occurred to authors Karl Binding and Alfred Hoche† that "a doctor or other assistant [can give] a person suffering from serious cancer of the tongue a lethal morphine injection."[2] Prior to 1939, such individual requests by relatives or patients themselves provided a basis for accelerated preparation of state extermination of the chronically ill. The department of the Führer's Office that would later organize this extermination was in charge of responding to such pleas for mercy, which came more and more often

* At first, in educational films and slide shows, the Nazis had propagated an image of psychiatric patients as disgusting and unworthy of living. When popular reaction indicated in 1940 that murder of the sick, while accepted, did not enjoy active support, the Führer's Office and the T-4 functionaries changed their strategy.

An aesthetically accessible film was made this time to appeal to emotion rather than reason. The script was drafted by Hermann Schweninger, a documentary filmmaker and schoolmate of the euthanasia official Brack. As a GEKRAT transport leader, he had had practical experience in the deportation of thousands of southern German patients to killing institutions. Wolfgang Liebeneiner directed; the main roles were played by Heidemarie Hatheyer and Matthias Wiemann. *Ich klage an* (*I Accuse*) premiered in Venice in 1941.

This film was intended to disseminate the two main points of the draft law on active euthanasia that had existed since 1939: death on demand and the destruction of "worthless lives." The director collaborated closely with the Führer's Office on the details of production, language, and scenes; at the premiere, the Reich Ministry of Propaganda prohibited reviews of the film from employing the word "euthanasia." The plot involves a beautiful woman who becomes ill with multiple sclerosis and, after nearly asphyxiating, asks that her suffering be ended. After experiencing terrible pangs of conscience, her husband, a doctor who has devoted all his research to curing her, decides to give her an overdose of medication. This killing out of sympathy and great love is contrasted with the suffering of a child who has become blind and deaf as a result of meningitis. The film leaves the audience with the idea that it might be necessary to make euthanasia legal.

† In 1921, Karl Binding, professor of criminal law in Leipzig and a liberal reformer of German penal law who is still respected today, and Alfred Hoche, a Freiburg psychiatrist, laid the propaganda foundation for the later murders. Together they wrote the book *Die Freigabe der Vernichtung lebensunwerten Lebens: Ihr Maß und ihre Form* (Destruction of worthless life: Its extent and form).

from an increasingly fascist middle class. It is not widely known that the institution responsible for killing handicapped children after August 1939—the Reichsausschuss zur wissenschaftlichen Erfassung erb- und anlagebedingter schwerer Leiden (Reich Committee for the Scientific Processing of Serious Genetic Diseases, or "Reich Committee")—also arranged killings upon request. In northern Germany, such killings were carried out in Uchtspringe Mental Hospital near Stendal.[3]

Those involved in implementing the euthanasia program were generally between 30 and 40 years old. To the extent they had thought at all about their own death, it was to be quick and uncomplicated. A heart attack, a bullet to the head—the ideal end, quick and painless. It could hardly be called dying. We happen to know exactly what Assistant Secretary Herbert Linden, the official in the Reich Ministry of the Interior responsible for supervising institutional killings, thought of this. In 1941, an unmarried Catholic Viennese woman, the mother of a handicapped half-Jewish child, managed to force her way into his office and take him to task: "Please, Dr. Linden, that may be a Berliner's view, but a Viennese perishes at the thought. Imagine if you were sick and knew you were being taken away to die." Dr. Linden responded with a laugh: "Oh, I'd be quite happy about it."[4] Linden shot himself on 27 April 1945.

Orienting the euthanasia discussion toward the individual case suits a modern, secular society attempting to overcome its inability to deal with death. Lobbyists for relaxation of the laws pertaining to "mercy killing" can be found in all political parties, now as ever, regardless of otherwise conflicting ideological positions. The discussion itself has both subjective and objective effects on the will to live and on societal estimates of the value of the life of the seriously ill and handicapped. Support for relaxation of the law increases conspicuously in times of economic crisis. In no society does a wish to die arise simply from the depths of the individual's soul. The woman Dr. Hackethal helped poison herself mentioned that she no longer dared go out on the street because her face was so disfigured; yet the public debate completely ignored this aspect of her life and death.

Death wishes depend upon material conditions, as well as upon whether a society classifies suffering and death as superfluous misery. The Nazi campaign against "worthless life," like Julius Hackethal's television campaign for quicker death, created its own demand. Such debates produce desperate, self-destructive desires that are transformed into new, apparently individual arguments in an expanding campaign for the destruction of life. In the years after 1939, thousands of German parents and relatives demanded euthanasia for their children, siblings, spouses, or parents, or accepted it half-knowingly as a "deliverance."

The fascist ethos of achievement and extermination was fashioned not only through orders from above but also through impulses from below. Binding's formulation was quite characteristic: "I, too, would say that the mother who does not cease to love her child despite its condition should be allowed to object, as long as she herself takes on its care or bears the costs of it."[5] Beginning in 1943, such mothers were registered at employment offices by the euthanasia authorities; state financial allowances for handicapped children had already been cut off in 1941.[6]

Silent Consent

What the Nazis still lacked in their arsenal of domination was public opinion research. In the summer of 1939, when Hitler's personal physician Theo Morell wrote a memorandum, "Extermination of Worthless Life," he attempted to compensate for this lack by analyzing earlier surveys. His memorandum was intended as the basis for a decision by his powerful patient, and was probably written at Hitler's express wish. A draft has been preserved. After formulating the first paragraph of a possible law on the extermination of worthless life, Morell immediately turned to the "question of implementation." In his opinion, such a program would require a "government operation": "Should the measures be based on a published law, or should they be implemented by way of a secret directive? The latter course may at first seem incomprehensible. However, I consider it justified to treat it in this context. It touches upon a factor expressed in Meltzer's statistics."[7]

Morrell was referring to a questionnaire by Saxony's chief medical officer, Ewald Meltzer,[8] director of the Katharinenhof (the Saxon State Home for Non-Educable, Feeble-Minded Children in Grosshennersdorf). In 1920, "shortly after the appearance of Binding's report," Meltzer had asked the parents of children in his sanitarium what they thought of Binding's ideas. For this purpose, in autumn 1920 he sent a four-part questionnaire to the male parents or guardians of the two hundred children then living at the Katharinenhof:

> 1. Would you give your consent in every circumstance to a painless shortening of your child's life, after an expert had determined him incurably imbecilic?

2. Would you give your consent only if you could no longer care for your child, for example if you were about to pass away?

3. Would you give your consent only if your child were suffering serious physical and mental anguish?

4. What is your wife's opinion on questions 1–3?[9]

After learning that the first questionnaires to arrive had "worried some of the parents," Meltzer subsequently assured parents in a note that the questions were purely theoretical and that they need not fear for their children's lives; the children would continue to receive the same conscientious care they had been given in the past. Meltzer was surprised by the results of his survey, and he kept them to himself for five years. Of the 200 questionnaires, 162 were returned. Of these, 119, or 73 percent, contained at least one yes response, and 43, or 27 percent, contained at least one no. Among the 43 respondents who answered no to the first question, only 20 answered no to all four.[10]

The majority of those responding in the affirmative had answered with a simple, apparently effortless yes. Some justified their position, as well as their doubts, in brief sentences. Among them, Meltzer highlighted a particular group of parents with similar arguments; this was the line of argument that would be of great interest some twenty years later to Theo Morell and Adolf Hitler:

It is an interesting fact that many of those who answered "yes" expressed themselves as follows: "what should I, a single woman, do? It's up to you, do what you think best! It would have been better if you hadn't asked me at all, if you had just put the child to sleep." "As a former nurse, I consider the question inappropriate, as you just make it difficult for the parents"; her profession and her Christian feelings told her that all incurable patients . . . should be released painlessly from their sufferings and that the relatives should be informed only that they have passed away. "I would have preferred not to have been bothered with this question. If it had been news of sudden death, we would have accepted it. The child would have been at peace a long time ago if something had been done right at the beginning." "I would have preferred not to know anything about it." "Agree in principle, but parents shouldn't be asked; it is difficult for them to confirm a death sentence for their own flesh and blood. But if it were said that he died of some illness or other, everyone would have accepted it."[11]*

* A minister described to American interrogators what happened to the children after 1939, and how the parents and Meltzer were treated: "I know further that in Saxony,

From these statements, Morell concluded for Hitler, "Many parents express the following: If you had simply done it and said that our child died from some illness. One could take this into account. We should not think that we cannot undertake beneficial measures without the *placet* of the people, our sovereign."[12] Meltzer interpreted the parents' attitude thus: "They would like to free themselves and perhaps the child as well from a burden, but they want to do it with a clear conscience."*

Thus, the policy of secrecy—based partly on the results of the questionnaire—was not a matter of careful concealment but an opportunity for the population to agree tacitly to government measures. A similar procedure was followed with the doctors who were occupied with laying the bureaucratic groundwork: "We were told nothing about the operation officially; unofficially it was assumed that everyone had somehow already been sufficiently informed."[13] This was written in the winter of 1940–41 by an assistant physician from the Rhineland, in the most private possible context: her diary. This "secret Reich matter," which was in fact public, essentially was an offer to the population to seek individual ways of avoiding responsibility—an unconfessed complicity that eased the conscience.

On the other hand, the physicians involved in execution through euthanasia demanded legal cover. In Werner Catel's words, "What we are doing here is murder." A euthanasia law, public procedures, legality, and norms were necessary. At the same time, those relatives wishing to take up the Nazi offer, out of conviction or despair and under extreme pressure from pseudoscientific propaganda and economic exigency, must have wanted the most informal, ambiguous type of killing possible. The absence of public norms, which left doctors in a moral dilemma, was in fact

---

euthanasia was practiced upon children in Grosshennersdorf by Löbau. I know for certain from relatives in my parish who lost children in this program that the parents' agreement to the killing of children in the euthanasia program was not obtained. The director of the institution where the killings were carried out, Dr. Meltzer, told me that parents were not informed. Because Meltzer opposed the killing of the children, the institute, which was the property of the church's Inner Mission [its charitable arm], was confiscated and placed under state supervision, and Meltzer was retired" (Nuremberg documents, NO 3817, affidavit of R. Schäfer-Wienecke).

* Meltzer's investigation may have been important to Morell and Hitler for another reason. The majority of the patients at Katharinenhof were the children of Saxon industrial workers—workers who, if they corresponded to the Saxon norm, voted heavily left-wing. Thus, less religiously based popular resistance to "officially secret, beneficial" extermination could be expected here, in the industrial center of the German Reich (Ewald Meltzer, *Das Problem der Abkürzung "lebensunwerten" Lebens*, Halle a.S., 1925, p. 52).

a concession to the uneasy consciences of close relatives of potential euthanasia victims.

Over the years, the Führer's Office cleverly turned this conflict of interest to its advantage. The more euthanasia was practiced, the less it was talked about publicly. At first, in response to inquiries by doctors, bishops, and lawyers, it was claimed that a euthanasia law existed; later, such a law was in fact drafted and discussed extensively by interested parties. Yet it was never officially adopted. In the minds of the perpetrators of euthanasia and their innumerable assistants in health and welfare agencies, a proper law really did exist, though it remained unpublished, supposedly due to "the war and foreign propaganda." This state of affairs allowed them to sleep peacefully at night—and continues to do so to this day. In the absence of an actual published law, however, it was possible to speak of "treatment" to the parents of handicapped children, for example, or "defense of the Reich" to wives of alcoholic men. These mutually accepted euphemisms remain effective today. The combination of a law behind the scenes, on the one hand, and "treatment" and "transfer" in public, on the other, was the best way for the Führer's Office to lay to rest two absolutely contradictory types of moral conflict.

The film *I Accuse* would formulate precisely the same two-track procedure, soothing to the consciences of the various protagonists: the absolute privacy of the situation, a law that should exist but does not, a discreetly "assisting" government. *I Accuse* reflects precisely this tension.

It was not organized resistance that prevented the euthanasia law's adoption. The authorities preferred to legitimize institutionalized killing informally, while at the same time, through propaganda and control of terminology, making such killing an absolutely private matter, a knotty problem that each person was expected to wrestle with on his or her own. In order to carry out euthanasia, the Nazis had to assure there would be no *public* debate over it. This was how so-called secret Reich matters functioned. Thus in general, when considering Nazi Germany, we must ask not How much did the Germans know? but Why didn't they want to know?

This technique of achieving unspoken, passive complicity makes it difficult to judge the degree of popular acceptance or rejection of euthanasia. Acceptance was broad; resistance fed upon popular religiosity and local traditions that the Nazis would only later succeed in destroying through "total war." It was crucial to the strategy of administrative extermination in Germany whether protests remained private or became public. Herein lay the difference between the well-known Protestant pastor Friedrich Bodelschwingh and Clemens August Graf von Gahlen, the Catholic bishop of Münster. Bodelschwingh wrote a few letters but remained outwardly loyal; Gahlen preached from the pulpit. He spoke out publicly, if belatedly, against murder.

During the planning trips they took to all German mental institutions starting in autumn 1941, the killing organization's physicians and rationalization experts took note of the way in which they were received by heads of medical departments and asylum directors. Out of several hundred asylums, only twice did they encounter some form of protest. The attitude of Chief Physician Ernst Lüdemann is representative, though his is the only view recorded:

> During our stay in Ricklingen [an asylum in Schleswig-Holstein run by the charitable arm of the Protestant church], I was introduced to the asylum's doctor, Dr. Lüdemann. . . . I explained clearly that our visit pertained only to the asylum and not to the sick; nevertheless, he mentioned the rumors that were circulating. When I responded that the rumors were less interesting than the rumor mongers, he said that he himself spoke out against rumors whenever he was aware of the facts. He pointed out that difficulties arose precisely because the whole operation was not based on a law. . . . Because of his Nordic-Germanic ethos and his medical work, the operation is understandable to him and in many cases welcome; but, as had been mentioned, without a law, inadequate processing, etc. [Achieving] greater popular support through the movement's propaganda would be desirable.[14]

An exception was the warden of the asylum for deaf-mutes in Wilhelmsdorf (near Ravensburg); he was the only one to disconcert the planning commissioners:

> The only thing interesting about this old asylum, which has nothing special to offer, is the warden. He returned the questionnaire that had been sent out beforehand, because he had been at the Stetten Asylum earlier and knew that patients were to be "killed," as he persisted in putting it. The board then compelled the warden to answer the questionnaire, as he had acted without their knowledge. The warden then filled out 69 of the questionnaires. Nineteen patients were transferred from his asylum, of which eighteen were "killed." The patients were examined by Dr. Mauthe, the senior medical officer. In October 1941, Dr. Straub visited the asylum and determined that another ten were incapable of working. None of those remaining were to be "killed." These are the warden's own words. The warden, Heinrich Hermann, is a fa-

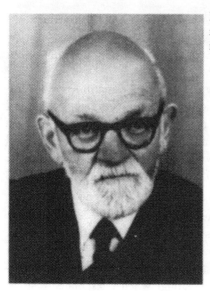

Every asylum director "shared responsibility for the euthanasia issue"—except Heinrich Hermann.

natical opponent of euthanasia. It is important to note that he is a Swiss citizen. This is absolutely unacceptable! No foreigner may occupy this position, which shares responsibility for the euthanasia question—especially not one with a negative attitude.[15]

These institutional murderers with civil servant status were not equal to a confrontation with the naked word "killing." The attack took them completely by surprise, leaving them essentially defenseless. None of the German asylum directors, described in the above document as "sharing responsibility for the euthanasia question," had the courage and moral strength of Warden Heinrich Hermann.* He remained head of the Wilhelmsdorf asylum until 1947.[16]

* On page 221 of Klee is a letter from Hermann dated 6 August 1940, addressed to his superior: "I know the aim of this planned registration. . . . I am simply convinced that the authorities are doing wrong by killing certain patients . . . by exterminating such a patient, or a member of the family or the asylum who is simply abnormal, we are acting against God's will. That is the reason I cannot go along with this. I am sorry, but we must obey God more than human beings. I am prepared to accept the consequences of my disobedience."
    My work owes much to Ernst Klee's *Euthanasie im NS-Staat: Die Vernichtung "lebensunwerten Lebens"* (Frankfurt, 1983). Because I also had access to the sources used by Klee, I have generally cited the source itself; however, Klee's work is important as a reference and as a check on my own work. More especially, without this

The Administration of Euthanasia

Unnatural deaths in German asylums began as early as 1938. Death rates rose markedly; in some cases (for example, at Schwerin-Sachsenberg, Stadtroda, and Großschweidnitz),[17] there is evidence that the centrally run extermination program begun in the summer of 1939 was merely the continuation of an existing practice, with bureaucratic formalities now attached. Starting in 1942, rather than being carried out in special facilities as before, euthanasia was reintegrated into daily asylum routine. A planning commission charged with linking mass murder to modernization of the asylum system as a whole wrote at the time: "With few exceptions, death by euthanasia will hardly be distinguishable from natural death. That is the goal to be striven for. That it can be achieved is proven by the fact that certain active psychiatrists with positive attitudes were already practicing medical euthanasia extensively in their asylums in completely inconspicuous form even before the Operation; today, even in a Catholic *Gau* [a Nazi party administrative region, or district], an asylum can use medical euthanasia for some time without its being recognized at all."[18]

Philipp Bouhler, who, along with Dr. Karl Brandt, was empowered to implement the euthanasia program, "feared the possibility that during a war individual *Gau* leaders here and there would take up this issue and carry it out uncontrolled in their *Gaus*."[19] At the same time, pressure from below provided a sufficiently solid basis for the imminent centrally supervised program of institutional murder.

From the beginning, external blitzkriegs were combined with domestic ones. Like its international counterpart, the domestic political status quo was to be violently altered. This is symbolized by the date—1 September 1939—on Hitler's authorization of euthanasia. This authorization, backdated in its written form but undoubtedly previously issued orally, was not an order; described as "legal authority" in 1940,[20] its vague formulation set into motion the planners' ambition and practical imagination, as well as a systematic bureaucratic procedure. The center of planning was composed of the Führer's Office, the security service, the Ministry of the Interior, and psychiatric practitioners.

With the outbreak of war in September 1939, SD killing units (the Einsatzgruppen) began to shoot asylum inmates by the thousands, not only in occupied and later annexed areas of Poland, but also in Pomerania

---

excellent overview, which historians failed to provide for 20 years, I could not have devoted myself in good conscience to deeper research on this subject.

and West Prussia, the provinces on the eastern border of the German Reich. In October 1939, large groups of Pomeranian patients were transported to a location near Danzig and shot to death.[21] Two offices were apparently in charge of the bureaucratic aspects of these murders: the Central Office for Patient Transfer in Kalisch,[22] and the Central Office for Patient Transfer in Posen headed by Medical Officer Hans Friemert.[23] The former Central Office was most likely responsible for Pomeranian victims, the latter for Polish ones.

At this time, preparations were made for more exact implementation within the German Reich. On 18 August, the Reich Committee for the Scientific Processing of Serious Genetic Diseases was created, as part of the health administration, to function as a collection center for data on "deformed etc. newborns." It was not long before the committee began organizing the killing of handicapped toddlers and infants in so-called Pediatrics Departments.[24] Soon after—on 21 September 1939—Department IV (responsible for the health care system and public welfare) of the Reich Ministry of the Interior drew up a list of "all asylums located within the territory of the Reich in which the mentally ill, epileptics, and the feeble-minded are held more than temporarily."[25] On 3 July, the same department had already succeeded in raising the per diem rate received by "psychiatric experts" for "visiting provincial asylums" to 20 RM, a considerable sum in the context of the times.[26]

On 9 October, the inmates of all mental hospitals began to be "registered for wartime economic purposes";[27] a large majority of inmates, though not all, were registered by 1942. Registration criteria included length of stay, particular diagnoses, and subjection to preventive detention, in addition to ability to work.

On the same day, a "supervisory body" for the planned killing program met in the Führer's Office. Participants included Viktor Brack, Werner Blankenburg, Dr. Hans Hefelmann,* and Reinhold Vorberg of the Führer's Office. Blankenburg was Brack's permanent deputy and at times took charge himself.

Professors Werner Heyde and Paul Hermann Nitsche were the heads

* In the 1960s, Hans Hefelmann gave hundreds of pages of testimony to the Frankfurt prosecutor and judges. He was a roving piece of state's evidence at all trials concerning euthanasia of children. Hefelmann lied consistently on one decisive point, which becomes apparent here. He always acted as though he had had merely organizational responsibility for the killing of handicapped children, as a low-level official. In fact, however, he was not only involved in all other killing programs but ranked above Heyde and Nitsche in the hierarchy.

of the newly created, privately organized, yet in fact government-run killing organization. Heyde was an SS member who for years had visited concentration camps and issued recommendations for forced sterilization; Nitsche was the official government psychiatrist in Saxony and liaison to the German Society for Psychiatry and Neurology. In contrast to the careerist Heyde, Nitsche was a man of the old school, highly regarded by his Saxon patients.

Doctors Gerhard Bohne and Herbert Linden represented Department IV of the Reich Ministry of the Interior. Bohne had been delegated by this department to the killing center as an administrative expert responsible for administrative procedure. In 1941 he was replaced by the substantially more clever Dietrich Allers.* Herbert Linden efficiently and quietly ensured cooperation between state health officials, the authorities in the Führer's Office, and the newly created clandestine special organizations. In September 1941, he moved far up the killing hierarchy, to rank immediately below Blankenburg. The Reich Criminal Investigation Department was represented by senior government councillor Dr. Paul Werner, who organized killing techniques.[28] Karl Brandt and Philipp Bouhler—close collaborators and personal advisers of Hitler's—supervised this body, along with the Berlin professor of neurology and psychiatry Max de Crinis, an SD agent and Heydrich's representative. He had no organizational function but was included in all important decisions.[29]

The SD was also involved in the daily routine of killing, through a number of experts who selected "patients unworthy of living." For example, from 28 February to 14 October 1940, Karl Heinz Rodenberg was expert adviser to T-4. Rodenberg, an SD agent since 1937, was named "honorary member of the security services of the SS Reich Leadership" in 1940; he was put in charge of sexual psychology issues in the Reich Criminal Investigation Department in 1942 and became scientific director of the Central Reich Office to Combat Homosexuality and Abortion in 1944.[30] The director of asylums in Graz, Oskar Begusch, was also an expert adviser and a member of the SD.[31]

The meeting on 9 October concerned the questions of who and how. Following consultation with toxicologists from the police forensic institute, the "how" became clear. Patients were to be killed painlessly—"disinfected," as it was termed—with carbon monoxide. Target figures were also established: "The figure is yielded by a calculation based on a ratio of

---

* After the war, Allers coordinated the evidentiary strategy of T-4 perpetrators in West Germany; Ernst Wentzler did the same for those on the Reich Committee.

1,000:10:5:1. This means that of 1,000 people, ten require psychiatric treatment, five of these as in-patients. Of these, one patient will be involved in the euthanasia program. This means that out of 1,000 people, one will be included in the program. Applied to the population of the Greater German Reich, we must therefore expect 65–70,000 cases. This determination should answer the question 'who?'"[32]

Although Organization T-4 or Central Office T-4 were the cover names—derived, as mentioned above, from the address of its headquarters on Berlin's Tiergartenstrasse, number 4—for a single killing authority, the names in fact stood for a fluid conglomeration of state and quasistate asylums. The name used by Operation T-4 on its letterhead was the Reich Association of Mental Hospitals (RAG). This letterhead suggested a supposedly voluntary centralization of the system of asylums that was actually far from complete. In addition, there was the Public Foundation for the Maintenance of Asylums, the important legal authority involved in the killings; it was responsible internally for work contracts covering 300 to 400 employees, and externally for sales and leases. Its address was Berlin W 35, 4 Tiergartenstrasse. Transport was seen to by the Public Ambulance Service Ltd. (GEKRAT). The last organization to be founded was the Central Clearinghouse for Mental Hospitals. It settled all cost issues and financial problems raised by the death of asylum inmates; thus, it controlled the entire course of the killing to an ever-increasing degree. At the same time, by way of partly faked bills to insurance companies and welfare organizations, it allowed T-4 to finance itself comfortably through social insurance contributions.

These organizations were controlled by the Führer's Office. Specifically, they were led by the department that, under the name of the Reich Committee for the Scientific Processing of Serious Genetic Diseases, implemented the killing of handicapped children in a manner that would serve as a partial model for the later practice of euthanasia on adults. From September 1941 on, the office of the Reich Commissioner for Mental Hospitals became part of this hierarchy. This was the cover name for none other than Department IV of the Reich Ministry of the Interior's medical administration—which, as stated above, was responsible for the health care system and public welfare. Until September 1941, this department mainly assisted in registering asylums and asylum inmates; thereafter, however, it became the leading institution among the T-4 organizations. From this point on, T-4 lost its self-directed, extrainstitutional form; it reintegrated into normal state activity to such an extent

TABLE 1. Killing institutions

Institution	Dates of Operation	Number of Deaths
Grafeneck near Stuttgart	Jan.–Dec. 1940	9,839
Brandenburg	Feb.–Sept. 1940	9,772
Bernburg	Sept. 1941	8,601
Hadamar	Jan.–Aug. 1941	10,072
Hartheim near Linz	May 1940	18,269
Sonnenstein in Pirna	June 1940–Aug. 1941	13,720

Source: NAW, T 1021, Roll 18.

that, toward the end, there were serious plans to rename it the Reich Office for Mental Hospitals.

When, on 24 August 1941, the mass killing was temporarily stopped and then transformed, the target of 70,000 victims had been exceeded by 273.[33] When one of its organizers was nominated for a war medal in 1942, the certificate of nomination read, "Without his decisive contribution, it would not have been possible to complete this special assignment, so important to the war effort, on such a broad basis and with the necessary speed."[34]

The number of psychiatric beds was to be reduced by some 50 percent, to two thousand per million Germans. In order to accomplish this, the average length of a patient's stay was to be drastically shortened; this required "more active therapies," which at the time meant primarily shock treatment. At the same time, long-term patients were to be destroyed. "Cure and care" was to become "cure or death."

The gassing facilities at Bernburg and Hartheim were still operating after 1 September 1941. Concentration camp inmates who were unable to work, criminals, and "psychopaths" continued to be killed there. In Hartheim the number far exceeded 10,000; in Bernburg it was significantly lower. On 15 January 1943, the latter asylum noted: "The Public Foundation for the Maintenance of Asylums, and therefore all asylums, have been idle since 24 August 1941. Since then, only a very small number of disinfections has occurred. A very limited number will continue to occur."[35] At Hadamar, execution of "useless" people—through lethal injections rather than gas—resumed in 1942. Once again, the number exceeded 4,000. After the gassing facilities at Sonnenstein were demolished, it became the site of the first German Reich administrative school; from

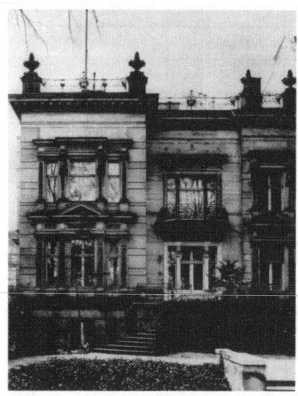

Photograph of the villa at Tiergartenstrasse 4, destroyed during the war. Officially it was bought from its Jewish owners; in reality, it was confiscated.

then on, all candidates for the professional civil service and domestic administration would take their examinations there.[36]

Following their initial experiments and early bureaucratic mistakes, those responsible for euthanasia began to structure the procedure more carefully and more flexibly. Starting in April–May 1940, the T-4 administrative authorities no longer listed by name the absolute number of inmates to be removed; instead, the lists contained some 25 percent more patients than could be deported: "The list contained 94 names, but only 65 patients were taken away, leaving a discretionary margin for those who were transferred, died, etc." This discretionary margin was controlled by the director of the asylum. He was no longer merely an accessory to murder who was sworn to secrecy; he could now share in the decision making, removing from the list patients he found particularly interesting or likeable, or those whose labor made them indispensable.[37]

The second step, taken at the same time, was the establishment of

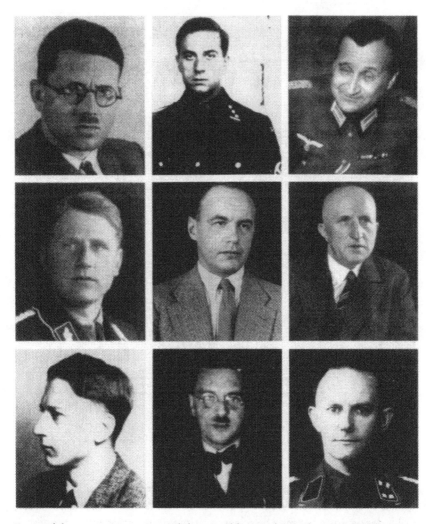

Faces of the perpetrators: (*top*) Philipp Bouhler, Karl Brandt, Max de Crinis; (*middle*) Leonardo Conti, Werner Heyde, Paul Hermann Nitsche; (*bottom*) Georg Renno, Oskar Begusch, Karl Heinz Rodenberg.

intermediate asylums. Transports no longer led directly to death but were interrupted by a stopover of several weeks at another asylum. It is commonly held that this procedure served only as camouflage. However, the period of several weeks between death sentence and execution also provided an opportunity to reduce the number of bureaucratic errors and safely absorb protests. On 9 August 1940, a directive to an intermediate

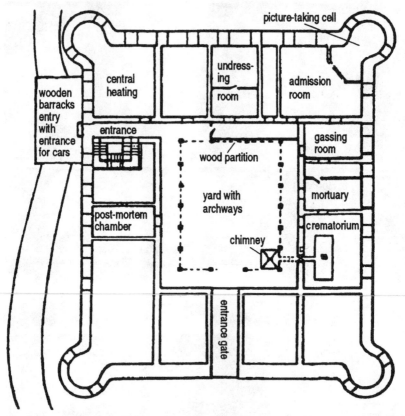

Floor plan of Hartheim Palace, near Lienz, which was turned into an extermination camp.

asylum in Neuruppin responsible for patients from Berlin stated: "In response to the question whether patients on the Public Ambulance Service, Ltd.'s deportation list may be released before deportation at the request of relatives, etc. without the assistance of the Service, the asylum was informed that applications for release must be complied with in every case, unless, as in other cases, there are particular reasons, such as police instructions, preventive detention or danger to the public, which justify rejecting the application for release."[38]

This directive provided a disguised period during which relatives could object. The protagonists waited to see whether relatives would in fact speak up, or if they would instead allow the deadline to pass, thus offering unspoken complicity. At Hadamar, these principles were still strictly applied as late as 1944. Naturally, some institutional directors lied to or turned down concerned relatives. However, the Central Office was not interested in rigid implementation of its intentions; its aim was to make the procedure as smooth as possible. In any case, the drafting and discussion of a euthanasia law legitimized the operation, making it nothing more than an anticipation of future legislation.

The difficulties of the procedure as they appeared, quite realistically, to the perpetrators are described in notes taken by State Court President Alexander Bergmann. Bergmann took these notes at a meeting on 23 April 1941, at which Viktor Brack and Werner Heyde finally convinced leading representatives of the German legal system to take a constructive role in the mass murders:

Brack—Department Head
Euthanasia problem—1 September 1939 proposal by the Führer to Bouhler and Brandt through increase in doctors indicated by name. Grant of mercy killing to the incurably ill.

Not responsibility of state authorities. New problem without precedent, therefore preliminary investigation necessary before law. State authorities not suited for work like this, which appears illegal to outsiders.

It is not a question of the destruction of worthless lives, but an act of mercy for the seriously ill and their relatives.
Law on final assistance by doctors.
§1 At their own wishes for the incurably ill (shortening of death throes).
§2 Painlessly ending the lives of the incurably ill, not at their own wish.
Organization
Must be disguised under neutral names—best psychiatrists—special mental hospitals specially equipped for humane implemenatation.

Find men with courage to implement and nerves to endure.

Registration form from Reich Ministry of the Interior to asylums with patient reports. Return to Reich Ministry of the Interior. Photocopied by Reich Association. Send to several (3) experts independent of one another. After return, transfer 3 recommendations to new photocopies; these to main expert. If he agrees to liquidation, patient transferred to another home; here patient examined based on personal knowledge. After observation, taken to liquidation facility. Here, too, implementing doctor retains a veto.

Discussion with relatives. Discussion on assets. At first, unfortunate choice of means to inform relatives. Value of operation not merely pecuniary. Important commitment of valuable personnel to care of patients.

Dr. Heyde—Prof.
Question of earmarking patients. Naturally only the incurably ill, but limits here too. At first only mentally ill considered, because community life generally impossible for them.

Prerequisites therefore:

1. incurable mental illness
2. not useful for productive communal life even within the asylum.

Illnesses to be considered at all:

Schizophrenia (70 percent of the institutions).

Epilepsy—disease of the central nervous system through syphilis, congenital feeble-mindedness, result of encephalitis, additional pathological changes.

Senile illnesses are excepted for the present.

Registration form includes the former illnesses, as well as persons who have been in the asylum for 5 years, the criminally ill.

Check against patient reports (also against false registration forms)

Possible processing of patients by special commissions in the case of unreliable asylums. The initial recommendations are purely medical; the main recommendation is not only medical, but also political (for ex., whether injuries from the World War may also be included—negative; in addition, old people excepted).

Following approval of prerequisites, photocopies go to Public Ambulance Service, Ltd. Patients to intermediate asylums, renewed observation. Then to liquidation asylum, which is largely closed off from the outside world.

Patient dies of fabricated causes; reason: Führer's call for secrecy. Death certificate. Date and cause of death incorrect. In addition, however, a true registry will be kept. Now the estate is carefully processed, which is generally most important to the relatives. In 80 percent of the cases, the relatives agree; 10 percent protest, 10 percent are indifferent.[39]

These minutes, from April 1941, do not indicate the slightest hesitation on the part of these protagonists of euthanasia. Although they saw resistance, they believed it could be kept within bounds; thus they now decided to expand their extermination operation.

In the summer of 1940, all Jewish mental patients were murdered on the basis of a transfer decree from the Reich Ministry of the Interior. As with criminals, Jews were not selected because of the seriousness and duration of their illness; instead, they were killed without any prior selection because of "biological inferiority."[40] On 8 March 1941, in strictest confidence, Blankenburg wrote to the *Gau* leadership concerning registration of the "antisocial":

> On this occasion, I ask you to send a complete index of all workhouses and other asylums located in your *Gau* and other asylums where the antisocial are kept. At the same time I ask you to indicate who runs the asylums involved and how many inmates are accommodated there.
>
> Because experience shows that inmate groups are quite varied, I would be interested in receiving information on these if possible. I am particularly interested in learning whether, as I have been informed in the case of certain asylums, incurable cases of mental illness and idiocy are also being housed there when other accommodations are not available.[41]

On 10 March 1941, on the basis of a discussion in Berchtesgaden, the two "euthanasia commissioners" tightened up the guidelines for selection.[42]

At about the same time, in April, Operation 14 f 13 began in the concentration camps. It did not differentiate among inmates imprisoned because of race, religion, lifestyle, or political convictions. However, there was one difference: for Germans categorized as Aryan, the T-4 doctors carried out a superficial physical examination; for those categorized as Jews, they reached a decision based upon the files.[43]

On 22 June, Germany began its campaign of extermination against the Soviet Union. Once again, it was the SD killing units that set new standards in the practice of mass murder and the criteria upon which it was based. The campaign was similar to the attack on Poland, but far more extensive; it aimed to kill not tens of thousands, but millions of people.[44] At the same time, the "Final Solution of the Jewish Question" went into effect. It was linked in many ways to the employees and technical experience of T-4.[45] And at this point, the decision had also been made to starve millions of Russian prisoners of war to death.

An assessment of Dr. Curt Schmalenbach on 21 June 1941 indicates the extent to which T-4 doctors were involved in expanding the killing to include unproductive, supposedly inferior classes and segments of entire populations: "He was only recently appointed a senior government councillor, and is constantly rushing off on secret assignments (for example to Paris, Warsaw, Prague, Vienna, etc.). In addition, he has an identification card from the Führer's private office (Bouhler), with which he is authorized to refuse any information on his activities and the purpose of his trip."[46]

When Hitler halted Operation T-4 on 24 August 1941, he did so for a number of different reasons. Protest had come for the first time not in writing but publicly, in a sermon by the Münster bishop Clemens August Graf von Gahlen. The film *I Accuse* was completed at the same time, and it seemed a good idea to allow a pause to give the propaganda time to spread. A second possibility is simply that Operation T-4's aim—the killing of 70,000 "useless eaters"—had been achieved, and the specialists in human extermination in the Führer's Office sought new and greater responsibilities.

Though the physicians involved were at first surprised, they took advantage of the period of relative calm to "raise the reputation of psychiatry," carry out medical research, and engage in long-term planning and reform of the entire asylum system. They hoped to use the extra space and personnel resulting from the mass murders for modernization. Only at first glance does it seem contradictory that these medical executioners also worked actively and energetically to develop new methods of therapy and transform mental hospitals into clinics.

On 23 October 1941, Reich Minister of the Interior Frick appointed Herbert Linden to be Reich Commissioner for Mental Hospitals.[47] Linden from then on ranked above Heyde and Nitsche in the hierarchy of killing. With this step, the practice of mass murder was reinstitutionalized following its initial breakthrough phase. T-4, the GEKRAT, and the Central Clearinghouse became auxiliary organizations to Department IV of the Reich Ministry of the Interior. The activists at T-4 reminisced about the "period of the Operation," not without nostalgia; at the same time, they adapted constructively to the new situation and worked to secure their own positions. In August 1944 Hans Joachim Becker, chief of finance of the Reich Association, described a positive side of the increasing pressure to act in the face of looming defeat. In an almost reformist tone, he wrote to Linden, "As I have already stated, I consider the present time—in which we are seeking new, simpler methods—to be perhaps quite suited to tackling the area of responsibility that is important to us." Becker proposed creation of a Reich Office for Mental Hospitals.[48]

Although Hitler's order led to a definite reduction in killing in German psychiatric institutions, at the same time it varied and extended the range of victims. After August 1941, the murders continued along specific, precise lines. Criteria included "public menace," "criminality" (requiring preventive detention), a "psychopathic condition," "antisociality," and racial and social "inferiority." Added to psychiatric criteria, these additional characteristics became a death sentence for the mentally ill. In addition, patients were commonly killed for research purposes, and killing through starvation was also permitted.[49]

At the same time, a new, even more systematic "processing" of potential victims began. In the years that followed, patients in old-age homes and hospitals for tuberculous patients and inmates of workhouses and correctional institutions were caught in the bureaucratic nets of the Reich Association.

At the beginning of 1942, a letter on empty beds contained the following: "It has proven increasingly necessary to place the openly tuberculous antisocial in asylums. However, the number of beds made available for this falls far short of the demand."[50] In 1942, T-4 started on old age homes. On 21 August, Nitsche wrote to Herbert Linden:

> The medical commissions of the Reich Association of Mental Hospitals have determined that a very large number of old-age homes in the Reich, almost exclusively belonging to the Catholic Caritas association and the Protestant Innere Mission, and their inmates are still not known to either the supervisory or the medical authorities. . . . most of these homes are also unknown to the Reich Association, although it has been shown that a large number of inmates are required to register on Registration Form I. In addition to the infirm and physically frail, the feeble-minded and chronic mentally ill are almost always found in these homes.[51]

The Reich Committee for the Scientific Processing of Serious Genetic Diseases expanded its killing jurisdiction to include children up to 14, and later up to 17 years old.[52] On 20 June 1941, the Reich Ministry of the Interior published a decree entitled Planwirtschaftliche Verwendung von Anstalten und Heimen zur Unterbringung Minderjähriger, insbesondere für die Zwecke der erweiterten Kinderlandverschickung (Wartime Utilization of Asylums and Homes to Accommodate Minors, Especially for the Purpose of Increasing Transfers of Children to the Countryside).[53] The extent to which T-4 included these welfare cases in its planning is evidenced, first of all, by the later killing of mixed race children from homes in Hadamar, and second of all by an excited note from Nitsche: "Dr. Hebold informs me that the Hitler Youth in Saxony has created numerous homes for delinquent youngsters that have been occupied for the last three to six weeks. Patients processed by us have also been transferred to these homes. The question now arises whether these homes and their entire stock of patients are to be processed by our doctors again, or whether only patients already processed are to be sought by our medical commission."[54]

This phase of institutional killing, based on careful systematization and long-term planning and reform, came to an abrupt end early in 1943. This cessation was brought on not by internal opposition but exclusively by the course of the war. From this point on, emergency medical care for the bombed-out cities was organized by the Reich Ministry of the Interior under the leadership of Karl Brandt, who was appointed General Commissar for Health and Medical Services. Killing once again increased sharply, but it was now organized on a new, decentralized basis. Recently developed distinctions eroded in face of the need to make beds available for the physically ill; from then on, the mentally ill were killed as needed.

In 1945, Dr. Richard Schäfer, pastor of the Risa Parish on the Elbe, told American investigators, "In 1940 and in 1943 and 1944, urns were sent more frequently. In 1942 deliveries became less frequent, but never ceased entirely." [55]

All German cemetery authorities were informed from the beginning that urns would be sent. This happened at a meeting of the German *Gemeindetag* (conference of mayors) on 3 April 1940, and was personally noted by Plauen's mayor Wörner. He subsequently informed his cemetery inspector, Hopfe, "regarding urns to arrive in the near future." The meeting was headed by the mayor of Munich, *Reichsleiter* Karl Fiehler; the head of Department III—Social Policy (including the institutional system) of the German *Gemeindetag,* Dr. Georg Schlüter, was responsible for any questions that might arise. He had already held this position in the Weimar Republic. The wording of the invitation is also interesting; it indicated that the meeting was taking place "at the behest of a higher office," and that the agenda would not be announced until the meeting itself. The mayors of all German cities were present. The minutes read as follows:

Secret Reich Matter
For the secret files of the administration
Only Chief Inspector Hopfe to be informed.

On 3 April 1940, a secret meeting of the German *Gemeindetag* took place in Berlin. It was chaired by Herr *Reichsleiter* Fiehler; an old party comrade, Brack, spoke on patients in city mental institutions. He explained:

In the many mental institutions in the Reich there are an infinite number of incurably ill patients of all kinds who are completely useless to humanity; in fact, they are nothing but a burden, their care creates endless expense, and there is no possibility that these people will ever become healthy or useful members of human society. They vegetate like animals, and are antisocial people unworthy of living; but otherwise, their internal organs are healthy and they could live on for many decades. They only take nourishment away from other, healthy people, and often need two to three times as much care. Other people must be protected from these people.

If, however, we must already make preparations for maintainance of healthy people, then it is all the more necessary first to eliminate these beings, even if only to better maintain curable patients in mental hospitals.

The space that would thus become free is needed for all sorts of things important to the war effort: military hospitals, regular hospitals, and auxiliary hospitals.

Thus those seriously ill, that is, incurable patients who are involved must be *packed into very primitive special asylums*. In these specially created asylums, nothing must be done to maintain these seriously ill patients; on the contrary, everything must be done in order to have them die as quickly as possible.

In order to carry out this operation, a *commission of physicians has been appointed* to sift through all asylums involved and decide which patients should be sent to such asylums.

A High Commission superior to this commission will make final decisions in special cases.

The entire problem is very difficult, and it is necessary to act very cautiously, for the public must not learn of it. It is difficult above all because of the church, which is absolutely opposed to cremating the dead; a dispute now with the Pope is completely undesirable. It is also dangerous because of the Americans, who could enter the war against us for such a reason.

One can keep the entire problem secret from the population; that is not such a big problem.

Much more difficult is the question of the asylums themselves. It would be best if those involved were to be placed in very bad barracks where they could contract pneumonia; in other words, accelerate their death rather than artificially maintaining them.

Those who die in this way would have to be cremated to prevent disease, not in city crematoriums, but in the asylums' own ovens. When doing this, it is necessary to consider the dispute with the church, namely with the Catholic church, and to avoid any tensions. Nor must it be forgotten that most of the relatives are still against cremation.

In practice, the entire operation would have to proceed more or less as follows: Those involved are sifted through by the commission, and then evacuated to other institutions, so that cremation of the corpses can proceed in these asylums.

The best way to deal with the relatives of the patients involved is for the asylum to inform the relatives of the deceased with the notation that [cremation] of the patient has already occurred to prevent disease, and *the urn with the mortal remains is available to the family and will be sent at no cost;* however, if there is no place to store the urn in their hometown or its surroundings, the urn will be sent to the nearest cemetery office free of charge for temporary storage, *where the urn will be available at any time to the relatives whenever they would like it.*

When such urns are sent to the cemetery offices, the cemetery office must keep no files on them. And no cost lists for expenses that may arise, so that no traces of the operation can be found. The *storage of such urns* should occur simply and without any extravagance, primitively and functionally. All such urns should be stored in *one* place, so their purpose can be recognized at any time; for the name of the patient, dates of birth and death, and home community are on the urn, so that if the relatives want the urn it can be found immediately. Relatives should not be brought to the site of the urns; instead, the urns should be picked up by the cemetery administrator.

The practical procedure at the cemetery should occur as follows:

One fine day, a package will arrive at the cemetery with more or less the following accompanying letter:

Enclosed please find an urn for the deceased person involved, name, dates of birth and death, name of home community. We request storage of the enclosed urn.

The cemetery administration will bring this urn to a predetermined site, at which all urns sent later in the same way will be stored, and there the urns remain. That takes care of the entire ceremony.

Few expenses can arise for the communities, as the cost of cremation will be paid by the Reich. Otherwise, the Operation relieves the communities to a great extent, as future costs of care are eliminated in each individual case.

Questions should be addressed to Herr Deputy Dr. Schlüter at the *Gemeindetag* in Berlin.

Leipzig death notices, 1940:

"We received the painful news of the sudden death of our dearly beloved daughter, sister, and sister-in-law Edith Francke. Cremation has already occurred in Grafeneck. Leipzig, Gustav-Adolf-Strasse 47a, Rothenberg t. Odenwald, 1 October 1940.

In silent mourning,
Paul Francke and wife, née Consentius
Gisela Francke
Pastor Dr. Lucius and wife, née Francke
We ask that you refrain from expressions of sympathy."

"Otto Rees-Koch, recipient of the Cross of Honor for soldiers at the front 1914–18 and other honors. Born 11-26-84; died 9-15-40. After weeks of uncertainty, I received the incomprehensible news of his sudden death and subsequent cremation at Linz on the Danube. Leipzig o 5, Ob. Münsterstr. 2.v.

In deep mourning
Emma, widow Theilemann
In the name of all who knew him.
Urn funeral Wednesday, 10-15-40, 9 o'clock A.M., Johannis cemetery."

"Relieved of his great suffering. With pain and disbelief, we received the news of the passing on of my dear husband, my kind father, our dear son, son-in-law, and brother-in-law, Martin Vogt, at the age of 48. Leipzig S. 3, Adolf-Hitler-Strasse 77.II.r.

In silent mourning
Marie Vogt née Reck
Charlotte Vogt
in the name of all his relatives
Cremation has already taken place at Hartheim near Linz on the Danube."

The next two sections provide a background for Dr. Schäfer's evidence. They concern planned extermination of the antisocial within the framework of euthanasia and T-4's emergency medical practices during the bombardments.

Social Inferiority as Grounds for Euthanasia

"Aliens to the Community" and Psychopaths

The concept "alien to the community" (*gemeinschaftsfremd*) was at the time a sociological term, corresponding more or less to today's concepts of marginality, deviance, and nonconformity. The definition was geared toward prevention—a socio-educational and policing goal that was not invented by the Nazis.[56] A law "on the treatment of the *gemeinschaftsfremd*," which was completed in 1945 but never actually took effect, defined it as follows:

> An "alien to the community" is:
> 1. One whose personality and way of life renders him incapable of fulfilling the minimum demands of the national community through his own efforts, especially as a result of extraordinary defects in judgment or character.[57]

This definition included dissipation, rowdiness, drunkenness, and loafing on the job; it also covered those with disorderly lifestyles—beggars, those remiss in paying support, thieves, swindlers, and of course criminals.

On 18 July 1940, the Reich Ministry of the Interior issued the little-noted "Guidelines for Evaluating Genetic Health." These guidelines divided all Germans into four categories: (1) antisocial, (2) acceptable, (3) average citizens, or (4) persons of particular genetic value. Under this edict, the antisocial were excluded from all financial allocations.[58] In March 1941, the regulations covering allowances for children stated:

> Children's allowances relieve family burdens in order to promote healthy German families worthy of the community. The aim of this population policy is to strengthen the German people. Therefore, considerations of charity and social welfare must be avoided in decisions on granting or refusing children's allowances.
>
> Children's allowances must be granted in accordance with the aims of children's allowances. This is not the case if children's allowances are granted:

1. to antisocial (alien to the community) families as defined in the decr. of the Reich Min. of the Int. of July 18, 1940—*RMBliV*, p. 1519–; . . .

7. to a head of household who cannot guarantee effective utilization of the children's allowance . . .

8. for children of single mothers whose progenitor is unknown.[59]

The sociological and ideological concept "alien to the community" was supplemented and its groundwork laid by the psychiatric concept of the "psychopath," under which any form of individual resistance, often simply desperate nonconformity, had long since been declared an illness. In the Third Reich, this became grounds for extermination. In 1942, T-4 expert Hans Heinze defined who was to be considered "unstable," "emotionally impoverished," "moody," "insecure," "querulous," or "sexually deviant":

> Prostitution, vagrancy, and professional criminality are, according to Linden, without exception states of behavior that in themselves justify an assumption of unfitness for marriage. This commentary also mentions pimping and so-called pauperism for endogenous reasons. According to Rüdin, others obviously unfit for marriage are those who have been punished for psychopathy, so-called born criminals and enemies of society, swindlers, cheats, frauds and confidence tricksters, hysterical scoundrels, provenly unstable and thus antisocial psychopaths, the common emotionally impoverished, particularly those who are serious and incorrigible criminals by nature; also confirmed prostitutes, pimps, incorrigible and active confirmed homosexuals, and incorrigible shirkers.[60]

Even after he had begun making diagnoses that effectively sentenced people to death, Heinze still spoke publicly of forced sterilization. He demanded it "urgently" for "antisocial and recidivist criminal psychopaths whose hereditary deviance of character can be inferred from their genealogy." This definition concerned the lowest class of public welfare recipients, "elements tending toward parasitism." "We hope," continued Heinze, "that after the war, the fight against or extermination of subhumanity through purposeful measures will take its honored place as a further great deed beside those already accomplished."[61]

The Reich Committee

Forced sterilization was anticipated by the Law on Aliens to the Community and its preparatory propaganda. Since the beginning of the war, this type of "maintenance of genetic health" had been greatly restricted, if only because of the amount of time and legal bureaucracy it involved. The killing of those who might otherwise have fallen victim to the sterilization law was quantitatively more significant. There was, however, a precursor to the planned legislation—a secret decree of 19 November 1940.[62] It involved "abortions [in cases] in which it can be assumed with great probability that the birth of additional children would be undesirable." Such abortions were permitted until the end of the sixth month. On the basis of a "special authorization"* granted Brandt and Bouhler orally by Hitler, the section of the Führer's Office that supervised the entire euthanasia program (and implemented it itself where children

* Some German historians continue to seek a written order by Hitler on extermination of the Jews. If this order had been made in writing, as was the case with the written authorization of euthanasia, it would prove Hitler's personal responsibility for, and control over, the extermination of the Jews. Wolfgang Scheffler, a historian who knows the material better than most, objects: "Such a written commitment by Hitler is quite improbable, particularly in light of the problems caused by his authorization of euthanasia." The discussion of "special authorization" of extralegal abortion strongly supports Scheffler's argument. The secret decree on abortion was dated 19 September 1940; the Führer's Office (Reich Committee) made the decision, and the Reich Ministry of the Interior (Linden) carried it out. A conflict developed with the Reich Ministry of Justice, which asked Linden on 16 April 1941 to "inform us of the text of the 'special authorization.'" On 24 May, Linden wrote to the Reich Ministry of Justice: "The text of the authorization is not known to the Reich Ministry of the Interior. *Reichsleiter* Bouhler is keeping it to himself. . . . The authorization is from the Führer."

On 24 September, the Reich Ministry of Justice asked for a meeting with the responsible members of the Ministry of the Interior and the Führer's Office. Undersecretary Roland Freisler wrote: "To prepare for the meeting, I would wish to become familiar with the text of the authorization upon which the procedure is based." On 7 October 1941, the Reich Ministry of the Interior responded that "the Führer's assignment [had been] made not in writing, but orally."

On 26 November—that is, more than a year later—the meeting of the three administrations occurred. The Ministry of Justice noted on the meeting: "The Führer's Office is of the opinion that it is not the right time to ask the Führer to put the authorization in writing. It is certain that the Führer stands by this authorization."

If Hitler refused to put this authorization in writing, it is not possible that he ever gave an "order" (or, more likely, a "special authorization"), in writing, for the physical extermination of the Jews. The discussion described above shows that the backdated written order on psychiatric murders was only provided by Hitler out of necessity, as a result of medical and ministerial pressure, and that the complications that followed, as well as the concrete responsibility for additional, written authorizations or even orders, kept him from making the same mistake again (Geheimerlaß des Reichsministerium des Inneren [RMdI] [Secret Decree of Reich Ministry of the Interior], 19 November 1940, BA, R 22/5008).

were concerned) also authorized abortions for "eugenic, racial, and ethnic reasons."

The Reich Committee was responsible for these decisions; the only consultant involved was Ernst Wentzler, a pediatrician who also participated in the murder of children. The actual abortion procedure was restrictive. On the one hand, it functioned as a loophole for the wives of Nazi leaders; on the other, it anticipated later categories. In the first 10 months, the Reich Committee reached a positive decision on only 53 applications, while rejecting 61. Criterion No. III, established internally, was an important part of the attack on the right to life of those not conforming to German concepts of order: "Inferiority of character, recidivist criminality."[63] All six applications based on this criterion were granted. For example, a report by the local Viennese health officer Hermann Vellguth to the Reich Ministry of the Interior stated, in regard to the family of Marie F., "Of the five children of the married couple F., three have already proven difficult. . . . In sum, there is no doubt that the expected child will be genetically damaged by its antisocial, psychopathic and seriously alcoholic father. Although Marie F. does not suffer from a hereditary illness under the G.z.V.e.N. [Gesetz zur Verhütung erbkranken Nachwuchses; Law for the Prevention of Genetically Diseased Offspring, 1933], and her condition does not require an abortion for health reasons, the birth of an additional child to the couple F. must be considered undesirable."

Viktor Brack authorized the abortion, at the same time offering a choice of two ways to destroy the "antisocial" husband: "Because I still intend to order the husband's admission to a concentration camp, I request that you inform me whether, in your opinion, this seems to be a good idea or whether, given his mental condition, F. requires permanent institutional care."[64]

Thus, the Reich Committee began to exterminate "undesirable" children even before birth, refining and modernizing euthanasia. Viktor Brack specified how far intrauterine prevention of "worthless" life should be pursued, but he also advised caution, pointing out: "Should a child with a hereditary defect be born in a case in which abortion was not ordered, alternatives are available through the Reich Committee."[65]

The criteria of "social behavior" and "generally worthwhile lifestyle" played a decisive role in Reich Committee killings from the beginning. In 1942, 17-year-old Gertrud N. of Kiel died on the Special Treatment Ward of the Reich Committee in Schleswig-Stadtfeld. The left side of her body was partially paralyzed, but she could walk, suffered attacks relatively rarely, and completed a school for the handicapped with some success. She did not require institutionalization. Official medical comments on her social behavior were the decisive factor leading to her commitment to a psychiatric clinic and the clinical execution that followed: "She was always difficult, but now she is impudent, disobedient, no longer listens at all, goes out in the evening, hangs around the barracks, comes home late at night, has already had sex with several men. When her mother locks the door to keep her from leaving in the evening, she yells and makes enough noise to wake the entire house, and invariably runs out as soon as anyone opens the door to check on her."[66]

Particularly when the medical prognosis was not clear, social integration became an additional criterion of inferiority in the files of the Reich Committee asylums. Examples from the Pediatrics Department in Ansbach include:

—Father apparently an adventurer and member of the Foreign Legion, and has a previous record.

—Father professional showman. . . . According to the files, the child's mother exhibits defects of character and ethics.

—Illegal child. Birth of child normal, on time. The mother of the child is currently in prison (Frau Düthorn, the social worker, indicates this is because of contact with prisoners of war). The grandmother comes from a Gypsy family.

—Diagnosis: a high degree of congenital feeble-mindedness with an antisocial streak. [The 15-year-old boy thus categorized attended the institutional school for the handicapped in Kaufbeuren, and was transferred to Ansbach after attempting to escape. The two final entries are: "August 20, 1944: engages in sexual behavior with young girls on the ward, must therefore be kept in isolation. August 27, 1944: became ill with a lung infection several days ago, to which he succumbed today."][67]

The Reich Committee also implemented the sterilization of children registered as mixed-race Gypsies (*Mischlinge*).[68] All this was part of the program of "extermination of subhumans" formulated by Heinze in 1942. The "public health" goals of the Reich Committee went far beyond the killing of individual patients and suffering children.

T-4 and "Aliens to the Community"

Reinhard Heydrich had already taken part in discussions of the euthanasia law at the beginning of July 1940. During the ensuing months of

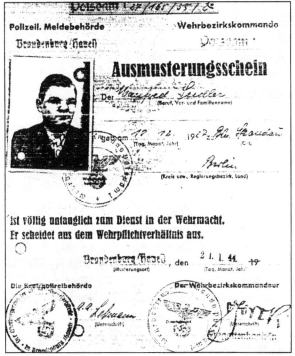

Discharged by the Wehrmacht at 17, killed by the Reich Committee. The Brandenburg-Görden Asylum wrote to his mother, "We are unfortunately unable to give you any good news of your son Manfred's behavior. Our repeated attempts to integrate him into the ward community have failed completely. . . . Therefore, there is nothing left to do for now but to continue to isolate him. Perhaps he will be able to write you in the foreseeable future. At the moment we cannot permit this for the reasons given." The boy died at the beginning of 1945 in Ansbach Asylum.

apparently irrevocable Nazi control over the "greater European area," the Main Reich Security Office, in cooperation with the Reich Criminal Investigation Department, planned to exterminate all nonconforming social minorities. In the summer of 1940, Heydrich apparently believed the time was ripe to work euthanasia into the catalogue of measures he intended to implement against subproletarian minorities; these already included forced sterilization and preventive detention at police discretion. To the Main Reich Security Office, and in terms of genetics and racial hygiene, no essential difference existed between chronic illness and ongoing nonconformist behavior. The draft law was temporarily given an explosive title, Law on Euthanasia for those Incapable of Living and Alien to the

Community. Hans Hefelmann commented, "It had become clear from additions to the draft law that Heydrich wanted to go beyond the scope of those originally affected."[69] This link also seemed quite natural to the euthanasia doctors themselves. Doctor Irmfried Eberl, whose career took him from the Berlin Health Office to Brandenburg, Bernburg, and finally Treblinka, commented on the planned regulation, "Of course, all criminals requiring institutional detention are also covered by this law."[70]

In fact, in the course of the debate over the euthanasia law, social nonconformity and medically diagnosable insanity were again distinguished from each other. However, limitation of the euthanasia law did not mean that the so-called antisocial were removed from the killing program.

In 1941, ability to work became the central criterion for selection: "Elimination of all those incapable of productive work, even in the asylums; that is, not only of those who are mentally dead," was the brief description.[71] The only exceptions were senile inmates, who were to be killed only "in extreme circumstances, such as criminality or antisociality." "Antisociality" thus became an additional characteristic for selection. In practice, Operation 14 f 13, which now went into operation in the concentration camps, made medical and social grounds interchangeable. This was what Heydrich had hoped for in the euthanasia law.

Purposeful terror in the occupied Eastern European countries set the standard in this area as well. In December 1940, for example, the *Gauleiter* (regional party head) of West Prussia had district leaders organize a "special evacuation of antisocial non-Germans." It would include the "following antisocial elements":

1. Persons with criminal records who have been convicted repeatedly by courts of law. Courts of law include the former Polish legal authorities.

2. Persons who, because of constant excessive use of alcohol, are no longer capable of successfully handling their economic and domestic relationships.

3. Female persons who give themselves, for money, to an unlimited number of different persons (prostitutes).

4. The remaining widows and children of persons liquidated for just cause because of their political or criminal background, where activities against the state can be expected of them.

5. Shirkers who persistently refuse to do physical labor assigned to

them and suited to their abilities, despite repeated requests from the authorities.

    6. Persons who are completely degenerate or particularly inferior in appearance.[72]

In 1941, the SD killing units active in the East reported with barbaric regularity that in addition to "Soviet commissars," Jews, and the mentally ill, they were shooting capital criminals, beggars, and "troublemakers." In July 1942, the "Führer of the German population of Slovakia" expressed his thanks for the deportation of seven hundred "antisocials" from the German population: "We succeeded in including the mentally inferior, drunkards, antisocial elements, and to a small extent people who had fallen into need through no fault of their own and could not pull themselves up by their own efforts."[73]*

The fundamental legal step that later made possible the killing of nonconformists, defined socially rather than medically, was the Gesetz gegen gefährliche Gewohnheitsverbrecher und über die Maßregeln der Sicherung und Besserung (Law against Dangerous Habitual Criminals and on Regulations on Detention and Corrections) of 24 November 1933. This law defined the concept of the "dangerous habitual criminal," adding it to the Reich Penal Code as §20a: A person convicted twice within five years to prison sentences of more than six months each could be sentenced the third time to up to five years' imprisonment, even if "the most recent crime is not subject to heavy penalty." The increased sentence could be tripled to fifteen years if the crime itself were punishable as a felony (at least five years' imprisonment). A person who had committed not only two, but "at least three intentional crimes" could be subject to the increased penalty for each new crime, even if he had been sentenced to less than six months for the previous crimes.[74] Despite all the nationalist, racist propaganda of the times, this law treated foreign and domestic convictions equally.

In §42b, this unique addition to the penal law regulated detention in mental hospitals for crimes committed in a state of diminished responsibility. Paragraph 42c provided for placement in a detoxification or treatment center; §42d governed compulsory commitment of those convicted of misdemeanors under §361 of the Reich Penal Code (vagrancy, begging, prostitution) to one of the 26 workhouses in the German Reich. The aim

---

* The deportations took place by ship from Bratislava, probably up the Danube to Mauthausen-Hartheim.

of this measure was to "encourage [the victim] to work systematically and accustom [him or her] to an ordered way of life." Beggers were only to be committed to workhouses "if the perpetrator begged professionally, or because of refusal to work or dissipation"—a regulation that protected war veterans. The euthanasia operation would later, to a certain extent, offer the same protection. The paragraph closed with the provision that "those incapable of working whose committal to a workhouse is ordered may be committed to an asylum."

The prerequisites for these three types of committal—insane asylum, detoxification center, workhouse—were established quite simply in §42e: In addition to the usual punishment, the court could order detention "when necessary to protect public security," as well as, under §42f, "for as long as required." Initial committal to a treatment center, a workhouse, or an asylum was limited to two years. Committal to a mental hospital was "not subject to any time limit"; neither was the second and any further committal to a workhouse or asylum.*

Just as the registration and stigmatization procedures of the July 1933 Law for the Prevention of Genetically Diseased Offspring defined those who would later become victims of the euthanasia operation, the Detention Law defined and distinguished the particular group of people who would be persecuted and killed in workhouses, detoxification centers, and psychiatric institutions.

When a large number of patients were transferred out of the Bedburg-Hau Asylum in the Rhine Province at the beginning of the war, a doctor noted, "Soon after the evacuation from Bedburg, rumors spread that most of the Bedburg patients sent farther into Germany were no longer alive. In particular, of those committed to detention, only one war wounded was still alive (brain-injured officer)."[75] Registration Form 1 asked, "In preventive detention for criminal insanity? . . . Crimes?" These questions targeted additional reasons for killing, a combination of various "inferiorities." Medical and social criteria were already combined in selec-

* The Regulations on Detention and Corrections added 14 new paragraphs (42 a–n) to the Reich Penal Code. They were a confused collection of repressive measures against the lower classes, borrowed from the stock of the Weimar administration: §42k governed forced sterilization of sex murderers and exhibitionists; §42l prohibited people from following their trades if they had served sentences of at least three months which were connected with the trade; §42m governed expulsion of foreigners from the German Reich if they had received prison sentences of over three months and represented "a danger to others or to public security;" §42n provided for a combination of individual measures for certain persons.

tions. Each criminal inmate of an asylum was subject to the registration requirement and was thus doubly endangered. Those in preventive detention in psychiatric institutes were among the first victims.

Public prosecutors were responsible for implementing preventive detention. Extermination was apparently not coordinated with them. Often, prosecutors discovered only during routine checks on length of detention that prisoners they had committed to asylums were already dead. In August 1940, Dresden's public prosecutor complained to Undersecretary Roland Freisler:

> The piano tuner Arnold K., born in 1892 in Jersitz near Posen, was charged with treason in case 4 a Js 37/39 before the State Court of Appeal in Dresden. He had 12 previous convictions; in the most recent case, he had received one year's imprisonment for recidivist fraud from the state court in Bautzen, which also ordered him committed to an asylum. K. had been injured in the war by a shot to the head and was 70 percent incapable of gainful employment. In the treason case, the Waldheim asylum confirmed on 29 November 1939 that K., who by then had been admitted there, was an unstable criminal psychopath; he was not, however, covered by §51 of the Penal Code.
>
> The prosecutor for the State Court of Appeal then brought an indictment, and on 21 February 1940 the State Supreme Court requested it be served on the accused by the Waldheim district court. On 22 February, however, they were informed that service could not occur, as K. had been transferred from Waldheim by the Public Ambulance Service, Ltd., Berlin. When the prosecutor then requested that the above-mentioned company inform him of K.'s present location, he received the following letter:
>
> Brandenburg State Asylum
> Re.: File number 4 a Js 37/39 g.
> Your letter of 27 February to the Public Ambulance Service, Ltd., Berlin W9, Potsdamer Platz, has been forwarded to us. The piano tuner Arnold Karl Ernst K., born on 7 November 1892 in Jersitz near Posen, was transferred here on 8 February 1940 from the Waldheim asylum. K. died here on 16 February 1940 of a heart attack. Heil Hitler!
>
> Signed for
Dr. Meyer

Such cases were often reported to the Reich Ministry of Justice—for example, cases from Chemnitz, Stuttgart, and Naumburg (Saale). A case of 12 October 1940 is horribly typical: With the agreement of the Reich Ministry of Justice, the Dresden prosecutor scheduled the execution of a death sentence for six o'clock in the morning—only to discover that the delinquent had already "died of traumatic fever" three weeks earlier in Sonnenstein.[76]

At the regional level, meanwhile, the authorities communicated with each other much more effectively. On 12 June 1940, Heidelberg's chief prosecutor, Dr. Haas, asked the prosecutor's office in Karlsruhe about the transfer of four patients committed to Wiesloch under §42b of the Reich Penal Code; the asylum had informed him that it was a "secret Reich matter." The answer came promptly. After consultation with the chief prosecutor, the Ministry of the Interior instructed the director of Wiesloch: "It is all right for you to inform the prosecutor that transfer to the Grafeneck State Asylum occurred in the interests of the war economy."[77] But this procedure remained the exception; Undersecretary Franz Schlegelberger, the acting Minister of Justice, eventually lodged a formal complaint with Hans Lammers, head of the Führer's Office, that "abuses" had arisen in penal jurisdiction:

> Trials were initiated and carried out, although the defendants were no longer alive, because prosecutors were not aware of this fact. Indictments and new trials could not be brought to a conclusion because perpetrators or witnesses were "deceased" in the meantime. It has repeatedly turned out that convicted persons committed to asylums have been removed from the prosecutors' continued supervision, transferred from asylums without a hearing, and later eliminated. This has proven particularly awkward when the court must decide on continued commitment under §42f of the Penal Code. The fundaments of criminal procedure have been shaken to such an extent that medical experts declare they can no longer in good conscience determine a defendant's diminished responsibility in borderline cases, thus creating the basis for commitment to mental hospitals, because such commitment means execution of a death sentence without trial.[78]

Soon after this intervention, on 23–24 April 1941, prosecutors and presidents of the state courts were summoned to Berlin and officially informed of the euthanasia program by Viktor Brack and Werner Heyde. At this meeting, the assembled legal experts all accepted, from both legal and political points of view, the directive that every "existing legal norm" was to be interpreted and applied "according to the wishes expressed by the Führer."

After a round of irritated questions, the experts began to offer suggestions for improvement. The prosecutor from Jena proposed, "It would be a good idea to introduce a requirement that liquidation facilities keep correctional authorities informed."[79] The Düsseldorf prosecutor reported on 16 May that the Wuppertal prosecutor, "incorrectly interpreting" instructions, had investigated the whereabouts of all preventive detainees in his district, and remarked:

> In itself, these conclusions would not require a report, as the fact that persons committed in this way are killed provides no cause for measures to be taken. In my opinion, however, it is not clear that it is necessary for the prosecutor to be informed of the transfer of such persons. . . . This directs the attention of officials and employees who deal with the files to the transfers, the frequency of which may in fact prove conspicuous; this seems to me unnecessary and perhaps even a cause for concern. . . . In order to ensure necessary camouflage of the procedure, I consider uniform treatment necessary; this means not reporting transfers, but indicating deaths in the files without a cause of death and within a suitable time period, so that such reports do not accumulate within a short span of time.[80]

Undersecretary Roland Freisler shared this view; but in June 1941, after a one-month period, he had to admit, "The Office of the Führer of the Nazi party has told me . . . that it is not possible at this time to inform the prosecutors immediately."[81]

One point of friction and conflict was eliminated just before the mass euthanasia program ended. The judiciary overcame its normative scruples; instead of demanding a legal basis for the program, it now participated constructively in the mass murders. Freisler's remark hinted at a forthcoming reorganization of the killing organization.*

---

* Based on these documents, which he used but inadequately cited, the historian Lothar Gruchmann argued in 1972 that the judiciary "restrained" euthanasia, even if it did not succeed in "surrounding [the euthanasia procedure] with all *necessary* normative protections." This distortion, with its implied justification of normatively secured murder, sheds light on the intentions of Gruchmann's employers, the Munich Institut für Zeitgeschichte (Institute for Contemporary History): production of legends that help legitimize governmental continuity. In his essay "Euthanasie und Justiz im Dritten Reich" (Euthanasia and the judiciary in the Third Reich), Gruchmann completely fails to discuss the process by which, beginning in 1942, the German judiciary carried out and "normatively surrounded" the extermination of inmates in psychiatric preventive detention.

The following works exist on the behavior of the German judiciary in connection

Rummelsburg — Questionnaire on "Aliens to the Community"

Directly following the supposed suspension of euthanasia in August 1941, the inmates of German workhouses and detention centers—beggars, prostitutes, those delinquent in paying support, thieves, and vagrants—were caught in the nets of Operation T-4; more specifically, those of the Reich Association of Mental Hospitals. The pause in killing ordered by Hitler did not apply to them. The Reich Association and the Reich Commissioner for Mental Hospitals in the Ministry of the Interior, Herbert Linden, were working feverishly on new registration techniques for people not categorized primarily as medically inferior, who instead exhibited social defects. Ingeborg Seidel, a secretary sent to Hadamar by the Frankfurt labor office, was transferred to the Berlin headquarters in 1941, at the end of the mass gassings. In 1946 she testified: "I was assigned by the Foundation to duty in the Rummelsburg workhouse. Here files were prepared that would process the so-called antisocial elements for extermination."[82]

On 12 January 1942, a model evaluation was made of the inmates of the communal workhouse at Berlin-Rummelsburg. The following officials were invited: Herbert Linden (of the Reich Ministry of the Interior); Hans Hefelmann (of the Führer's Office); Prof. Heinrich Wilhelm Kranz (a researcher on antisocial behavior from Giessen); Prof. Metzger; Frau Knorr (a criminal biologist); Hermann Vellguth (the chief medical officer in Vienna); Erwin Jekelius (the former director of a sanitarium for alcoholics in Vienna); Robert Ritter (a Gypsy specialist and forensic biologist for the Reich Criminal Investigation Department); and Hans Heinze (a T-4 expert and psychopathy specialist).[83]

The commission thus brought together psychiatrists who, like Heinze, had worked for years on the concept of the "deviant character" with leading criminal biologists (Kranz, Metzger, Knorr) and mass-murder strategists (Hefelmann and Linden). Hermann Nitsche, Gerhard Wischer, and Robert Müller from the central office of the Reich Association were also invited. Each member of the commission evaluated the in-

---

with institutional murder: Helmut Kramer, "Oberlandesgerichtspräsidenten und Generalstaatsanwälte als Gehilfen der NS-'Euthanasie': Selbstentlastung für die Teilnahme am Anstaltsmord," *Kritische Justiz* 17 (1984): 25ff.; Lothar Gruchmann, "Euthanasie und Justiz im Dritten Reich," *Vierteljahreshefte für Zeitgeschichte* 20 (1972): 235–79; Lothar Gruchmann, "Dokumentation: Ein unbequemer Amtsrichter im Dritten Reich, Aus den Personalakten des Dr. Lothar Kreyßig," *Vierteljahreshefte für Zeitgeschichte* 32 (1984): 463–88.

mates of the workhouse on the basis of a new registration form for "aliens to the community." At the top it asked for the "consecutive number," followed by "camp name, etc."—in this case, "workhouse"—and its location, Rummelsburg. This was followed by personal data—marital status, number of legitimate and illegitimate children, religion, race, citizenship, whether the inmate had fought at the front or been disabled in the war. After all this general and personal data, the form asked who would be responsible for the costs. It then asked about the inmate's "relationship to relatives," his profession, whether a "frequent change of job" had occurred, and finally, the "reason for commitment" and "committing office." Questions on "problems in the family," "time spent in mental hospitals," previous convictions, alcoholism, begging, pimping, prostitution, and "behavior in the asylum" completed the form. The experts were then expected to make a prognosis that would spell the difference between life and death: "assessment of possible future social usefulness, possibility of release." In connection with this question, "physical condition"—in other words, ability to work—was also to be judged, as well as "addiction" and "compulsive sexual activity."[84]

The evaluation was organized as a sort of competition between the various members of the commission; they assessed each inmate separately, then determined the degree of consensus, apparently in order to develop uniform criteria. The result of this investigation was noted by Erich Straub, one of Nitsche's medical assistants in the Berlin central office, in the "Report on the Work in Rummelsburg":

> Registration forms for the inmates were issued in prescribed form; based on attendance lists, a list was made of all inmates present on the 13th of the month and compared with the registration forms issued, in order to ensure complete processing. In this way we could guarantee that all inmates were processed.
>
> Number of completed registration forms: Women: 449; Men: 975.
>
> Of these 975 men, 35 could not be examined, as they had been quarantined due to the danger of epidemic. These 35 must be examined later. The registration forms issued for them are on file with the resident physician in Rummelsburg.[85]

The head of the Reich Association, Dietrich Allers, expressly noted beneath this report, "In cases in which old registration forms were used, tranfer to new (three-page) ones has occurred." Under the date 11 April in Nitsche's files is a handwritten notice of the results of the experimental evaluation in Rummelsburg. The experts agreed that 314 of the inmates, one-fourth, should be killed. For an additional 765 detainees, at least one of the experts involved advocated killing.[86]

Examination of those detained in Rummelsburg was preceded by an economic analysis of the asylum. On 17 December 1941, Administrative Inspector Ludwig Trieb, in charge of efficiently organizing the institutions in the Reich Association, issued a detailed report:

> The Rummelsburg workhouse and house of detention in Berlin-Lichtenberg is owned by the city of Berlin. In the budget for the city of Berlin, the asylum is listed under "General Welfare."
> The following costs are expected for accommodation:
> of welfare cases   per day   1.75 RM
> of workhouse inmates assigned
>   by the judiciary   per day   1.50 RM
> charitable associations   per day   1.75 RM
> . . . Normal occupancy is given as 1,574, although the target figures for 1940 were expected to be:
>   600 persons   workhouse and asylum for tardy support payers
>   450 persons   incapable of work, in house of detention
>   800 persons   able to work, in house of detention
>   150 persons   hospital
> total 2,000 beds
> The maximum figure was, in fact, attained, with an occupancy of 1,879.
> . . . In an asylum like Rummelsburg, which accommodates a number of people incapable of working, the inmates must be subdivided accordingly. I have thus created three groups, divided as follows:
> Group 1: Occupational therapy (up to 1.00 RM pocket money per month) in the form of housework. The income of 9,000 RM from this section is . . . insignificant. The work to be done is:
> potato peeling,
> hemp plucking,
> feather stripping,
> sorting metal, rags, paper, etc.
> The people employed are primarily those known as "incapable of working," of which 450 are found in the house of detention.
> Group 2: Household businesses such as a carpentry shop, shoemaker, tailor, locksmith, mason, painter, upholsterer, machine room, large bakery, garden work, housecleaning, hospital cleaning, kitchen work, laundry, sewing hall producing underwear, clothes, etc.
> Valuable work is done here. . . .

The large bakery, which is very modern and run with machines, bakes bread for 31 city enterprises such as orphanages, hospitals, and other asylums. . . . The large laundry does the entire laundry for 20 city asylums, although the equipment is not modern. The laundry itself is also spatially limited. The laundry's achievements are to be commended. . . .

Even though services may be cheaper on the free market, the city of Berlin receives significant advantages. In addition, given the present situation on the labor market, it must be taken into account that suppliers are not interested in granting large discounts.

The other workshops do mainly internal work.

Group 3: City work details supervised by city offices and work details in other enterprises:

4 details in city forests

1 detail in the construction office

1 detail in the heating office

4 details in the gardening office (central cemetery)

1 detail in street cleaning

For this group of details, the city of Berlin pays 1.60 RM wage per man per day.

1 detail in the large Klingenberg power plant

1 detail in the Knorr brake factory (80 men)

1 detail in the Gaedige construction firm

1 detail in the Gast Signale factory (50 men)

1 detail in a canned-food factory (50 women)

1 potato-peeling detail that prepares the potatoes for large Berlin factories (80 women)

The firms pay a wage of 5.00 RM per man per day.

Some 500 high-quality workers are employed in these city work details. The asylum pays only up to 5.00 RM pocket money per month. Some of these city work details also work on Sundays.

In Trieb's opinion, working group 1 should be "reduced"; that is, the inmates should be killed. Departments 1 and 2 of the workhouse should be made more efficient and their work intensified:

Working Group 1: can be reduced accordingly. The remainder must achieve increased performance.

More efficient procedures will also compensate to some degree.

Working Group 2: can be reduced to a limited extent.

Here, too, compensation is possible through intensive division of labor and efficient procedures.

Working Group 3: must be preserved as long as the labor market provides no replacement or other compensation.

Large-scale intervention with the supply of city work details cannot be justified at the moment. Neither the city of Berlin nor other essential enterprises in the defense economy could withstand such a loss. Where intervention with the supply of city details cannot be avoided, an attempt must be made to supplement from Group 2.[87]

The actual consequences of the Rummelsburg review for the inmates and detainees, and the extent to which similar commissions filled out the new selection questionnaires in other workhouses in the Third Reich, have not yet been investigated. However, it is probable that responsibility for detention in workhouses was withdrawn from T-4 in the early summer of 1942. With the end of the blitzkrieg, the concept of "extermination through work" gained priority. The workhouse inmates, largely committed on the basis of court decisions, may have been transferred to concentration camps by the judiciary. Camp statistics from Mauthausen, for example, indicate that 4,031 German preventive detainees were sent there between 8 December 1942 and 17 January 1943.[88] At this time, "corrective detainees" from Rummelsburg were probably also deported, and their work taken over by prisoners from the Berlin subsidiary of the Sachsenhausen concentration camp.*

* For purposes of further research, it will be necessary to investigate the fate of inmates of various German workhouses. The following is a list for the year 1926: Coswig (Anhalt: men and women; attached to the prison); Kislau (Baden: men and women); Rebdorf (Bavaria: men); St. Georgen-Bayreuth (Bavaria: women); Wolfenbüttel (Braunschweig: men and women; attached to the state prison); Hamburg-Fuhlsbüttel (Hamburg: men and women; attached to the prison); Dieburg (Hesse: men and women); Detmold (Lippe: affiliated with the prison); Lübeck-Lauerhof (Lübeck: men and women; attached to the prison); Güstrow (Mecklenburg-Schwerin: men and women); Strelitz (Mecklenburg-Strelitz: men and women; attached to the state prison); Vechta (Oldenburg: men and women; attached to the prison); Colditz (Saxony: men and women); Gotteszell (Württemberg: women; attached to the state prison); Vaihingen a.E. (Württemberg: men); Benninghausen (Westphalia: men and women); Brauweiler (Rhine Province: men and women); Breitenau (Hesse-Nassau: men and women); Glückstadt (Schleswig-Holstein: men and women; the state of Bremen accommodated men and women transferred to the workhouse at its own expense); Bad Salzelmen (Saxony: men and women); Moringen (Hanover: men and women); Schweidnitz (Silesia: men and women); Tapiau (East Prussia: men and women); Ückermünde (Pomerania: men and women; administered by the provincial correctional institute and asylum); Rummelsburg (Brandenburg, Berlin: men and women); Stralsund (Pomerania: men and women) (Verzeichnis der deutschen Arbeitshäuser nach dem Stand von 1926: Heidelberg, 1927).

The Judiciary's Extermination Program

It is certain that a reorganization took place soon after the extermination of criminals in asylums ceased. This time, the Ministry of Justice assumed control. On 6 February 1942, a decree from the Reich Minister of Justice for which Franz Schlegelberger was responsible demanded the concentration of Jewish prisoners committed to mental hospitals in specific collection asylums (there were very few such prisoners left, but the procedure itself was significant). The decree at the same time expanded the list of persons to be executed without a death sentence to include those Jewish prisoners "who [were] mentally ill while serving their sentence and are not or are no longer suited for commitment to the psychiatric section of a penal institution"—in other words, "inconvenient" persons who could be collected almost arbitrarily under the heading "psychopath":

The Reich Minister of Justice	Berlin W 8, 6 February 1942
4424-III s 1 59	Wilhelmstrasse 68
	Tel: 11 00 44
	outside: 11 65 16

To the Prosecutors
(near Prague: through the Reich Protector
in Bohemia and Moravia in *Prague*)

Re.: Commitment of mentally ill Jews to mental hospitals

I request that Jews whose commitment to an asylum has been ordered under §§42a no. 1, 42b of the Penal Code, as well as Jewish prisoners who become mentally ill while serving their sentence and are not or are no longer suited for commitment to the psychiatric section of a penal institution, be brought from the districts

Braunschweig, Celle,	to the	Hamburg-Langenhorn
Düsseldorf, Hamburg, Hamm,		Asylum
Kiel, Oldenburg, Rostock		

In addition, there were—at least—the Farmsen nursing home in Hamburg and the Lainz city nursing home in Vienna.

For this list, I thank Wolfgang Ayaß, author of the important work "'Es darf in Deutschland keine Landstreicher mehr geben': Die Verfolgung von Bettlern und Vagabunden im Faschismus" ("There must be no more vagrants in Germany": Persecution of beggars and vagabonds under fascism), Paper for Kassel Polytechnic, 1980).

Berlin, Hamburg, Jena, Dresden, Breslau and— only the women—from the districts Danzig, Königsberg, Marienwerder, Posen, Stettin	to the	Görden-Brandenburg (Havel) State Asylum
Danzig, Königsberg, Marienwerder, Posen, Stettin (only the men)	to the	Tapiau Provincial Asylum
Graz, Innsbruck, Kattowitz, Leitmeritz, Linz, Prague, Vienna	to the	Wagner von Jauregg Asylum (Asylum am Steinhof)
Bamberg, Darmstadt, Frankfurt a.M., Karlsruhe, Kassel, Cologne, Munich, Nuremberg, Stuttgart, Zweibrücken	to the	Eglfing-Haar Munich Asylum

I ask you to see that mentally ill Jews who have until now been committed to other mental hospitals be transferred to those now responsible for them.

Signed
Marx[89]

After the Jews in detention had been dealt with, it was the turn of the "Aryans." In a discussion with Heinrich Himmler on 18 September 1942, the newly appointed undersecretary in the Ministry of Justice, Curt Rothenberger, and SS Major General Bruno Streckenbach came to a decision on the "delivery of antisocial elements from prisons" to Himmler's SS "for extermination through work."[90] The minutes continue, "Preventive detainees will be delivered without exception." Four days earlier, the new Minister of Justice, Otto Thierack, had already secured agreement to this program elsewhere. In a note on the discussion, he wrote: "With regard to extermination of antisocial lives, Dr. Goebbels' point of view is that all Jews and Gypsies, Poles who have served prison sentences of around 3–4 years, and Czechs or Germans who have been sentenced to death, life in prison, or preventive detention should be exterminated. The best idea is extermination through work."[91]*

---

* The idea was not a new one. In 1937, the president of the Thuringian State Race Office, Karl Astel, had already suggested bluntly to Heinrich Himmler: "I would like to take on such an extensive job, which in addition provides a standard for use of preventive detention and possibly extermination, that is, killing of criminals"

A memorandum from 10 October 1942, in which a new abbreviation was established for use in evaluations, shows the immediate effect that this decision had on T-4 practice: "*KZ* means the evaluating doctor submits that the patient should be transferred to a concentration camp (KZ)."[92] On 2 October 1942, the T-4 doctors Curt Runckel[93] and Kurt Borm had already begun to tour German mental hospitals to evaluate those committed there under §42 of the Reich Penal Code, particularly with regard to their ability to work. T-4 reported the results of this investigation to the Reich Ministry of Justice, which made lists of criminal patients who "no longer need treatment in mental institutions and are capable of working." The report read, "In agreement with the *Reichsführer* SS and the Chief of the German Police in the Reich Ministry of the Interior [Heinrich Himmler], the Reich Minister of Justice has decided to place these people at the disposal of the police for accommodation in police labor and disciplinary camps."[94]

This recommendation resulted in the compilation of lists that were then sent by the Reich Ministry of Justice through its prosecutors to the various mental hospitals.[95] This is probably one reason why the trail left by this branch of institutional murder is so extraordinarily faint. The judiciary made no effort to follow it after the war.* Yet it is certain that, for example, the 12 men from Neustadt Mental Hospital in Schleswig-Holstein who were deported on 25 March 1944 "into criminal police custody

---

(Zentrale Stelle der Landesjustizverwaltungen, Ludwigsburg [ZStL], USA 2, Film 1 [Astel Complex]). Astel had formulated this idea in order to secure funds for his ambitious research project in eugenics involving "4,600 criminals jailed and . . . registered in Thuringia."

* The extermination of prisoners in psychiatric care with the help of the legal and police apparatus has been the subject of only two trials: (1) an investigation by the Frankfurt prosecutor (Js 10/65) of Dr. Curt Runckel (suspended in 1968); and (2) a jury trial of four officials of the Reich Ministry of Justice for having transferred thousands of "antisocial" prisoners to police custody, to be murdered in concentration camps (Sta.Wiesbaden, 2 Ks 2/51; the acquittal on 24 March 1952 is published in Rüter, *Justiz und NS-Verbrechen* [Amsterdam, 1968], vol. 9, pp. 269ff.). When asked the whereabouts of the files on this particular trial, the Wiesbaden prosecutor informed the author on 4 January 1985, "Only fragments of the 26 volumes of files are available—that is, volumes 18–20, 22, and 24–26. The remainder, including the reference files, have been missing for many years. For a long time, the proceedings acted as supplementary files to the well-known RSHA [Main Reich Security Office] trial by the prosecutor at the Berlin Supreme Court. We have never been able to determine whether they failed to be completely separated from this monster trial or were unintentionally destroyed later on, here in the archives, in which we sometimes employ untrained temporary workers."

in Kiel"[96] were among the very same protective detainees examined by T-4—not on its own, but as an adjunct of the judiciary.

The example of 50 deported Hamburg men at the beginning of 1943 reveals how little coincidence was involved in the composition of deportation lists following these evaluations. The choice of those to be deported lent practical significance to the link between extermination by euthanasia and killing of the antisocial, between the Euthanasia Law and the Law on Aliens to the Community. Other decisive criteria in this intermediate phase of institutional killing were noted meticulously in patient histories:

—Committed to the Langenhorn Asylum in 1935 for attempted rape, by a decision of the Hamburg Superior Court.

—Assigned to the Langenhorn Asylum in 1939 by the Hamburg Superior Court for immoral conduct in a state of insanity.

—Committed to the asylum in Hamburg-Langenhorn in 1938 by the Hamburg City Court for various robberies committed in a state of insanity. . . . Broods over plans to escape.

—Committed by the Hamburg City Court in 1937 for homosexual prostitution committed in a state of insanity.

—Sent back from Rickling Asylum in an exchange, because he is too aggressive there.

—Transferred in 1934 from the Alsterdorfer Asylum to Langenhorn. Reasons given: psychopathy and antisocial behavior. Dangerously insane, with considerable previous record. Sentenced to two years' imprisonment in 1937 for extortion and continued intimidation, and subsequently committed to Hamburg-Langenhorn by a decision of the Hamburg District Court.

—The patient became a loafer; he was convicted in 1928 for immorality and sent to a reformatory in Göttingen. Prison sentence for misuse of weapons and fraud. He was sterilized in 1935, and committed to the Hamburg-Langenhorn Asylum as of August 1938, by order of the Hamburg Superior Court. Chronic alcoholism and querulousness.

—Arrested in 1936 for attempted murder; subsequently committed to Langenhorn because of insanity.

—Delivered to Langenhorn because of insanity. Shot his mother and aunt with a pistol.[97]

The files of inmates deported from the prison at Hamburg-Fuhlsbüttel to Langenhorn and then to Hadamar can be found at the former Hadamar extermination facility.[98] A decree from the Ministry of Justice on

22 October 1942 stated, "A final arrangement for mentally ill prisoners has not yet been made";[99] the Hadamar death site made clear what this "final arrangement" would be.

It was not only those with penal convictions who were transferred from psychiatric asylums to concentration camps for extermination through work; as of 1944, the psychiatric category "psychopath," corresponding to the concept "antisocial," would also suffice. Nitsche wrote to T-4 consultant Otto Hebold that these people did not require psychiatric institutionalization, but actually belonged in concentration camps; they had been sent to mental hospitals as a result of incorrect application of legal regulations.

On 29 August 1944, Nitsche wrote the Berlin central office in a similar vein: "Enclosed please find two registration forms sent to me today from the Gugging Asylum regarding Franz J. and Erwin L., with my endorsement re: transfer to police custody for placement in a concentration camp."[100] The two patients were not committed by a court; the director of Gugging, Erich Gelny, had furnished the diagnosis "feeble-minded psychopath" for one, and characterized the other's condition as a "depressive reaction by a mentally inferior, excitable person."

Nitsche concluded: "Neither case requires psychiatric treatment. Both would be disruptive in a mental hospital, and cannot be detained with sufficient security; thus the Gugging Asylum requests transfer as quickly as possible. I request accelerated forwarding to the responsible police precinct, with the asylum's wishes particularly emphasized."

To the extent that the German judiciary's murder program involved prisoners in mental hospitals and workhouses who were capable of working, a strange constellation emerged. In his camps, Himmler hoped to work to death those still capable of working—to make productive use of them. Under no circumstances did he wish to burden these camps—gigantic forced labor enterprises—with people incapable of working, with the sick and the infirm. Conversely, the directors of mental hospitals particularly wished to send their unproductive patients to be killed; those capable of working—and these included criminals in particular—had long since become the mainstays of asylum activity. The tug of war that emerged as a result is revealed in a petition from the administrative director of the Wiesloch Mental Hospital on 19 March 1943, addressed to the Karlsruhe prosecutor:

> In addition to the mass of unsocial, strictly supervised patients accommodated here under §42b, [we also have] a number of patients who have

long behaved well in every respect and are a great help to the asylum. . . . The positions of many employees of the asylum who have been drafted into the Wehrmacht have already been filled by patients committed here under §44b of the Reich Penal Code, with positive results. . . . Given this situation, we ask the Reich Ministry of Justice to investigate the matter once again and, if at all possible, in the interests of the asylum, the reserve hospital, and the entire population, to leave the suggested patients in the asylum.[101]

The administrative director at Wiesloch, Wilhelm Möckel, had no qualms about passing this letter off later as an act of resistance. In fact, two differently constructed killing programs collided here. The extermination of "worthless life" demanded a nucleus of patients capable of working, in order to keep the machinery of selection and killing in motion; whereas extermination through work aimed at the attainment of quick profits, which the sick could only hinder. There must have been a serious dispute over this procedure between the Reich Commissioner for Mental Hospitals, on the one hand, and the Reich Ministers of Justice and the Interior, on the other. As a result, on 2 July 1943 the Minister of Justice wrote his prosecutor: "Based on renewed negotiations with the Health Department of the Reich Ministry of the Interior . . . I declare the list sent to you to be invalid."[102] Herbert Linden had gotten his way. The Ministry of Justice had to "issue new lists"—lists of psychiatric prisoners who were also "suited from a psychiatric standpoint for transfer to police custody." In addition, the Ministry of Justice had to establish a limitation: "Neither are these new lists conclusive. . . . Still excepted from delivery to the police are those employed in important work either within or outside the mental hospitals, whom it is either impossible or inexpedient to replace with other workers. I request that those who must therefore be removed from the lists be determined in cooperation with the mental hospitals involved."[103]

A month later, Herbert Linden informed the asylum directors of the outcome of the negotiations and granted them additional decision-making authority. It was "up to the director to decide" whether or not to surrender a patient. In addition, in the future there would be no more central evaluations; the head of the asylum would decide whether to send inmates to concentration camps or keep them. As a result, the Wiesloch Mental Hospital could retain criminals capable of working, while sending those deemed sick or infirm to Hadamar.[104]

NERVENKRANKENHAUS des Bezirks Unterfranken in LOHR A. MAIN

An das
L a n d g e r i c h t
Untersuchungsrichter IV

6 Frankfurt/Main
Klinger-Str. 25/I

Bankkonto:
Stadt- und Kreissparkasse Lohr Nr. 148

Postscheckkonto: Nürnberg Nr. 8173

Telefon: (09352) 576, 577

Akt.-Z.: N/V - 1520

8770 LOHR, den 15.4.1965

Betr.: Voruntersuchungssache R ▬▬▬▬▬ wegen Mordes,
. AZ.: Js 15/61 (GStA)

Bezug: Ihr Schreiben vom 7. April 1965

Auf Ihre Bitte hin haben wir unsere Unterlagen über die 8 in dem
beiliegenden Schreiben vom 27.1.1944 angeführten Kranken durchge-
sehen. Dabei konnten wir folgende Feststellungen machen:

(...)

Am 30.3.1944 wurden weiterhin auf Anordnung des Reichsministers
der Justiz in das KZ.-Auschwitz verlegt:

W▬▬ Charlotte   geb. 9. 1.1916
W▬▬ Emma   geb.27. 4.1909
P▬▬ Hertha   geb.25.11.1911
D▬▬ Dorothea   geb.21. 9.1891
M▬▬ Maria   geb.13. 7.1901

Über das Schicksal dieser Kranken ist hier nichts bekannt.

In das Konzentrationslager-Mauthausen wurde am 30.3.1944
R▬▬ Josef verlegt. Über sein weiteres Schicksal ist hier
nichts bekannt.

Aus einem Schreiben der Staatsanwaltschaft Aschaffenburg
vom 28. Juni 1949 - es betrifft die Unterbringung von Geisteskranken in KZ.-Lager, AZ.: 4 Js 19/49 - konnten wir noch die
Namen der anderen von Ihnen gewünschten Kranken feststellen.

Am 30. März 1944 wurden weiter noch in das KZ.-Mauthausen verlegt:

S▬▬ Karl   geb. 14. 8.1894 zu Kirchheim, Bezirksamt
                                                Heidelberg
W▬▬ Alfred   geb. 16. 1.1923 zu Schweinfurt
R▬▬ Ernst   geb. 14. 2.1919 zu Schweinfurt
K▬▬ Richard   geb. 15. 8.1899 zu Bamberg

Nervenkrankenhaus des Bezirks Unterfranken in Lohr am Main

B▬▬ Alfred   geb. 13.11.1901 zu Krefeld
K▬▬ Ludwig   geb. 21. 2.1915 zu Heidingsfeld
K▬▬ Anton   geb. 2. 9.1905 zu Bischofsheim v. d. Rhön
M▬▬ Paul   geb. 4. 2.1915 zu Dipach, Landkrs. Kitzingen
S▬▬ Anton   geb. 3. 2.1915 zu Kirchzell Landkrs. Miltenberg

Am gleichen Tag wurde in das KZ.-Auschwitz verlegt:
R▬▬ Maria   geb. 17. 2. 1901 zu Neresheim/Wrttbg.

(...)

Weitere Angaben über das Schicksal der angeführten Kranken nach
ihrer Entlassung aus der hiesigen Anstalt vermögen wir nicht zu machen.

(Dr. Nützel)
Bez. Obermedizinalrat
Stellv. Direktor

The ticket to Auschwitz and Mauthausen for German psychiatric patients.

The end to general euthanasia in August 1941 shifted the focus of domestic murder in the Third Reich to marginal social groups. So many tramps, beggars, swindlers, peddlers, and prostitutes were exterminated during the Third Reich that it is difficult in both western and eastern Germany to imagine how these people lived at the time, and how many of them there were.

"Operation Brandt": Emergency Medicine and Institutional Murder

Auxiliary Hospitals

On 28 July 1942, after hopes for a blitzkrieg had been dashed in the winter of 1941–42, Hitler appointed Karl Brandt—who with Philipp Bouhler had been responsible for organizing institutional murder since 1939—as his Commissioner for the Health Care System, responsible only to Hitler and bound only by his instructions. Brandt was responsible for "special assignments," as it was formulated in the Reich legal bulletin, and for "balancing the need for doctors, hospitals, medication, etc. between the military and the civilian sectors."[105] Immediately following Brandt's appointment, in August 1942, the Reich Commissioner for Mental Hospitals, Herbert Linden, undertook a survey on the use of asylums as auxiliary hospitals. The responsible authorities were asked to answer the following questions within ten days:

> Recently it has become apparent that it will become increasingly necessary to fall back upon mental hospitals to obtain hospital beds in case of emergency. Since responsibility for beds gained in asylums through the economic precautions that have been taken so far lies elsewhere, additional measures are necessary to meet further demand. I therefore request that you inform me by 15 August of this year (deadline is to be met on time)
>
> 1. how many mental patients can still be accommodated in the district's asylums (incl. charitable and private), assuming the most efficient possible use of available beds,
>
> 2. how many additional mental patients could be admitted in case of emergency if emergency camps were to be set up in
>
> a. heatable corridors, common rooms, etc.
>
> b. asylum chapels . . .

3. (*only for areas threatened with air raids*):
which mental hospitals are to be evacuated in specific emergencies
and employed as auxiliary hospitals. I request, where possible, provision
of names of asylums that are not particularly endangered from the air.

Should an emergency occur, I will ensure immediate evacuation of
these asylums, so that patients made homeless can be transferred within
a short period from evacuated hospitals to the auxiliary asylums to be
created. It must be left to local authorities to consider measures now to
ensure that the vacated asylums can be adapted for use as hospitals.

Because, in the above concept, mental hospitals will represent a significant emergency reserve of additional beds, they can no longer be
used in the future to accommodate the homeless. I further request that
you desist from demanding the evacuation of mental hospitals lying on
the periphery of endangered cities, as vacating these asylums would
limit my flexibility should an emergency actually happen.[106]

The legal basis for these plans was the Reich Air-Raid Protection
Law of 1935.[107] Linden concluded from the results of this survey, "By
crowding asylums and providing emergency beds for the mentally ill,
enough room can definitely be made available in emergencies, within each
state at first, . . . to temporarily house the physically ill and freshly
wounded."[108] On 23 September 1942, Linden's superior, Fritz Cropp, indicated how he imagined the procedure would function in "emergency
situations": "The discomforts that will arise from crowding the mentally
ill and creating emergency camps in some asylums will have to be accepted
for a few days. However, in cooperation with the Reich Commissioner, I
would endeavor to remedy this by deporting the mentally ill to asylums in
less-endangered states, Reich *Gaus,* and provinces in order to eliminate
temporary overcrowding. I therefore request that I be informed, case by
case, of the number of mentally ill patients that can be considered for
transfer. I ask that applications for precautionary evacuation or relief of
asylums be avoided."[109]

In these plans, mental patients functioned as placeholders in case of
need. They kept beds warm; that is, as long as there were patients to care
for, the entire asylum remained functional, the personnel were indispensable, and the asylum could not be turned into a barracks. The Reich Association had learned a lesson from its negative experience during the first
phase of the killing, when 50,000 of the 70,000 beds that were "freed up"
were ultimately used for other purposes. The Association's institutions no

longer killed according to a predetermined plan dependent upon killing capacities; they now eliminated patients based on local necessity, in decentralized fashion.[110] Various criteria for killing no longer existed; all that counted was ability to work, plus the extent of the medical consequences of air raids. These factors alone determined the number of persons to be deported by the Reich Association. The title the perpetrators gave this combination of institutional killing and high-quality medical care for the physically wounded was not "uncontrolled euthanasia" but—quite correctly—"Operation Brandt." *

Therefore, according to a decree by the Reich Ministry of the Interior, as of 1 February 1943 it became necessary to "process" not only selected long-term patients and those with particular illnesses, but all inmates. In his new registration order, Linden wrote: "For technical reasons and genetic stock-taking, it is important to me that the patient population in each asylum be registered in full. I request in future that *all* [underlined in original] patients be reported who have been admitted to the asylum since the last semiannual notification, regardless of type or length of illness." [111]

Although Linden had all patients reported, he still opposed their indiscriminate starvation and physical and psychological neglect. On 26 February, he argued with the Reich Minister of the Economy over whether the mentally ill deserved the same amount of soap as the physically ill. Cutting their soap rations, he argued, was only justified if the illness had caused "idiocy" (mental death) and inability to work. He further felt that

---

* A word here on Dirk Blasius' essay "Psychiatrischer Alltag im Nationalsozialismus," in D. Peukert and J. Reulecke, eds., *Die Reihen fast geschlossen* (Wuppertal, 1981). Blasius—who accused Ernst Klee of lacking "responsible historical implementation" in his important book (*Die Zeit* 49, 1983)—got nearly everything wrong on the two relevant pages of his essay: "Only a small group of about 50 persons was aware of the significance and extent of the killings" (p. 379). Fifty persons was about the size of the staff of a single extermination center, not to mention the numerous documents attesting to public and official knowledge. Elsewhere Blasius writes, "One can no longer precisely reconstruct the extent to which medical directors of insane asylums shared responsibility for the killing program." This claim ignores the historic fact that T-4 evaluations were available to numerous directors. This type of allegedly "responsible" writing of contemporary history is part of a tradition of reconstructionism and ideologizing that must be overcome by looking at and carefully analyzing historical sources. Equally incorrect, as I show in this chapter, is the explanation for "uncontrolled euthanasia," quoted approvingly by Blasius: "Many directors, accustomed to the killing, were independent enough to have patients eliminated at their own discretion and without creating a stir" (p. 380). This supposed individual "independence" is part of the usual repertory of excuses for the central administration.

defamation of the mentally ill could "impede patients' receptiveness, and thus significantly endanger the community."[112]

At the beginning of 1943, Undersecretary Conti, the Reich Health Leader, appointed Permanent Secretary Fritz Cropp to be General Commissioner for Air-Raid Damage. Cropp had been director of Department IV of the Ministry of the Interior since 1940; he had been Herbert Linden's superior, responsible for his activities in the various euthanasia operations. When the air war against the German Reich intensified dramatically at the beginning of 1943, he was responsible for emergency medical care in the hard-hit cities. Starting in June 1943, "all civilian hospital beds (excluding insane asylums and homes for the infirm)" were to be reported monthly, as were the "number of (a) hospitals destroyed and (b) hospitals badly damaged as a result of air attacks"; at the same time, the "number of (a) mentally ill, (b) infirm, (c) other patients transferred or admitted (to or from where?) in adjustments between districts" was also to be reported.[113]

On 24 June, because he could not reach Conti, Karl Brandt spoke directly with Cropp on the telephone regarding accelerated transport of the wounded from Mühlheim and Oberhausen in the Ruhr region. Cropp took the following notes on the conversation:

> Prof. Brandt further mentioned that he had spoken with Ass't Secy. Dr. Linden on the report of his trip, the general proposals he had made, and especially on the evacuation of insane asylums. He generally agrees with him in his assessment of the necessary measures, but does not believe it advisable in every case to leave the mentally ill in the mental hospitals. I thereupon told him that I had spoken in a similar vein with Dr. Linden several days previously, and that he had already explained to me at that opportunity that Prof. Brandt's views and intentions regarding organization of the asylum system correspond with the measures taken and planned by the Reich Ministry of the Interior.[114]

It was already clear before this that the euthanasia program would once again be expanded. In March 1943, the husband and wife team that administered the gassing facility at Bernburg, Hans and Margot Räder-Grossmann, wrote to former T-4 consultant Friedrich Mennecke, now assigned to the eastern front: "Nothing at all has happened here as yet. It is said that we will soon get a lot of work, and by the beginning of May we should know whether yes or no. Aside from several men who were released to the Wehrmacht, no one is let out of here."[115]

The strategy employed later—without gas chambers—must have

taken concrete form immediately after this. In a letter to the medical officer of the province of Hanover on 4 April 1943, Linden was already push-
ing to have deserving psychiatrists from the central office of T-4 installed
in directorial posts in the provinces, "now that, because of decisions at a
higher level, wartime economic measures in mental hospitals are being
discontinued." Even during total war, the central authorities could not do
this so easily. Linden had to resort to begging and explaining his reasons
precisely.

> Because the Reich itself has no insane asylums of its own . . . I permit
> myself to inquire whether your administration may wish to take on a
> psychiatrist with suitable qualifications in a leading institutional posi-
> tion in the administration. . . . I am certain that the measures imple-
> mented by the Reich Association will be revived at the right time, al-
> though the method of implementation may be different; in particular, it
> may be necessary to include public mental hospitals to a greater degree
> in the execution of the measures. Especially in such a case, however, the
> availability of a director who unconditionally supports these measures
> will be of extraordinary importance.[116]

At the end of June 1943, after some delay, the described form of
decentralized and individual killing could begin.

In May, Cropp had organized a large-scale transfer that the public
apparently immediately interpreted correctly. According to Cropp, "Experience has shown that relatives attempt to avoid such transfers, taking
the patients home for a short time even against the doctors' advice, and
bringing them back after the transfer operation." Cropp feared that premature release would lead to undesirable conditions, especially in areas
in danger of bombardment. "The presence of mentally infirm persons in
air-raid shelters, etc., can easily lead to unhealthy situations, since their
behavior is unpredictable."[117] Therefore, the premature release of patients
not yet considered cured had to be prevented—if necessary with the help
of the police. The state administration's fear of an outbreak of "psychological epidemics," of incalculable despair, of people proving unrespon-
sive to Nazi leadership and influence—the old Nazi fighters' fear of
revolution—was their reason for keeping patients in asylums. Conversely,
this later became the reason for forcibly committing and killing people
who panicked during large-scale attacks and fled inwardly into insanity to
escape the external catastrophe.

The evacuations began in Germany's westernmost region, the
Rhineland, continued in Hamburg and Westphalia, and were soon ex-

tended to Berlin. Of course, the hospital beds gained in this way were not available equally to all the physically ill. In a report on an inspection tour, Conti stated succinctly, "No special measures need be taken for medical care of prisoners of war and Eastern workers."[118] Under the heading "Internal Measures for Hospitals," an express letter of 5 July instructs chief medical officers to admit only "those patients truly in need of hospitalization and suited for hospital treatment": "During total war, the urgent need for hospital beds rules out their use as homes for the aged or infirm. It also generally does not permit the admission of the hopelessly ill to spend their final days. Further, it must be stressed that only absolutely essential operations and treatments can be carried out."[119]

The authorities later referred only to a "prohibition" on "admitting the infirm to hospitals." In addition, "hospital trains made available for the transport of the sick and wounded" were not on any account to be filled with the infirm.

Centrally Planned, Decentrally Executed Euthanasia

On 25 August 1943, Nitsche wrote to the psychiatrist Max de Crinis from the Heidelberg University Surgical Clinic, where he was recovering from complications after an operation, "Regarding our operation with Prof. Br. [Brandt] . . . he has authorized me, through Herr Blankenburg, to proceed along the lines of the suggestion on E. that I made to him orally."[120] "E" and "Eu" were the usual abbreviations for euthanasia. A good two months later, on 30 October, Nitsche again wrote to de Crinis: "You will recall that I made a very concrete suggestion on the E issue to Prof. Br. at the end of June, when we both visited him." After Brandt accepted this proposal, he, Nitsche, "in accordance with Prof. B's E assignment," had "summoned [a number of] specially selected practical psychiatrists" on 17 August.[121] At this meeting, the participants settled upon decentralized, routine killing by injected overdose. Quotas and lists of those to be killed would no longer be centrally determined; instead, they would be based entirely on need. From 1939 to 1941, the Reich defense commissars' supposed instructions had been nothing more than an administrative illusion that transferred bureaucratic responsibility to an institutional phantom; now, commissars actually did make decisions on their hospital bed requirements, taking into consideration the size of the mentally healthy population that was physically endangered by air raids. The first phase of institutional killing had involved implementation of an ideological position—extermination of supposedly worthless life, elimination of visible suffering and visible poverty; it had been favored by the euphoria of the blitzkrieg. As of 1943, however, all unproductive people in general were to make room for those who could be "restored to health." The mentally ill, infirm, and chronically ill had become part of an overall triage. They were transferred and murdered whenever necessary—whenever local authorities needed sickbeds, blankets, sheets, stretchers, and basic medical equipment.

Apparently referring to the Berlin meeting of 17 August 1943, the director of the Waldheim Asylum, Gerhard Wischer, wrote to his mentor Nitsche: "Otherwise, the work discussed in Berlin is proceeding smoothly. I expect a monthly average of 20 to 30 patients; there have been no difficulties until now, either with personnel or relatives. . . . New patients are admitted nearly every day, so that we must step lively to keep up."

A few weeks later, Wischer reported further: "I . . . have plenty to do, as almost all new patients from the area between Leipzig, Chemnitz, and Meissen come to me. Of course, I could never accommodate these patients if I were not taking the necessary measures to make room, which are going very smoothly. However, I very much lack the necessary medications."[122]

On 29 December, Wischer reported to the "honored Herr Professor" on "a terrorist air raid on Leipzig that has brought a great deal of confusion. At the same time, there are many departures that are taken care of smoothly." Apparently, the medications had arrived in the meantime. On 2 December, Nitsche had once again inquired of his director Allers: "Above all, I would like to know whether the directors who received the E assignment based on the meeting held by me on 17 August (re: E assignment Prof. Br.) have received the necessary medications. And approximately when. Then I will be able to calculate more or less how long each one has been working along these lines."[123]

Provision of pharmaceutical poisons was the task of the Forensic Institute of the Reich Criminal Investigation Office. Albert Widmann, a chemist, was responsible. Written fragments have survived[124] on deliveries to the following asylums: Uchtspringe, Stuttgart North Children's Hospital, Görden, Ansbach, Eichberg, Gross-Schweidnitz, Tiegenhof, and Kalmenhof-Idstein. In addition, the Forensic Institute supplied the Reich Committee, the Reich Association, and the Reich Commissioner for Mental Hospitals. These central institutions then distributed the poisons through their courier systems to an unknown number of asylums. Until the end of 1944, as a business partner of IG Farben (Ludwigshafen), the Forensic Institute also ensured a regular supply of carbon monoxide to

```
Ich bestätige hiermit, von Herrn Prof. Nitsche

  3 000 Ampullen Morphium
  3 000    "     Scopolamin
erhalten zu haben:


Vorstehende Mengen werden dem Direktor der Anstalt
Meseritz - Obrawalde Herrn Grabowski übergeben.



Weissenbach,den 30. März 1944.
```

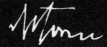

Pharmaceutical poison was supplied centrally through the Reich Criminal Investigation Department and distributed to the killing asylums by the Reich Ministry of the Interior, or T-4.

"I hearby confirm having received from Professor Nitsche:
3,000 ampules of morphine
3,000   "   of scopolamine
The above quantities will be delivered to the director of the Meseritz-Obrawalde asylum, Herr Grabowski.
Weissenbach, March 30, 1944."

Hartheim. In addition to these central deliveries, resident physicians in the asylums, for example at Hadamar, obtained supplies through local pharmacies. Toward the end of the war, physicians increasingly turned killings into undisguised executions, using air and gasoline injections.

In January 1944, Nitsche announced an intensification of the extermination program to his friend Carl Schneider in Heidelberg: "In this context, I still have to inform you today that on my next visit to Berlin I intend once again to summon to Berlin all the colleagues I summoned to Berlin on 17 August in accordance with Professor Br.'s E assignment—I told you in detail about the whole thing, and you couldn't come to Berlin at the time—to continue to promote the matter and to determine the present situation."[125]

Starting in mid-1944, still more people became victims of the decentrally organized killing program. On 24 July 1944, T-4 doctor Curt Runckel wrote to Nitsche that he had spoken with Professor Brandt about a plan to evacuate reformatories. Apparently, one of the issues involved was at least partial transfer to particular psychiatric institutions. Runckel further reported: "Professor Brandt asked me to inform you of these things, and at the same time to make the suggestion whether it would be possible for you inconspicuously to prepare the activation of our specific therapy."[126] A few days later, Nitsche remarked to Blankenburg on this inquiry, "In this way, they are, as we had hoped, complying with our wish . . . to discuss the E question as soon as possible along the lines of our negotiations in Vienna with Prof. Br." Nitsche asked for such a meeting as soon as possible, "including Prof. de Crinis."[127] The subject of the Vienna meeting on 3–5 July 1944 was a further escalation of institutional killing.

Restoring the Useful to Health — Killing the Useless

Evacuations began from the Rhineland in early 1943. Because the new form of killing had not yet been authorized, several hundred patients were deported from there to death centers in the Generalgouvernement (General Government: the Nazi term for occupied Poland), such as the Kulparkov Asylum near Lvov and the Tvorki Asylum near Warsaw. The patients from the Rhineland all died there within the next year and a half (the director of Kulparkov was the psychiatrist Max Rohde, who had served as expert adviser to the Galkhausen transit center in 1941).[128]

Starting in August 1943, a large number of psychiatric patients in Westphalia fell victim to the new wave of deportations. In September, the provincial association in charge of psychiatric care instructed the Gütersloh Asylum to separate into three groups all patients who had spent two years there relatively unmolested. Patients in groups 1 and 2 needed constant care and were incapable of working; patients in group 3 were useful in maintaining the asylum. The asylum included 457 of its wards in categories 1 and 2, 816 in category 3. According to the director, however, only 600 patients capable of working were necessary to maintain the asylum—which, like all large psychiatric institutions at the time, included a reserve hospital. In November and December, 712 Gütersloh inmates were taken away—in other words, slightly more than the asylum's administration, which had probably rounded the figures up, had claimed as necessary labor.[129]

In Bethel, Karl Brandt—who shared a mutual admiration for Friedrich Bodelschwingh—would also create hospital space in this way; in any case, in 1943 the "Mahaneim" house was evacuated. The patients were taken through Gütersloh to Meseritz. Patient Hildegard F.'s brother described this transfer in 1947 to the Berlin prosecutor: "Without the knowledge and against the wishes of her relatives, my sister . . . was transported in 1943, during the process of making room in hospitals, from Bethel hospital near Bielefeld, 'Mahaneim' house . . . first to the Gütersloh sanitarium near Bielefeld, and shortly afterwards, also without authorization, from there to Meseritz-Obrawalde. . . . The chief physician at the Gütersloh Asylum explained to me at the time that this was all carried out to make room in the hospitals, and had been ordered by the 'Führer.'"[130] This brother also told of a large number of other patients sent at the same time from Bethel through Gütersloh to the same mass grave.

The trials of Nazi doctors at Nuremberg began the process of investigating the link between air raids and the creation of hospital space, but neither the final decision nor the report by Alexander Mitscherlich and Fred Mielke referred to it. An interrogation of Medical Officer Hellmut Wex of Bremen yielded the following:

> When the Bremen institution was hit in an air attack on 26 November 1943, it became necessary to evacuate the bulk of the patients. Dr. Wex got in touch with Dr. Linden, an assistant secretary in the Ministry of the Interior, who on 9 December 1943 offered space for 341 patients in the Meseritz-Obrawalde Asylum; after some difficulties, a special train of coaches with wood seats was made available, most of them unheated and otherwise inadequate, and a number of patients (380, according to Wex; 305, according to Koster—this figure is also supported by documents) were shipped to Meseritz. One patient died on the train trip. Of the others, 242 died by 2 February 1944.[131]

By 1944, it was no longer a question of hospital beds but of making room in general. When most of the buildings of the University of Kiel were destroyed in a heavy air raid on 26 August 1944, the university had to be moved elsewhere. One of the ministerial officials involved testified in 1947: "The State Mental Hospital in Schleswig was considered for this. . . . To decide where the approximately 1,000 patients should be transferred, the administrative director of the university, Dr. Kinder, and the rector, Professor Holzlöhner,* and I came to Berlin to see Dr. Brandt." There they were promised that 1,000 patients would be transferred to other asylums: "Prof. Brandt could not yet tell us where. . . . Following my return, I informed Dr. Grabow of the Schleswig-Stadtfeld State Mental Hospital on the results of the Berlin meeting. For some two to three weeks,

---

* Ernst Holzlöhner was a professor of physiology who was directly involved in the hypothermia experiments in Dachau (see Mitscherlich and Mielke, *Medizin ohne Menschlichkeit,* Frankfurt, 1978).

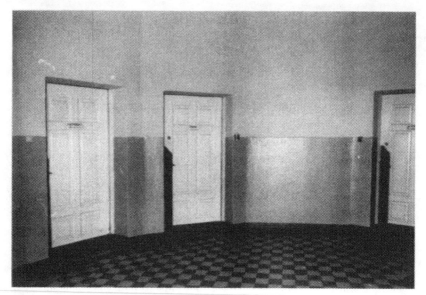

Meseritz-Obrawalde

we heard nothing at all on the deportation of patients. One day, the news suddenly arrived that 700 patients would be deported within twenty-four hours. Soon after the deportation was carried out, the first patient death notices from Meseritz-Obrawalde appeared in the newspapers."[132]

On 24 July 1943, a large-scale, one-week attack on Hamburg began that literally burned the city to the ground, claiming some 44,000 lives.[133] On 7 August, a group of 97 mentally ill women departed for Hadamar. The patient and personnel files that remain indicate that some 20 percent of the women deported to their deaths lived alone, with no relatives to care for them. Unable to cope with the inferno of the firestorm, they lost their wits and were thereupon committed to the Langenhorn Sanitarium. They were committed by family doctors, medical officers, and general hospitals. The fate of these euthanasia victims points to a completely unknown and as yet unresearched dimension of the Nazi practice of killing. Some of these cases can be documented based on medical histories:

> Amalie K., née Beckmann, born 29 August 1866 in Lüdingworth, died 16 August 1943 in Hadamar. She was 77 years old. On 1 September 1943, her son wrote to Hadamar: "My mother was separated from her daughter on 31 July 1943, and had lost everything in the air raids on Hamburg at the time. My mother was mentally active to the end and

could manage the household without any complaints, so that admission to a home cannot be explained. I ask to be informed of the illness my mother had and the cause of her death."

The answer from Hadamar was: "Frau K. was so frail that she had to be kept in bed constantly. Rapid degeneration began several days before her death. A weak heart in addition to this caused her death. She expressed no special wishes."

Marie R., born 28 December 1860 in Fichthorst, West Prussia, was admitted to the Hamburg-Langenhorn Mental Hospital without diagnosis at the age of 82 and transferred to Hadamar on 7 August 1943. An entry in her file indicates that she died during the transport of exhaustion accompanying mental illness.

Anna W., née Musfeldt, born 9 November 1851 in Blomischenwildnis, was admitted on 27 July 1943 as an air-raid victim in a state of confusion. She died on 26 August 1943 in Hadamar.[134]

Similar stories of bombed-out Hamburg residents can also be found in letters sent by relatives in 1946–47 to the Berlin prosecutor investigating the employees of the Meseritz-Obrawalde Asylum. A Hamburg engineer attempted to learn the fate of his daughter:

According to Death Certificate no. 1838/1943 in the Meseritz-Obrawalde registry office, my daughter, procurator Elfriede Friederike Auguste W., born 28 June 1908 in Hanover, died on 4 December 1943 at 8:30 in the clinic at Meseritz-Obrawalde, supposedly of a weak heart. After a bomb fell near my property in August 1943 and the top floor, where my daughter's room was, was heavily damaged, my daughter became very nervous and complained of headaches and sleeplessness. She was admitted to the Eppendorf Hospital in Hamburg as a private patient; from there she was deported without my knowledge to the clinic at Obrawalde-Meseritz. Upon inquiry at the office of the Eppendorf Hospital, I was told that because of the air raids on Hamburg the patients had been transferred to less endangered areas, in order to make room for victims of the Hamburg air raids.[135]

The chief physician at the Hamburg University Psychiatric Clinic who had transferred these patients to Meseritz-Obrawalde was the distinguished doctor Hans Bürger-Prinz, who would remain a respected figure after the war.

These entries in the patient files were confirmed by the testimony of a driver from Meseritz-Obrawalde. This man—originally imprisoned as a Communist from 1936 to 1940—was interned as a psychological case in Hamburg and deported to Meseritz-Obrawalde in April 1943; he survived by working for the asylum: "I recall a transport from Berlin of patients who had suffered severe shock as a result of the air raids on Berlin. These patients were not even distributed among the various houses, but instead were brought directly from the train to the hospital, where they were killed the same day. I know this for certain, because mass graves were later filled with corpses. I could also see the hearse, which collected the dead from the hospital without pause." [136]

After the air raids on Hamburg, occupants of old-age homes became the victims of euthanasia. Manfred Asendorf describes a group of 284 mainly older, bedridden Hamburg residents that left Arensburg on 6 August. After a two-day odyssey, 150 of the train's passengers were unloaded at the Neuruppin Mental Hospital. This asylum functioned as an "intermediate asylum" for the Brandenburg and Bernburg gas chambers. There, nine Hamburg residents died in the first fourteen days following their arrival. On 20 August, the director of the Neuruppin asylum "redefined" 38 men and, five days later, 16 women from the Hamburg group as mentally ill. For this purpose, he sent identical reports to the administrative head of the Brandenburg region, stating that "further accommodation was no longer possible" for these cases "because of a change in psychological condition." Later, the elderly people were placed in psychiatric care without additional formalities "in the interests of simplified administration." By 6 November, Neuruppin had been evacuated to make reserve beds available for Berlin. [137]

Occupants of old-age homes were also deported to Meseritz-Obrawalde. In the complaint that led to the prosecution of Doctor Hilde Wernicke and Head Nurse Helene Wieczorek, the plaintiff described the following: "In June 1944, Head Nurse Erdmann from House 6 received a transport of little old ladies who had been bombed out in Stettin. They were around 500 old, broken women. Erdmann had to eliminate them on instructions from Dr. Motz and Dr. Wernicke. After so many difficult experiences, through no fault of their own, following a life of hard work, this was the end." [138]

There was still another road to the euthanasia extermination camps. In 1946, a woman in Berlin-Moabit inquired as to her husband's whereabouts: "On 21 September 1943 my husband, Seaman Arthur P., was admitted to the Meseritz-Obrawalde State Sanitarium from the marine hospital in Bedburg-Hau. His file number was 12363." [139]

The groundwork for this type of extermination, which the Nazis aseptically called "removal," was laid by the head of the military medical service, Siegfried Handloser. In a 9 February 1943 order "on treatment of soldiers with hysterical and psychogenic reactions," he decreed, "War hysterics who cannot be cured of their symptoms through treatment are to be committed to the hospital sections of mental institutions."[140]

As an official of the Reich Ministry of the Interior, Linden directed the extermination in conjunction with his superior, Cropp. As General Commissioner for Air-Raid Damage, Cropp represented the positive side of the efficient rescue services. As Reich Commissioner for Mental Hospitals, Linden in his own way provided him with the necessary material resources.

The extent to which the resumption and progressive escalation of asylum killings were connected with emergency medical planning is indicated by the use made of six million reichsmarks earmarked in March by the Reich Ministry of Finance for auxiliary hospitals. On 21 September 1943, Cropp directed these funds in their entirety to the Reich Commissioner for Mental Hospitals, at the same time reminding Linden not to miss the deadline for applying for additional funding for the coming fiscal year. For the next 20 months, Linden corresponded with the office of engineer Albert Bremhorst, arguing about his large bills, under the heading "Erection of Emergency and Auxiliary Accommodations Using Wood-saving Construction Methods within the Framework of Measures to Make Western German Asylums Available."[141] The holder of the patent on this construction method, which would prove to be especially unstable and economical, was a Viennese architect named Neubauer; as Linden noted, his system, for which he demanded a 3 percent licensing fee, "in some ways resembles procedures that have already been employed successfully."

As a rule, during this period of the war a mental hospital included a reserve hospital, a hospital for the physically ill, nonmedical institutions, and, finally, those for whom the institutions had actually been built. These patients were now to make room by moving into concentration-camp-like structures. The asylums, recently pompously renamed "clinics" and "sanitaria" to emphasize their focus on healing, now obviously became camps; the directors, along with the physicians and chief physicians serving under them, turned into white-uniformed combinations of camp commandant and executioner.

Two criteria were probably decisive in selecting the location for Herbert Linden's barracks: first, the degree of air-raid danger, and second, the asylum director's willingness to treat patients concentrated in these new barrack asylums in such a way that their number would decrease as quickly as possible. Thus, to facilitate regional historical research, a list of asylums in which Linden had or wanted to have his barracks built may point to as yet undiscovered psychiatric crimes: Meseritz (6), Ückermünde (6), Sachsenberg (2), Pfafferode (2), Altscherbitz (2), Uchtspringe (5), Troppau (10), Schussenried (4), Winnental (8), Zwiefalten (2), Günzburg (2), Kaufbeuren (4), Plagwitz (3), Bunzlau (5), Lüben (5), Bergstadt (2), Loben (12), Rybnik (1), Hildburghausen (4), Stadtroda (2), Königslutter (3), Ansbach (2), Erlangen (1), Kutzenberg (3), Lohr (2), Mainkofen (2), Regensburg (2), Klagenfurt (2), Solbald-Hall (2), Conradstein (5), Tiegenhof (2), Wartha (2) (the number in parentheses refers to the number of barracks planned in 1943).*

Linden was able to implement his construction plans only with extreme difficulty. He insisted upon ignoring the objections of construction experts; he could, after all, call upon his powerful ally Karl Brandt, who, in the meantime, had risen through the ranks. On 27 October 1943, Brandt had already begun pressuring him to work toward "accelerated and if possible even broader activity . . . because of the loss of hospital space in the East."

On 27 December, Linden informed the Reich Ministry of Finance that he had already budgeted the six million reichsmarks allocated to him. He had ordered 145 barracks, each 42.5 meters long and 12.5 meters wide. "In order to meet rising demand for evacuation of mental hospitals," he applied for twelve million reichsmarks for the fiscal year 1944. Although the prefabricated units were still arriving at some asylums, the recipients reported that "a large number of the panels are completely destroyed or damaged," and there was not enough cement for the foundations.

In April 1944, Linden had to request that the asylums contribute mentally ill construction workers capable of working, so that he could put together a work detail to build barracks. Until then, Linden had cooperated with asylum directors to ensure deportation of patients incapable of

---

* This admittedly says nothing about the character of asylums located near large cities, those unsuited for barracks construction for reasons of space, and those in the western sections of the Reich thought to be particularly endangered. Even though no barracks were built, these asylums, such as Waldheim, Großschweidnitz, Wiesloch, Egelfing-Haar, Steinhof near Vienna, the Wiesengrund asylum near Eger, and Berlin-Wittenau, were very actively involved in the killing practice in German asylums that accelerated during the final phase of the Third Reich.

working; he knew he would have to overcome significant resistance and fears when—as with deportation of patients committed by the courts—the productive ones were involved. He expressly promised that "following completion of the operation, I will make certain mental patients are returned to the contributing asylums."

This fiasco did not bode well for the patients. In summer 1944, Linden further ordered installation of the notorious wooden bunk beds spread with straw in the asylums. The final construction measure, which must have been arranged by Linden, was consistent with this decision: crematoriums were to be built in German mental hospitals.

A crematorium was built in Kaufbeuren in July 1944; it went into operation soon after.[142] There is evidence that construction of such ovens also began in other asylums, such as Wiesloch near Heidelberg and Ückermünde. The director of the Pfafferode Asylum in Thuringia, Theodor Steinmeyer, hinted at central planning in a letter to his friend Friedrich Mennecke: "Incidentally, I am supposed to be getting the same building as Faltelhauser [director of Kaufbeuren]. You know what I mean. The state government has willingly assumed the costs, and it is now to be arranged from Berlin. I am curious whether all the difficulties to be overcome can be cleared up. But there is not much else I can do. The Eastern Workers' Office is very much in evidence [Pfafferode was an assembly center for mentally ill Eastern European laborers.]."[143]

At the beginning of March 1945, Red Army troops liberated the Meseritz-Obrawalde Asylum. In the period 16–26 March, the military medical leadership of the First White Russian Front carried out a forensic investigation, an exhumation, and a thorough interrogation of witnesses. The Red Army soldiers found "some thousand undoubtedly chronically psychologically ill people" still alive. They immediately realized that "the Obrawalde hospital was actually a national facility for the extermination of the German population." The investigating commission compiled a thorough hundred-page report with attached evidentiary photos, witness interrogations, and laboratory investigations. They also found the site of a crematorium under construction and an "oven door similar to the one in Maidanek" (in fact, the door in Meseritz was supplied by the same firm—Kori, on Dennewitzstrasse in Berlin-Schöneberg). The oven was not yet finished, but five thousand urns had already been prepared.[144] Assistant Secretary Herbert Linden of Department IV of the Medical Administration of the Reich Ministry of the Interior never had the chance to carry out his plans; he shot himself on 27 April 1945.

During the final two years of Nazi rule, the killing even of Germans

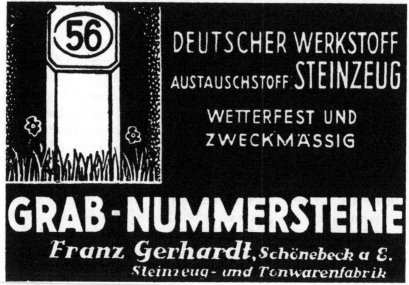

Advertisement in the newspaper *Cremation* (1942): "Numbered gravestones: German materials, substitute stone, weatherproof and practical."

unable to work reached proportions that have still to be investigated. To this day, Germans have shown themselves incapable of acknowledging what took place in 1943 in hundreds of large cities, affecting thousands of German families and technically implemented in large part by local administrators, welfare agencies, and insurance companies. Organized administrative murder of the unproductive and infirm must have become so natural that it was no longer an issue after 1945.

Operation T-4, the first National Socialist mass murder program that targeted an entire, carefully defined set of people, was in many ways connected, both institutionally and in its personnel, to the later murder of European Jewry. The most important connection, however, was the discovery made by its organizers that all levels of German administration, as well as the German people in general, were willing to accept such a procedure. Occasional remonstrance or resistance remained rare enough to permit a state policy of mass murder of people who had already been marginalized in various ways. The significance of Operation T-4 as a prelude to the gas chambers of Belzec and Auschwitz lies not so much in its development of techniques of camouflage and murder as in its undeniable political success—in the overt as well as tacit acceptance of the murder of marginalized, defenseless people by the overwhelming majority of all sectors of the population. It is thus hardly surprising that the national leadership drew the obvious conclusions, continuing its extermination policy and trusting that Germans would silently consent to this policy.

It is extremely problematic to ask "what if" questions when dealing with history; nevertheless, I am convinced that even limited protests against the euthanasia murders in 1940 would have hindered the development of systematic genocide in 1941. Even if we assume for a moment that intolerance and xenophobia, anti-Semitism, acquisitiveness, and arrogance are "typically German" qualities; even if we further assume that they were enormously reinforced—but only reinforced—by state policies; this still does not explain the single fact that numerous German families were prepared to accept the murder of their closest relatives without protest, even with approval. By so doing, they created the psychological conditions for the genocidal policies carried out in the years to come. If people did not protest even when their own relatives were murdered, they could hardly be expected to object to the murder of Jews, Gypsies, Russians, and Poles.

Notes

1. See Karl Heinz Roth and Götz Aly, "Das 'Gesetz über die Sterbehilfe bei unheilbar Kranken': Protokolle der Diskussion über die Legalisierung der nationalsozialistischen Anstaltsmorde in den Jahren 1938–1941," in *Erfassung zur Vernichtung: Von der Sozialhygiene zum "Gesetz über Sterbehilfe*," ed. K. H. Roth (Berlin, 1984), pp. 101–79.

2. Karl Binding and Alfred Hoche, *Die Freigabe der Vernichtung Lebensunwerten Lebens: Ihr Maß und ihre Form* (Leipzig, 1920), p. 17.

3. Testimony of Hans Hefelmann, quoted in the public prosecutor's files, StA Hamburg, 147 Js 58/67, Notebook "Aussagen."

4. Testimony of Anni Wödl on 1 March 1946, LG Wien (State Court of Vienna), Vg 2b Vr 2365/45.

5. Binding and Hoche, *Freigabe der Vernichtung*, p. 32. See also numerous examples in the files of local health offices—e.g., the "Arbeitseinsatz der Frau Alwine Janssen" (Work detail for Mrs. Alwine Janssen), a request sent to the head of the Oldenburg i. Holst Labor Office, with a copy "to the attention of the head of the killing department for retarded children in Schleswig-Stadtfeld, Dr. Hans Burkhardt." The document is in the files of the public prosecutor, StA Kiel, 2 Js 393/49.

6. Richtlinien des Reichsministers der Finanzen (Guidelines of the Reich Minister of Finance), 3 March 1941.

7. National Archives, Washington (hereafter NAW), T253, Roll 44, Morell file no. 81. Undated drafts. Duplicated in Roth and Aly, *Gesetz über die Sterbehilfe*, pp. 123–28.

8. Ewald Meltzer, *Das Problem der Abkürzung "lebensunwerten" Lebens* (Halle a.S., 1925).

9. Ibid., p. 86f.

10. Ibid., p. 88.

11. Ibid., p. 90.

12. Morell file (see n. 7).

13. Götz Aly, "Die wissenschaftliche Abstraktion des Menschen," in *Wege zum Menschen* 36 (1984): 276.

14. Bundesarchiv-Militärarchiv (Federal Archive–Military Archive), Freiburg [hereafter BA-MA], H 20, 463 ("Bericht über die Planung Schleswig vom 11–19.9.1941").

15. Ibid. ("Bericht über die Planungsfahrt Württemberg vom 21.10.1942–12.11.1942").

16. Response from the Wilhelmsdorf asylum administration to the author, 5 December 1984.

17. Testimony of Dr. Walter Medow, 5 November 1951, during the trial of Dr. Alfred Leu, prosecutor's files, StA Cologne, 24 Js 527/50. See also the trial, StA Schwerin, 1 KLs 3/46, documented in detail in the files of the Cologne trial. At the Großschweidnitz Hospital, the number of patient deaths in 1938 totaled 50; in 1939, the figure had already reached 141 (439 AR 3564/64, Zentrale Stelle der Landesjustizverwaltungen, Ludwigsburg [hereafter ZStL]). Hans-Ludwig Siemen reported on the Erlangen mental hospital: "From 1938 to 1940, the number of releases fell, although the number of admissions continued to rise. At the same time, the number of dead [the annual average] increased by almost 100" (Manuscript).

18. BA-MA, H 20, 463.

19. Nuremberg Documents.

20. Bundesarchiv (Federal Archive) Koblenz [hereafter BA], R 22/4209.

21. See Ernst Klee, *"Euthanasie" im NS-Staat* (Frankfurt, 1983), p. 95ff.; Jochen August, "Das Grab Nr. 17 im Wald von Piasnica: Die Tötung der Geisteskranken begann im besetzten Polen," *Antifaschistisches Magazin* 28, no. 193 (1984): 6ff.

22. Prosecutor's files, StA Berlin, 3 P (K) Js 134/60.

23. Archives of the Polish High Commission in Warsaw, Z 5/3.

24. See Klee, *Euthanasie*, p. 77ff.; Kurt Nowak, *"Euthanasie" und Sterilisierung im "Dritten Reich"* (Weimar, Göttingen, 1980), p. 77ff. (the book gives an excellent overview of the ideological and intellectual prerequisites to sterilization and euthanasia); Götz Aly, "Der Mord an behinderten Kindern zwischen 1939 und 1945," in *Heilen und Vernichten in Mustergau Hamburg*, ed. A. Ebbinghaus, H. Kaupen-Haas, and K. H. Roth (Hamburg, 1984), pp. 147–55.

25. Decree by Reich Ministry of the Interior, RMdI IV G 3487/39–5100.

26. Decree by Reich Ministry of the Interior, RMdI IV G 1510/39–5100 Westf.

27. Klee, *Euthanasie*, p. 98f.

28. Cited in Friedrich Karl Kaul, *Nazimordaktion T-4: Ein Bericht über die erste industriemäßig durchgeführte Mordaktion des Naziregimes* (Berlin, 1973), p. 63.

29. The role played by Max de Crinis has still not been sufficiently investigated; well-researched indications can be found in a series in *Quick* magazine that has also appeared as a book: Gerhard Jaeckel, *Die Charité* (Bayreuth, 1963), pp. 376–402.

30. Berlin Document Center (hereafter BDC), personal file of Karl Heinz Rodenberg.

31. BDC, personal file of Oskar Begusch.

32. Quoted in Kaul, *Nazimordaktion*, p. 64.

33. The exact statistics are found in NAW, T 1021, Roll 18.

34. BDC, personal file of Werner Blankenburg.

35. Author's archives.

36. *Ministerialblatt des Reichs- und Preußischen Ministerium des Inneren* (Ministerial Bulletin of the Reich and Prussian Ministry of the Interior, hereafter *RMBliV*) (1942): 37.

37. Staatsarchiv Potsdam (Potsdam State Archives), Rep. 55 C, no. 33 (Anstalt Neuruppin).

38. Ibid.

39. Handschriftenabteilung (Manuscript Division), Göttingen University Library, Lu-9, 24.

40. See Asmus Finzen, *Auf dem Dienstweg: Die Verstrickung einer Anstalt in die Tötung psychisch Kranker* (Rehburg-Loccum, 1984). This book succeeded in reconstructing for the first time the specific extermination of mentally ill Jews (pp. 23–60).

41. Nuremberg Documents, NO 781.

42. BA, R 96 I/2.

43. See the corresponding sections in Kaul and Klee that summarize the results of the investigation by the Frankfurt prosecutor. One source in particular is the letter from F. Mennecke; the original can be found in the Hessische Hauptstaatsarchiv (Main State Archives of Hesse).

44. In most of Czechoslovakia, which was called the Reich Protectorate of Bohemia and Moravia, the T-4 protagonists had to exercise restraint. After a very general preliminary informational trip, Herbert Becker reported on 15 September 1942: "No questions involving euthanasia—even sterilization under the Genetic Health Law— have yet been introduced into the Protectorate; they are not even to be discussed." A possible future inspection would have to be postponed until "later, calmer times." BA-MA, H 20, 463.

45. A well-informed work by Volker Rieß on this subject is forthcoming; see also Gitta Sereny, *Am Abgrund: Eine Gewissensforschung* (Berlin, 1980).

46. BDC, personal file of Curt Schmalenbach.

47. *Reichsgesetzblatt* (Reich Legal Bulletin [hereafter *RGBl*]) (1941): 653; *RMBliV* (1941): 1999.

48. BA, R 18, 3160.

49. Decree by Bayerisches Staatsministerium (Bavarian Ministry of State) on 15 December 1942, cited in Ernst Mader, *Das erzwungene Sterben von Patienten der Heil- und Pflegeanstalt Kaufbeuren-Irsee zwischen 1940 und 1945: nach Dokumenten und Berichten von Augenzeugen* (Blöcktach, 1982).

50. NAW, T 1021, Roll 11.

51. NAW, T 1021, Roll 12.

52. See Bundsarchiv (Federal Archives), Potsdam branch [hereafter BAP], Kanzlei des Führers (Führer's Office), no. 42.

53. *RMBliV* (1941): 1129.

54. NAW, T 1021, Roll 12.

55. Schäfer's testimony is recorded in the Nuremberg Documents, NO 3817. Information following in the text can be found in the Plauen City Archives.

56. See Bernd Wehner, *Dem Täter auf der Spur: Die Geschichte der deutschen Kriminalpolizei* (Bergisch Gladbach, 1983).

57. Cited in Detlev Peukert, "Arbeitslager und Jugend-KZ: Die 'Behandlung Ge-

96 ■ Götz Aly

meinschaftsfremder' im Dritten Reich," in *Die Reihen fast geschlossen,* ed. D. Peukert and J. Reulecke (Wuppertal, 1981), p. 416.

58. *RMBliV* (1940): 1519ff.

59. Richtlinien des Reichsministers der Finanzen (Guidelines of the Reich Ministry of Finance), 3 March 1941.

60. Hans Heinze, "Psychopathische Persönlichkeiten," in *Handbuch der Erbkrankheiten,* ed. Arthur Gütt (Leipzig, 1942), vol. 4, p. 286.

61. Ibid., p. 274f.

62. Secret decree by the Reich Ministry of the Interior (CRMdI), 19 November 1940, BA, R 22/5008.

63. Ibid.

64. Archives of the Polish High Commission in Warsaw, Reich Ministry of the Interior, vol. 4.

65. Ibid., vol. 2.

66. Prosecutor's files, StA Kiel, 2 Js 393/49.

67. Prosecutor's files, StA Ansbach, 1 Js 1147/62, Beiakten Krankengeschichten (supplementary file—patient reports).

68. Prosecutor's files, StA Cologne, 24 Js 429/61 (investigation of Dr. Maly), vol. 4, testimony of Wentzler. Corresponding indications can be found in the files of various health offices, as well as in the police files on Gypsies.

69. Testimony of Hans Hefelmann, 15 September 1960, GStA (General Prosecutor) Frankfurt a.M., Js 17/59.

70. Indictment of Heyde, Bohne, and Hefelmann, pp. 475–87, 6 StA Frankfurt a.M., Js 17/59.

71. BA, R 96 I/2.

72. ZStL, Ordner (Looseleaf) 349.

73. ZStL, Nuremberg Documents, vol. 246, NO-1660.

74. *RGBl* (1933, I): 995.

75. StA Düsseldorf, 8 Js 116/47.

76. BA, R 22, 4209.

77. NAW, T 1021, Roll 17.

78. See n. 76.

79. Ibid.

80. Ibid.

81. Ibid.

82. Testimony of Ingeborg Seidel, Main Hesse State Archives, Wiesbaden [hereafter HHStA], 461/32061/3 (Hadamar trial), vol. 3.

83. NAW, T 1021, Roll 12.

84. Ibid., Roll 10.

85. Ibid., Roll 12.

86. Ibid.

87. BA-MA, H 20, 463.

88. Hans Maršálek, *Die Geschichte des Konzentrationslagers Mauthausen* (Vienna, 1980), p. 123f.

89. BAP, Film 1648 (Reichsjustizministerium [Reich Ministry of Justice]).

90. Adelheid L. Rüter-Ehrlermann and C. F. Rüter, eds., *Justiz und NS-Verbrechen* (Amsterdam, 1968), vol. 9, p. 276 (see fn. pp. 63–64).

91. Ibid., p. 275.

92. NAW, T 1021, Roll 12.

93. Ibid., Gutachterliste (list of experts).

94. GStA, Js 10/65 Frankfurt a.M. (investigation of Runckel).

95. Ibid.

96. Prosecutor's files, StA Kiel, 2 Js 393/49 (Einstellungsvermerk [note of suspension], p. 15).

97. Prosecutor's files, StA Hamburg, 147 Js 58/67, vol. Anklageschrift (indictment), 620ff.

98. See Anstaltsarchiv Hadamar (Hadamar Asylum archives), personal files 430/2/1106; 430/2/2383; 430/2/2284; 430/2/1335; 430/2/509; 430/2/3120; 430/2/1198; 430/2/90; 430/2/2395; 430/2/4219.

99. Rüter, Justiz und NS-Verbrechen, p. 285.

100. NAW, T 1021, Roll 12.

101. Ibid., Roll 17.

102. Prosecutor's files, StA Hamburg, 147 Js 58/67, Beiakte Gesundheitsverwaltung (supplementary health administration file).

103. Ibid.

104. Compare the Wiesloch list of criminals incapable of working with the transport list in Hadamar: NAW, T 1021, Roll 17; Hadamar Asylum archives, transport lists.

105. RGBl (1942, I): 515f. Erlaß des Führers über das Sanitäts- und Gesundheitswesen (Führer's decree on the military and civilian health systems).

106. BA, R 18/5576 (express letter from the Reich Commissioner for Mental Hospitals, 5 August 1942).

107. RGBl (1935, I): 827.

108. BA, R 18/5576.

109. Ibid., 3768.

110. See NAW, T 1021, Roll 12.

111. Ibid., Roll 12.

112. Ibid.

113. BA, R 18/3791.

114. Ibid.

115. ZStL, Mennecke letters, vol. 2, sheet 177.

116. Letter of 4 April 1943, cited in Finzen, Auf dem Dienstweg.

117. BA, R 17, 3768.

118. Ibid., 3791.

119. Ibid.

120. BDC, personal file of de Crinis, personal file of Nitsche.

121. BDC, personal file of Nitsche. The discussion between Brandt, Nitsche, and de Crinis occurred on 23 June; see NAW, T 1021, Roll 10.

122. BA-MA, H 20, 465 (correspondence between Nitsche and Wischer).

123. Ibid. (correspondence between Nitsche and Allers).

124. BA, R 58/1059.

125. NAW, T 1021, Roll 12.

126. Ibid.

127. Ibid.

128. Prosecutor's files, StA Düsseldorf, 8 Js 116/47, vol. 2.

129. See Rudolf Hans, "Psychiatrischer Alltag im Nationalsozialismus: Eine Studie zur Anstaltspsychiatrie in Westfalen," thesis for state examination (Bochum, 1983), p. 68ff.

130. Prosecutor's files, StA Berlin, 11 Ks 8/46.

131. Nuremberg Documents, 630-PS.

132. Prosecutor's files, StA Kiel, 2 Js 393/49, vol. 1 (testimony of Illing).

133. See, for example, Olaf Groehler, *Geschichte des Luftkrieges, 1910–1980* (Berlin [GDR]), 1981), p. 376.

134. The patient reports on the women deported to Hadamar with the transport on 7 August 1943 are documented in the prosecutor's files, StA Hamburg, 147 Js 58/67, vol. 34.

135. Trial of Hilde Wernicke and Helene Wieczorek, prosecutor's files, StA Berlin, 11 Ks 8/46 (almost half the file is taken up with such letters from relatives).

136. Ibid., n. 134, vol. 25.

137. See Manfred Asendorf, who examined the files of the Hamburg welfare authorities in his article, "Als Hamburg in Schutt und Asche fiel und wie der NS-Staat die Krise bewältigte," in *Heilen und Vernichten im Mustergau Hamburg* (Hamburg, 1984).

138. Prosecutor's files, StA Berlin, 11 Ks 8/46.

139. Ibid.

140. BA-MA, H 20, 464.

141. BA, R 18/3707. The following citations are taken from these files.

142. Mader, *Das erzwungene Sterben*, p. 52ff.

143. ZStL, Mennecke letters.

144. Excerpts from the report of a colonel in the medical corps of the First White Russian Front, Faust Yosifowitsch Schkaravski, on the investigation of the Obrawalde Hospital, 16–26 February 1945. A German translation can be found in the prosecutor's files, StA Hamburg, 147 Js 58/67.

CHAPTER THREE

The Posen Diaries of the Anatomist Hermann Voss

Annotated by Götz Aly

Located in the archives of the West Institute in Poznań, Poland, is an important document from the time of the German occupation, document number Cyt.I.Z.DOK.I-752: the diary of Professor Hermann Voss. In 1941 Voss, an anatomist, was one of the founders of the so-called Reich University of Posen, where he served as dean of the Medical Department. In his flight from the Red Army in January 1945, he left behind the part of his diary covering the years 1932 to 1942.[1]

After the war, Hermann Voss lived in East Germany. He became chief anatomist in Halle from 1948 to 1952, and from 1952 to 1962 he was a professor of anatomy at Jena. After that, he remained active as a professor emeritus at the Greifswald anatomical institute; he later moved to Hamburg, in West Germany, where he lived until his death in 1987. German medical students know him for his anatomy handbook, popularly called "Voss and Herrlinger." This textbook was published simultaneously for almost 40 years in constantly updated editions by VEB Gustav Fischer in Jena and Gustav Fischer Publishers in Stuttgart, West Germany. The book's popularity most likely stems from the fact that, as stated in its first foreword in 1946, it "eliminates everything extraneous to actual practice." Going through 17 editions, a Spanish edition, and even an edition in Polish,[2] it has become a standard work.

Hermann Voss is also noted for co-editing the most important German journal of anatomy, the *Anatomischer Anzeiger,* published in East Germany from 1952 to 1974; from 1954 to 1980 he also established and directed the *Acta Histochemica,* a journal of international stature that publishes findings on delicate tissue studies. Students and doctors who

(*Above and opposite*) Extracts from the body record of the anatomical institute of the Reich University and from the notebook in which Voss recorded his trade in skeletons and bones.

have studied Voss for their exams and referred to his scientific works should be aware that they owe their basic knowledge to a man who in 1941 rejoiced over each Pole shot to death, who bought and sold the skeletons of resistance fighters, who had victims of the guillotine examined seconds after their death, and who, out of sheer racial hatred and fear, advocated "retaliatory" massacres of the kind that occurred in Lidice, Oradour, and many other places. The worse the situation became for the diarist in occupied Posen, the more he alternated between banality and bestiality.

The diary documents the psychological condition of a large segment of the German intelligentsia. They kept their distance from Nazism to the extent that it seemed unscientific and vulgar, but were not repelled by hatred of Communists, Jews, and Slavs. On the contrary, it was precisely the ideal and the practice of extermination at home and abroad, on the one hand, and the elevation of the Germans to the level of a master race, on the other, that had a profoundly integrating effect on men like Hermann

Voss. These factors granted him actual power, although he was by no means a 150 percent loyal, party line functionary.

The diary was discovered by Stefan Rozycki, an anatomy professor, as reconstruction of the Polish university began. As early as 1945, he cited an extract in the Polish biweekly *Medical News*.[3] The diary and the situation at the Posen anatomical institute, as well as Hermann Voss himself, were often mentioned later; they were used as evidence in the trial of Arthur Greiser, *Gau* leader and governor of the area of Poland known as the Warthegau.[4] Extensive excerpts from the diary were published in German in the fifties by Karol Marian Pospieszalski,[5] but they were barely acknowledged in West Germany, the self-proclaimed legal successor to the Third Reich. In 1964, Voss's diary crossed the Oder-Neisse border for the first time. The former concentration camp inmate and author of the "Song of the Moor Soldiers," Rudi Goguel, received a doctorate in history in

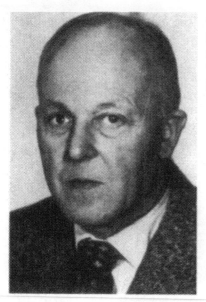

The title "Outstanding People's Scientist" was an honor bestowed by the East German Council of State for "contributions to the development of science in the service of peace."

East Germany in 1964 with an excellent thesis that unfortunately remained unpublished; in it, he mentioned and quoted these documents. His assessment: "It would be incorrect to assume that the Reich University's cooperation with the occupation regime was limited to traditional academic areas—teaching, research, and publication. We have shameful evidence that German 'scholars' at the Reich University had no reservations about taking part in the murderous excesses of the SS and the Gestapo, if not as actual assistants, then as profit-making accomplices."[6]

This publication had no apparent consequences for Voss, at the time the most respected and influential anatomist in East Germany. In West Germany, the textbook author's past was never acknowledged.

The diary consists of 225 loose, typewritten sheets covering the period from 13 October 1932, the author's 38th birthday, to 14 August 1942—almost 10 years. It does not bear Voss's signature; however, its precision, its detailed discussion of family and career, show the text to be authentic. In particular, it corresponds to the handwritten "Chronicle of the Anatomical Institute of the Reich University" that Voss also left behind in Posen.[7]

The text is part of a larger whole. In the first entry, Voss points out that he is beginning the fifth volume of his diary, and it is almost certain that he continued to keep the diary past August 1942. An enthusiastic typist, Voss most probably typed copies of the diary himself. Perhaps he intended to give one to his wife; perhaps, out of fear and skepticism, he wished to have a duplicate of this valuable document in case something happened to the original during the war. Voss had received the blank book in which he handwrote the original diary in 1932, as a birthday present. It "was unusually large and thick." "Only the gods know if I will live to reach the end of this diary," wrote Voss, who lived to be more than 90; he replied to his own question with the pessimism of those years of crisis: "I hardly think so."

The diary contains nothing really intimate; in several places it becomes clear that the author was writing at least partially for an audience. When he describes the purchase of a silver teapot—it cost 160 reichsmarks—he explains, "I mention the price here not to brag, but because it is often interesting later on to know how much such things cost when they were obtained." And after he joined the Nazi party in 1937, against his convictions and only so as not to have to give up his final, modest career dream—advancement from assistant to chief anatomist—he wrote without mentioning his opportunistic motives: "The reasons that moved me to take this step are many. However, I do not want to go into them here."

Voss kept the diary irregularly. The intervals between individual entries span several days to several weeks; sometimes they last more than a month, and once, as a result of illness, the pause covers three months. His subjects are essentially the banal facts of daily life; they rarely include thoughts or reflections. The author briefly mentions the books he has read, noting and commenting upon political events and those connected with his profession, his leisure time and, especially, his family.

Hermann Voss was born on 13 October 1894 in Berlin; he was the son of the lessee of a manor. He grew up in Warnkenhagen and Malchin in Mecklenburg. His studies in Munich, Heidelberg, and Rostock from 1913 to 1918 were interrupted by a year and a half of military service as an assistant army doctor in France—a period, he would recall 18 years later, that "was actually the best and most pleasant of my entire life." He studied with Dietrich Barfurth and received a doctorate in 1919 for a study of the experimental generation of parthenogenic frog larvae from unfertilized cells.[8] Starting on 1 May 1919, he became assistant anatomist at the anatomical institute of the University of Rostock, after marrying Eva, a woman four years his senior, in January. In November a son, Hermann, was born. Through the diary, the reader comes to know him as a severely handicapped, physically helpless child. The boy was intellectually developed far beyond his years, and his parents showered him with love and attention. Voss studied Sanskrit and Greek with him; the 17-year-old read Kant. All the family's care and energy were devoted to him until his death in June 1939 of suffocation. A second child, a daughter, Sabine, was born in 1933.

In 1926, Voss obtained a post at the anatomical institute in Leipzig. It was 12 years before he finally advanced to chief anatomist and associate professor in 1938. This embittered him; he felt he had been passed over, and he observed of other appointments that, despite National Socialism, "in this world, the rabble always wins." When, in 1934, a colleague five years his junior, Max Clara, was appointed his new superior, he noted, filled with resignation: "It is clear from this sort of appointment that we of the world war generation no longer count." In addition, a lecture he presented at an anatomists' convention was not well received, and it seemed inevitable that he would spend the rest of his life as assistant anatomist in Leipzig: "I will move heaven and earth to get my own home as soon as possible. I can do this now without concern, for I cannot imagine that I will ever leave this place." He built the house with devotion, cared for the garden, and was happy to put some distance between himself and the big city, which was alien to him.

In 1937 he hoped once again, like so many of his academic colleagues, to advance his career at the expense of an ousted Jew: "In Cologne, the position of department head has opened up because of the dismissal of the non-Aryan Veit. Clara told me today that he had recommended me for this position in C. and also in Munich." But once this hope, too, had been dashed, only the foreign aggression of the Third Reich remained to create new positions. The suppression of Czechoslovakia, the Anschluss of Austria, the annexation of Alsace-Lorraine, the opening up of Prague and Strasbourg, Vienna and Graz, brought some life to the bogged-down, Aryanized professorial market.

Not until early 1941 were Hermann Voss's long-buried hopes of obtaining a chair realized. However, the phantom Reich University of Posen, which existed only on paper, was the worst, least prestigious place he could have landed. While in his diary the personal catastrophe of this advancement, linked to a sort of exile, is clear, he also included a convoluted, dramatic sentence in the "Chronicle of the Anatomical Institute of the Reich University of Posen": "On 1 April 1941, I, Hermann Voss, associate professor of anatomy and chief anatomist at the anatomical institute of the University of Leipzig, was appointed temporarily by the Reich Ministry of Science and Public Education to the position of professor of anatomy and director of the anatomical institute of the Reich University of Posen."

Hermann Voss loved Johann Sebastian Bach, Wilhelm Raabe, his profession, and his family. He hated Jews, Communists, and Slavs:

> The English and French peoples do not want war, but the Jewish press in these countries is forcing them into it. (29 September 1938)

> Our beautiful German spring is once again, as it so often is, a "green-painted winter," as H. Heine, alias Chaim Bückeburg, or whatever his name really was, quite accurately put it. (19 April 1935)

> This afternoon I unfortunately heard only part of Hitler's great speech in the Reichstag. In it, the German people were informed of facts of world-historical significance. It is to be hoped that his earnest desire for peace will succeed in protecting the peoples of Europe from a future war and thus from destruction! It might well be possible, if Juda did not reign among all other nations! Until other nations achieve the same insights as we, the hope for uniting the European states is nil, for as long as Juda reigns he will agitate continuously for war against Germany. A battle of light against darkness! In the end, light will and must win! (7 March 1936)

> In Leipzig, the vote on Sunday [on the Anschluss of Austria] went particularly badly. Absolutely as well as percentally, there was a record number of no votes—and the Führer stated here in Leipzig: "I know that all of Saxony is behind me." Yes, the "dear Saxons!" In addition, it can be shown indisputably that the worst voting took place in the "settlements," where the people were given who knows what. Full of old Communists who are once again getting insolent. The whole crew should be sterilized. (13 April 1938)

> In the end, the entire conflict is one of Bolshevism against National Socialism, for in Czechoslovakia the Reds seem to be at the helm already. And only powder and shot are of any use against these beasts. (16 September 1938)

> The Polish people are multiplying twice as fast as the Germans, and that is decisive! The much more primitive Slavic peoples will devour the German people, which do not multiply fast enough by far. (23 June 1935)

> I think that one should look at the Polish question without emotion, purely biologically. We must exterminate them, otherwise they will ex-

terminate us. And that is why I am glad of every Pole who is no longer alive. (2 June 1941)

For Voss it was also clear that "there must be wars, otherwise nations would degenerate"; he was very glad to hear, in 1934, "that guns are once again being cast in Krupp's locomotive department"; he saw the German Reich's withdrawal from the League of Nations as a "true deliverance," and the reintroduction of military service as "excellent news." From this point of view, Voss appears to have been a typical national conservative.

But there are also very different elements in this diary that do not fit the cliché of the cheering *Untertan* (subject). Voss did not prefer private contact with his own kind, his academic colleagues. As shown in biting references in his diary, he kept his distance from them. He was the only academic on his volleyball team, and he tended to cultivate friendly contacts at the institute mainly with the employees. His diary describes lengthy bicycle tours with the dissector and the medical illustrator:

On Pentecost I went bicycling with Schäffner and Herschel[9] to Laasan near Jena. We left here on Saturday morning, shortly after four o'clock, and got there by around two o'clock in the afternoon. We left on Tuesday morning at seven o'clock and were back here by 5:30. On the way there we went through Zeitz-Mühltal-Klosterlausnitz-Thalbürgel-Jena-Kunitz, on the way back through Camburg-Naumburg-Weissenfels-Markranstadt-Lausen-Gr. Zschocher-Connewitz. The distance each time was some 90 km. We slept in a tent; however, I did so only for two nights—the last night I slept at the inn in Laasan in order to get a good night's sleep. We wandered around the area a great deal and saw many plants, especially the wonderful orchids—lady's-slippers, nest root, coral root, orchis purpurea—and many animals. My two companions know everything there that creeps and flies. (25 May 1937)

Voss studied Russian and took piano lessons. He ate yogurt every day, noting that "it tastes wonderful and agrees with me"; he did not buy a car, instead bicycling twice a day the four kilometers to the anatomical institute: "I have brought my steel horse up from the cellar and brought it into working order. It is a wonderful investment. Yesterday I made the following calculation. A monthly ticket for the electric streetcar costs 12.50 RM. I ride my bicycle eight months in the year and thus save exactly 100 RM. The bicycle cost 130 M. Thus it earns an annual interest of 77 percent."

The life of the Voss family is described extensively in the first part of the diary; it is an important part of the author's life, and the relationship between husband and wife, on the one hand, and parents and children, on the other, inspires respect and sympathy.

In contrast to these intense descriptions of the closeness of his family life in Leipzig, the author's descriptions of his professional life are meager. The "semester film" winds down again; the older he becomes, the faster courses and examinations follow upon each other. Professional satisfaction lies in the writing and publication of scientific works. The rest is duty. During a short period of military service in 1939, into which he was drafted "as a doctor, against my will" after 20 years of working in anatomy, Voss wrote the following verse: "Must is a hard nut / these words are true / and sound ever anew. / But even the hardest nut / has a sweet core. / Would you like to know where? / I will tell you: / change, loyally and quietly / the 'must' to your own 'I want to.'"

In April 1941, when Hermann Voss arrived, full of anxiety and depression, humiliated and dissatisfied, in occupied Poland, his previously latent aggressive, destructive characteristics were activated in perhaps typical form. His civilized Leipzig demeanor disappeared into thin air. The man who had once listened to the final chorus of the Saint Matthew Passion—"We cast off in tears"—whenever he left his home in Leipzig for the "wild east" now equipped himself with a whip with an iron core, in order to teach the Polish workers manners. Fear and aggression came to determine his entire way of thinking: "Here in Posen it is now a question of victory or death. There can be nothing else." For Voss, however, victory meant the death of the Polish majority, dangerous by virtue of their very existence. He profitably combined their extermination, which was then beginning, with the necessities and opportunities of his profession. Here the Posen diary entries will be quoted in detail, while the period between 1933 and 1940 will merely be touched upon.

The Diary

Thursday, 20 April 1933
Today Hitler's birthday is being celebrated throughout the Reich for the first time. On the houses one sees everywhere the swastika and the old black-white-red Reich flag, "pure" or with a swastika in the middle. We, too, have hung our new flag out the window for the first time. For me there is only one flag. It is the old Reich flag under which I grew up and

served in the war. This afternoon I saw a young man in front of our house examine our house and the neighboring buildings and write something down. He wore the insignia of the National Socialist Party! I am busy making a clear copy of my paper on nuclein synthesis in axolotlei. In these tumultuous times it is often difficult to collect oneself to do scientific work. Let us hope that at last, at last, more peaceful times are coming! The semester does not begin until 2 May. . . .

Saturday, 17 June 1933

Upon returning I found a card from Stieve* in which he announces the acceptance of my paper and calls its content "very valuable." I was very pleased with this. After all, these are the first words of recognition I have received for a scientific paper. The gods only know when the paper will appear; certainly not before next year.

Sunday, 16 July 1933

. . . Yes, it is much more difficult to check a revolution in full tilt at the right moment than to set it in motion in the first place. Hitler is fully aware of this. And that is enough, for I am convinced that with his iron will he is the man to prevent a slide into the abyss, to prevent chaos. There are probably very few Germans today who do not trust him in this way. I have always admired his energy; now I also admire his good sense. Kind fortune has once again presented the German Reich with the right man at the right time. And I am firmly convinced that things will get better now. Tremendous things have been achieved by our Chancellor: he has smashed not only the Reds, but also the Blacks, which I never would have thought possible. All parties have been eliminated; the situation that has been created might not always be good in all circumstances, but it is the only correct one for the German Reich in its present state. H. thus has unlimited power in his hands, more than any monarch has possessed for a long time. I believe he will use it well, for the good of the German people. . . . National Socialism has achieved great things, there is no doubt of that. But in order to really recognize this, one must turn one's eyes to the distance, the future. In these times, when viewed from up close, it is and has often been marred by many small blemishes, often disturbing, but—one must admit upon calm consideration—unavoidable during such a tremendous process; for people are not angels, nor Hitlers, but simply people, with all their weaknesses.

* Hermann Stieve (1886–1952), anatomist in Leipzig and Berlin.

I have always been national-social in my entire being and world-view, but I have never yet managed to dedicate myself completely to one political party. I always refused all invitations to join purely National Socialist organizations. In the end I will probably not be able to avoid it. At any rate, I will then be conscious of having resisted this connection for as long as possible. Many of my colleagues immediately threw themselves into the party for fear of losing their jobs. They were people with bad consciences who used to be Social Democrats and democrats. I saw this at our institute among the employees (not among my colleagues!). Those who had once shown not the slightest trace of national feeling were the first to join the party.

Sunday, 12 November 1933
    . . . Yesterday afternoon I was at a rally of German academia organized by the Nat.-Soc. Teachers Union in the Albert Hall. It went very nicely, with dignity. The event began with the processional. We all rose and greeted Hitler's banner with raised right arm. Then the "Volkunger" by M. v. Schillings was played, and following an opening speech by the *Gau* leader Göpfert, a series of university professors began to speak. The round was led off by our colleague Eugen Fischer, now anthropologist and rector of the University of Berlin. He was followed by the rector of our university, Prof. Golf, and by Prof. Heidegger, rector of the University of Freiburg, Prof. Hirsch,* theologian in Göttingen, Prof. Pinder, Munich, Prof. Sauerbruch, Berlin and Prof. Schumann, Halle. In my opinion, Prof. Hirsch is of Jewish extraction. His name was immediately suspicious. As I observed the row of speakers—the only one I knew by name was E. Fischer—I said to myself: Judging by his looks, that one must be Hirsch. And I was right, it was he! He spoke quite well, but was typically Jewish, especially in his posture and movements. After the speeches were over—each speaker could speak for only ten minutes—a resolution was read that is to be translated into three foreign languages and sent to all universities in the world, and in addition, a telegram of homage to the Chancellor. Then the Dutch prayer of thanks, the national anthem, and

---

* This refers to Emanuel Hirsch (1888–1972), a prominent Protestant theologian who actively supported Hitler. What made Voss, a fan of Theodor Storm, suspect Hirsch, who became a member of the Nazi party in 1937, of having a Jewish background was probably his intellectual acuity. See Robert P. Ericksen, *Theologen unter Hitler: Das Bündnis zwischen evangelischer Dogmatik und Nationalsozialismus* (Munich, 1986), especially the chapter "Emanuel Hirsch—Der Nazi-Intellektuelle," pp. 167–268.

the "Horst Wessel" song were sung. The ceremonial recessional formed the close of the assembly. When I arrived home shortly after seven, Hindenburg was speaking on the radio. This afternoon we voted for Adolf Hitler's government. After voting, one bought a "yes" insignia for five cents, which was pinned on by an SA man. It is a true deliverance that we are finally out of this League of Nations. How long I have awaited this! Incidentally, on Friday we all listened together at the institute to the Führer's great speech. One gains more and more confidence, and begins to believe that things will improve in Germany under this government. . . .

29 April 1934

. . . Yesterday I sent my first muscle work to Stieve. Hopefully more can follow; the next to come is to be the eye muscle, then the muscles of the extremities in human beings and then chimpanzees. Incidentally, chimpanzees reminds me to mention that I have just begun to collect literature on the apes: chimpanzees, orangs, and gorillas. I would like to give a lecture or, even better, write a book on them. In that way, one could create for oneself a *monumentum aere perennius;* but this is a pipe dream and will probably remain so. . . . *

Sunday, 17 June 1934

This morning I mounted my steel horse at 8:30 and rode off. Wonderful sunshine and a slight east wind. The ride past cornfields with beautiful blue cornflowers was a joy. One sits within these stone walls for days and weeks on end and sees absolutely nothing of the open fields, of all that is going on there, all the things that grow and bloom. I rode through Holzhausen, Seifershain, and Fuchshain toward the Naunhofer Forest. Before Köhra, I stopped in a corner of the woods and lay in the shadow of a birch for half an hour. It was wonderful! After this pause for rest I rode through Köhra and up to Belgershain, and from there back through the Oberholz, where I refreshed myself in a pub with a "Berlin white beer." This morning I determined that, contrary to expectations, the muscles that move the whole hand (M. flex. carpi radialis & ulnaris) have finer muscle fibers than

* It did not remain so. Voss later did in part create this monument, with a *Bibliographie der Menschenaffen (Schimpanse, Orang, Gorilla)* (Bibliography of the apes [chimpanzees, orangs, gorillas]). It was published in 1955 by VEB Gustav Fischer, Jena (GDR). In the foreword, he wrote: "I set myself . . . the task, some 25 years ago, of collecting anatomical writings on apes and compiling a bibliography, thus creating an essential prerequisite for monographic or textbook presentations of the anatomy of individual apes." He dedicated the work to the memory of his friend and colleague, Professor Curt Fahrenholz, who died in 1946.

the finger flexors (M. flex. dig. sublimus & profundus). Of all the arm muscles I have examined until now, these two hand flexors have the finest fibers, and can therefore also perform the finest movements. Determining such a new fact about the human body really makes one happy. . . .

Saturday, 15 September 1934

Yesterday Eva bought a little savings bank for 90 pfennigs to replace our old one. It was shaped unusually, like a church. It had been quite bent out of shape by our little daughter, and had thus outlived its usefulness. In the time we have lived here in L., almost 1,000 marks have gone through this "church." Hopefully the new bank will also attain this, or even more. It now stands in the music room on the telephone table. Anyone who talks on the telephone must throw a ten-piece in the bank. If you have not tried it yourself, it is hard to believe that in a few years several hundred marks can grow out of such small sums. Our little daughter is cute. She enjoyed this wonderful summer. There has hardly been a day since spring that she could not go outside because the weather was bad. Her day proceeds as follows. Of course she wakes up early in the morning and gets her first feeding. After we have our coffee, she is freed from the prison of her bed and may run around the room and the hall, which she naturally eagerly attends to, making all sorts of mischief in the process. Toward 10 she is bathed, then goes back to bed and sleeps until around noon. She has been eating lunch with us at the table for some time, sitting in her child's seat. She eats quite well, almost as much as an adult, and has recently gained a great deal of weight. After lunch she goes out to the garden with Dada— that's me. In nice weather—and as I said, when wasn't the weather nice this summer and fall?—she is dressed only in a pair of rompers and a little hat that covers her extremely thick head of light, almost white hair. I look after her for an hour so that E. can lie down and rest for awhile. Later she takes over the little one, or if necessary our girl, Ruth, whom the little one calls Elia after a song she has sung to her. Thus she is outside the whole afternoon, until she has dinner between six and seven o'clock and is put to bed. Her vocabulary is still rather small. . . .

Sunday, 31 March 1935

The paper today reports that Prof. Krüger has been appointed rector of the university; that is, a man who gained barely a single vote in the so-called rector elections. We could have had this without the fuss of the rector elections! Tomorrow the semester is supposed to begin; very little has been seen of the students so far. . . .

Sunday, 29 August 1937
. . . The struggle over my position continues. Now Herr v. Hayek, the little Viennese Jew* who was with my friend Elze† in R. [Rostock] and has now returned from Shanghai, is again being proposed as a candidate. I spoke with Clara about it yesterday, but he does not want him. It no longer makes any difference to me at all whether I get the position or not; I only wish that a decision would be made one way or the other, so I know where I stand. I find no recognition anywhere. It is sometimes difficult not to lose faith in oneself. But they can treat me as badly as they wish; I will not let them get me down. As long as I remain healthy I will continue to work. That is the main thing. . . .

Sunday, 12 December 1937
. . . On returning home Wednesday evening, I found a letter from London. I thought it would contain a request from an English colleague for some academic work of mine, but when I opened it, it proved to be a propaganda sheet from the so-called German Freedom Party. I did not even read it, I was so furious at the impudence of these Jews and emigrants. The next day, Eva took it to deliver to the police in Stötteritz, but they were not interested in it, as it had come from abroad. They said we should burn it, which we did immediately. Since then it has occurred to me that our Führer spoke once about the activities of this German Freedom Party. With me, at any rate, they are barking up the wrong tree.

18 August 1938
Another "love letter" today from the district military command. Report on 26 August, after first obtaining endless papers, certificates, etc.! And what is it all for? In order to prepare us for a second war 20 years after the end of the first! Yes, in the past, pestilence and epidemics decimated human beings; in the future, wars, which will not spare women and children, will do the same. Thus, everything remains the same; only the methods of mass extermination change. I am not at all an opponent of war. There must be wars, otherwise nations would degenerate. In addition to its terrible and horrible sides, which is all most people see, war also has much that is beneficial. Whether the two balance each other out, I do not

* This refers to Heinrich von Hayek (1900–1969). Since this anatomist held an associate professorship at the University of Würzburg from 1938 until 1952, he could only have been a "little Jew" in the racist fantasies, nurtured by competitive jealousy, of his colleague Voss.
† Curt Elze (1885–1972), professor of anatomy in Würzburg.

know. That is not the essential point. However, the fact that women and children are also killed is not one of the beneficial effects of war. This is completely un- and anti-natural. For even among animals, only the men fight. How is it possible that nations cannot agree that women and children should not be murdered? It is, after all, in everyone's interest.

In the coming weeks, the anatomists' assembly will be meeting here. If only it were already over! Unfortunately I must participate in this charade; otherwise, wild horses could not drag me there. It is too narrow-minded a company. And what a step backward compared with the past, especially in regard to persons and character! . . .

Sunday, 28 August 1938

We did it! The anatomists' assembly is over. Quite a hustle and bustle, especially for Eva, who had to participate in some of the tours for the ladies in the morning and afternoon. . . . On Friday morning, more lectures; in the afternoon, business meetings and elections to the board. In the morning, Clara gave me the election slogans. These came about as planned. Thus there are now two National Socialists on the board of the society. In addition to C. [Clara], Pernkopf* from Vienna. After the close of the business meeting I rode out to our house with Fahrenholz and Körner.† They looked over the house and had a cup of coffee with us, and then I had to change immediately for the banquet that took place at eight o'clock in the "Harmony." Sunday morning saw very pleasant presentations by "the younger generation," and finally, around one o'clock, farewells all around. Next year the assembly is to be held in Budapest. Assemblies of professional colleagues are a funny thing. They have little purpose for people like us; they are more for the young people and the professors.

---

* Max Clara (1899–1966) was, beginning in 1934, a professor and Voss's superior in Leipzig. One of the leading Nazis in the German Anatomical Society, he withdrew after the war to the University of Istanbul. He died in Munich.

  Eduard Pernkopf (1888–1955), anatomist in Vienna. Before Clara's appointment, he was the only National Socialist anatomist to hold a chair. After early anti-Marxist activity, fighting the Soviet movement at the University of Vienna, he was at the center of the dispute in the twenties between the German Nationalist–National Socialist students supporting his chair and the socialist, democratic, Jewish, and foreign students who supported Professor Tandler's competing chair; thus in 1938, he rose almost automatically to become the leading Nazi on the Vienna medical faculty. Until now, however, he has been acknowledged only as a brilliant representative of topographical and comparative anatomy.

† Curt Fahrenholz (1890–1946), anatomist in Leipzig and Berlin; Fritz Körner (1905–50), professor of anatomy in Jena. Voss succeeded Körner in 1952.

For them, it is like a market: some want to sell (the young people), others want to buy (the professors); that is, they want to meet young people in case they should need one of them as an assistant. . . .

Wednesday, 15 March 1939

Today is once again a great day in the history of the German people. This morning at nine o'clock German troops marched into Prague! It is still difficult to believe. It is hard to grasp that the old German states of Bohemia and Moravia will once again come under German rule. The oldest German university in Prague, the mother of Leipzig University, once again in the possession of the German Reich! It is inconceivable. What a blow to Slavdom, and what a plus for us. We are really living in great times and should be happy to be able to experience these things. What difference does it make if there isn't always as much butter as one would like, if sometimes there is no coffee, if one must do one or another thing that one does not really like, etc. These are ridiculous nothings compared with the progress of our people. . . .

Monday, 27 May 1940

. . . Here in Saxony, there are many who lament the fact that it appears we will defeat England, and not she us. For if the latter were the case, the National Socialism they so despise would disappear, and that is more important to them than anything else. Such pitiful blindness can probably be found to this degree only among these great people. And this is where I must live! We rejoice at every report of victory. Unfortunately, memories of 1914–1918 constantly mix a drop of wormwood with this cup of joy. Now, too, one can say: all's well that ends well. . . .

Friday, 17 January 1941

This afternoon I was summoned by the rector. He presented me with the silver medal of service. Actually I do not celebrate my 25th anniversary at work until 1944, but according to the regulations a two- to three-year training period is added on.

Saturday, 25 January 1941

Yesterday, Bargmann* was released by the military; he will take over his lectures in the coming weeks. Thus I have less work, but also less

---

* Wolfgang Bargmann (born 1906) was, like Voss, assistant anatomist in Leipzig. In 1942 he became professor of anatomy in Königsberg, and in 1946 a professor in Kiel; he later served as vice-president of the German Research Society and head of the Anatomical Society.

money. Yesterday Clara was in Munich at the Lecturers' Union. He told me there was a question from the Ministry about me concerning Posen. They took this opportunity to present him with a recommendation concerning me that he himself had made, of which the people in Munich of course knew nothing. I am now very curious as to how this will develop. *Rebus sic stantibus,* as the lawyers say, this would be the only chance for me to become a professor. All other opportunities have been blocked for me by Elze and consorts. I must swallow the bitter pill.

5 February 1941

Last year I earned 17,000 marks in salary, lecture, and testing fees. But this means paying extraordinary taxes this year. And the unpleasant part is that the income will now sink considerably, for the number of students has dwindled.

8 February 1941

This morning I found a letter in the mailbox containing the following: "Dear Herr Professor! The University of Posen is to be opened at the beginning of the summer semester. The Medical Department will be able to offer only preclinical studies at first. I intend to recommend you to the Reich Minister for the anatomy chair to be created there, and request that you indicate whether you would be willing to accept an appointment to the University of Posen. Heil Hitler! Scheer." Whether I want to or not, I must accept this appointment, which must be viewed with mixed feelings. We have to wait and see what fate will make of it, good or bad. I am not happy, but neither am I complaining. I am, as Wilhelm Raabe says, patient in everything. Incidentally, yesterday I bought W. Raabe's letters, which I am reading with great enjoyment. . . .

19 February 1941

. . . Another letter arrived from Berlin this morning in which I am requested to report on 26 February, that is, in eight days, in Posen to the administrative director of the university to view the institute. On the way I am to appear before Assistant Secretary Scheer in Berlin. This week I will not come to the institute very often, and during the coming weeks I will be traveling. Dr. Bargmann will take over my lectures. I see already how my ties to the institute are loosening. For over five years I have been little more than a stranger there anyway. Aside from a few employees, such as Schäffner, Knoch, and Herschel, the departure will not be hard for me. I hope to be able to leave by 1 April. If it has to be, then let it be as soon as possible.

Saturday, 1 March 1941

Yesterday I returned from Posen. On Monday the 24th I left at eight o'clock in the morning, traveling from here through Halle to Berlin. At noon I was in the Ministry, meeting with Assistant Secretary Scheer. I learned nothing new there. Ate lunch at Friedrichstrasse Station, then went to visit Herbert Bauer in Charlottenburg, where I spent a pleasant afternoon and evening. In the afternoon we took a short walk and viewed a house that had been hit by an aerial bomb. I left for Posen the next morning at eight from Charlottenburg Station, in terrible weather and an awful mood. I got a good seat, in first class, and the journey proceeded as planned, which is saying a lot these days. At a quarter to one the train arrived in Posen. During the last part of the journey we had clear weather and pleasant sunshine, which held the entire afternoon in Posen. Upon my arrival I went immediately to the administrative director, who of course had no time for me, so that I had to waste the entire afternoon. I found quarters in the Posener Hof, but had to share them with another colleague who arrived at eleven in the evening with a terrible cold or flu, broke down the next afternoon, and went to stay with his parents, Baltic Germans from Riga, so that I was alone the second night. In the hotel, incidentally, the food was excellent and available without ration coupons! There I met a Herr Olschewski, a potash chemical representative, who in the evening took me to a restaurant with the most wonderful and varied fish dishes. It made a great impression on me to see a fully lighted city once again, at least on the streets. The buildings were apparently darkened. There are still over 200,000 Poles in the city who are absolutely necessary as workers. However, they are only allowed on the streets until eight in the evening.

On Wednesday the 26th we assembled at the administrative director's; he made some general remarks, and then the tour began. The medical institutes are located in a large building containing the most modern equipment. The anatomical institute is the largest. It includes 35 rooms with over 2,000 square meters of space. It is really very respectable, and a great deal could be done with it in the future.* It is a good thing some

---

* The University of Poznań was established in 1919; the building housing the Institute of Anatomy and Forensic Medicine was completed in 1929 and still serves this purpose today. In 1939, the Germans expelled the Polish professors and killed some of them, in connection with the planned systematic extermination of the Polish intelligentsia. When the Reich University was founded in 1941, the Germans denied the previous existence of a Polish university and spoke of a newly founded institution. A few days after liberation in January 1945, the Polish university opened again. It was

personnel are already there, including a head dissector, von Hirschheydt, who used to be in Riga,* an old man who nevertheless makes a very good impression. Around three we finished viewing the various institutes. I then joined my physiological colleague, Dr. Eichler of Freiburg. We ate lunch together and then went to the university secretariat, where we spent at least an hour filling out various questionnaires in order to have our travel costs reimbursed. Then we went to the station to ask about trains, had dinner, and drew up plans.

The next morning at eight, another meeting with the administrative director, at which we gave our impressions of the institute. At nine I took my leave and was driven to the station in the director's car—his name, incidentally, is Dr. Streit.† My train was supposed to leave at 9:30; it was somewhat delayed, but thank God only a little, and left at ten o'clock. Contrary to my expectations, I got a very good seat, and the journey was smooth and uneventful. Around two we had already arrived at the Schlesisch Station in Berlin. I rushed to the Ministry again, where I was to make a report, had to wait a long time for the Assistant Secretary, and then learned nothing more than that final professional negotiations were to begin soon. I then went again to my friend Herbert's, where we spent a very nice evening with a half bottle of cognac and numerous childhood reminiscences.

Yesterday in the early afternoon I got back to Leipzig. Here everything is sick again, already, or as always, depending how one looks at it. Apparently these train rides with all the sitting do not agree with me. The

---

named after the Polish poet Adam Mickiewicz. In 1950, the medical faculty was separated from the university and became the Medical Academy of Poznań.

* Germans from Riga were resettled under the German-Soviet treaty of 1939. They formed almost a third of the academic personnel of the Reich University of Posen.

† About the administrative director, Goguel says (p. 95): "At the beginning of October 1939, the Ministry of Science had already sent SS Major Dr. Hanns Streit to Poznań, where he was to take the first steps towards creating a German university. Streit, who had been active for years in the leadership of the National Socialist Student Union and the National Socialist Lecturers' Association, had the right background for the task: Known as a fanatic fascist, tough and relentless in the pursuit of his goals, he additionally had the best of connections to almost all institutions involved. . . . In Streit's view, the 'popular struggle' and racism were to characterize the face of teaching. Thus he planned to introduce a series of 'new-style' chairs: racial politics, peoples' studies, including border and foreign Germanness, history and language of Judaism, agricultural and settlement history, farming and economic history, and finally [in place of theology, which was not included], history of the spirit and faith, a chair for which he had 'especially high hopes.'"

veins in my right leg seem to be acting up again. Perhaps a small embolism will relieve me of all my troubles and my horror of Posen! *Mors unica spes!* It is impossible to find housing in Posen. This will mean living there for a long time without the family. An awful thought. However, there is enough room at the institute; one could find very good living quarters in the histological wing on the third floor, facing the south, east, and west. The University of Posen is to be inaugurated on 20 April, the newspaper says today. As the director told us, it is being started for "political" reasons. At first, there will probably be no students at all. Where would they come from during the war? . . .

Tuesday, 11 March 1941

On Saturday I sent the letter containing my "wishes" to the Ministry. I am very curious how they will react to my personal wishes. I expressed four requests: (1) that housing be provided at the institute, should I so desire; (2) a separation bonus for as long as I have to live separated from my family in Posen; (3) complete transfer of my pay seniority to the new salary group that I will belong to as professor; (4) guaranteed lecture fees of 4,000 marks.

. . . In addition, I received a letter from the Reich Minister today: "I request that you temporarily occupy the chair in anatomy at the medical faculty of the University of Posen starting 1 April 1941." I will receive a salary of 9,300 marks; that is, 300 marks more than at present! On the journey to take over my duties I am to present myself at the Ministry in order to close the negotiations. Now I very much hope that I will at least be able to be here for the Easter holidays. Not a trace of joy at the chair. I accept it, like all other strokes of fate. Everyone tries to convince me of Posen's brilliant future. But what good does this future do me? Who is to guarantee that it will really come, and second, that I will live to see it! . . .

Thursday, 27 March 1941

Today I received the first letter addressed to Head of the Anatomical Institute of the University of Posen, and this evening the first inquiry about a position as assistant. Around eight o'clock, a young colleague from Jena called; he is interested in such a position and might be willing to come to Posen with me.* Unfortunately, I could give him no exact information, as I have not yet been informed officially as to the assistant positions at my institute. We agreed that he would come by during the Easter vacation so

* Apparently, this young man was his future colleague Robert Herrlinger.

we could discuss it all in person. I owe this inquiry to Körner. A few days ago I wrote him about the thing in Posen. I received in return a very excited letter of congratulations that did me a great deal of good.

Wednesday, 2 April 1941

I was in Berlin yesterday for the "close of professional negotiations," as it is so beautifully called. For where were the negotiations? Everything was simply dictated! They only guaranteed me 2,000 marks lecture fees, although they did improve my basic salary (9,900 instead of 9,300 marks!). A Herr Berger revealed these things to me. I only saw Prof. de Crinis* very briefly. I answered his question whether I was satisfied with a "no." On Monday I met with Professors Thomas and Gildemeister,† the two physiologists. Both were very pleasant and gave me a number of useful hints. Above all, they told me that I do not need to be in Posen by 1 April. It is enough if I am there for the inauguration of the university on the 20th. That of course pleased me very much, and as no one in the Ministry yesterday expected me to travel straight to Posen, I will stay here until Easter. Today I packed my last things at the institute. The two "men" can hardly wait to move into their new room. Yesterday I kept remembering the day I came to Dresden for the first time to negotiate my appointment. It was 1 November 1938. It was a beautiful day, and I had often dreamed of how nice it would be to travel to negotiate a chair. But how different it was yesterday! The one pleasant thing yesterday was that I could come back home! It is still winter. The new snow that fell especially heavily here a few days ago has not yet disappeared completely. Plus a gray sky and northeasterly wind. Miserable weather!

Thursday, 3 April 1941

And today the first beautiful spring day! This morning everything was all white again, but by nine o'clock the sun had come out, the snow melted in no time, and we had the most beautiful spring weather. This

---

* Professor Max de Crinis (born 1898) occupied a chair in psychiatry and neurology at the Berlin Charité Hospital. As a personal friend of Heydrich's and member of the SD, he was heavily involved in consulting on euthanasia. As head of the Office of Science of the Reich Ministry of Education, he was in charge of filling all German chairs in medicine. During the final months of the war he was, in addition, chief psychiatric adviser to the Wehrmacht. On 2 May 1945, he and his wife committed suicide.

† Martin Gildemeister (1876–1943) and Karl Thomas (1883–1969) were professors of physiology in Leipzig.

afternoon I worked hard in the garden. It was wonderful. Today I wrote to the administrative director of the University of Posen that I intend to arrive on the 17th, and inquired whether he has accommodations for me there. I am very curious what his answer will be. In addition, I wrote today to Insel Publishers about "Nala and Damajanti." If the work is accepted and published by this publishing house, it would make me ten times happier than the chair in Posen.

Easter Sunday, 13 April 1941

Yesterday I finally received word from Posen, not from the director, but from the head dissector at the institute, von Hirschheydt, to whom I had written on Monday. The inaugural ceremonies for the Reich University of Posen have been postponed to the 27th of April. From the 26th to the 28th of April I will have private quarters; afterwards they could set up a room at the institute for me to live in until I find another apartment. I am agreeable to that. He also wrote that there were people there who wanted to study medicine in the summer semester. These must be first-semesters, since, as I further learned from the letter, the physiological institute will not open for another year. There was good news today for Easter: Belgrade has been conquered, as well as Bardia in North Africa.

Sunday, 20 April 1941

In the meantime I have received an offical invitation to the inaugural ceremonies for the Reich University of Posen. We will have to endure a vast number of speeches. A uniform or tails are required attire. I will therefore have to take the latter along. We just had a "dress rehearsal," since I will have to buy various accessories. I hope I will not be the only one in this "attire" and will have other "comrades in suffering." We will be in the minority in any case.*

Monday, 21 April 1941

Everything in Posen seems to be topsy turvy. Yesterday evening I received an express letter which claimed that I had promised the director

---

* There is a richly illustrated volume on the founding of the Reich University of Posen which contains the speeches held at the inauguration: *Die Gründung der Reichsuniversität Posen: Am Geburtstag des Führers 1941* (Posen, 1942). On page 80 it states: "It is of deep symbolic significance that, on the instructions of the *Gauleiter,* a medal commemorating the founding of this first National Socialist Reich University has been struck out of the official chains of the former Polish rector and the deans. It is to be awarded to 200 men and women who have contributed the most to the creation of the Reich University."

that I would lecture in the coming weeks in a lecture series for the Germans in Posen on the occasion of the inaugural ceremonies for the university. I am asked to indicate the theme and content. At first I wanted to refuse completely, because I had not been informed of such a lecture; but then I thought it over and agreed after all, when the colleague who is heading the whole event called this morning from Posen. This afternoon I received a telegram from the director: "Presence required immediately. Accommodations available." So I will leave the day after tomorrow, assuming I get my permit from the police tomorrow, which is not at all certain. Well, then the gentlemen in Posen will have to wait another day. I wrote to the director twice, asking about accommodations and stating in the letter that I intended to arrive in Posen on the 17th of this month. I received no reply. And then today this telegram! Apparently they have lost their heads. Well, that's their problem. I will not let it upset me.

Posen, 25 April 1941

Evening, eight o'clock. As I write this I am sitting in the director's office of my institute. We set up this room and the library next to it yesterday and today. Now I would like to describe the most important events of the past three days. On Wednesday afternoon at one o'clock I left Leipzig. The trip was very complicated and difficult, because the express trains were all overcrowded. However, I was fortunate enough to get a seat, after standing for a short time, both before and after Berlin. I arrived at ten o'clock in the evening. In the morning I had sent Herr von Hirschheydt a telegram asking him to pick me up at the train station. At first I could not find him. I had quite a fright, as I did not know where I should stay for the night. It was really a relief when he appeared. He had been on the platform, but of course we missed each other in the crowd. We drove in one of those typical one-horse hackneys to the institute, where I am to live for the present. We then went out for a glass of beer, and I went to bed around midnight; but I could not fall asleep for some time, as the female students from Berlin who were serving here during their vacation lived on the same corridor and were making quite a bit of noise celebrating their farewell party. My "bedroom" is quite nicely furnished, the bed somewhat too short and hard, but otherwise very clean and neat.

Yesterday morning I reported to the director and was told to come again in the afternoon. He could not actually think of any reason for having had me come two days earlier. He also told me that in about 14 days the professors' house would be finished and I could then live there. Well, it will probably be two months rather than two weeks before that happens. The door to my room did not shut, and only Poles live in the institute. Then there were my overtaxed nerves. In short, before going to bed in the evening I pushed the wardrobe against the door. It was, by the way, reassuring to me that there is a guard standing right across from my window, in front of the building housing the *Gau* Air Command II. Incidentally, at the university yesterday I got the addresses of some rooms. Yesterday I only looked at the building in which one was located, but that was enough. This morning I saw another one that had been especially praised. It was impossible! I will probably have to give up the search and remain at the institute. Yesterday I went to the university bursar's and was informed that I will receive eight marks a day as a separation bonus. I can live on that here, so I will not have to use any of my actual salary. I quite like the city of Posen; one would only have to get rid of the Poles for it to be very pleasant here. Provisions are much better here than in Germany proper. You can get bread and rolls without ration coupons. Today I ate cutlets twice, in the afternoon and evening, without coupons! A fabulous state of affairs! But I hear that this is to end soon. Yesterday there was a stew: beans and sausage, very cheap, hearty, and tasty. Tuesdays and Saturdays, there are only meatless meals. I am very curious to see how many medical students will show up. At the university I heard from fairly reliable sources that around 20 are already registered.

Sunday, 27 April 1941
This morning was the inauguration of the Reich University of Posen. Many more or less good speeches were made. At any rate, medicine is the stepchild of the university. This afternoon there will be a banquet, to which I, as a so-called professor at this wonderful university, have not received an invitation! That is simply ridiculous! In fact, my "reception" in general by this pseudo-university is just wonderful. One is treated like a shoeshine boy. But I have definitely decided that I will take every opportunity that offers itself to speak frankly.

Tuesday, 29 April 1941
Yesterday evening I gave my lecture in the auditorium of the physiological institute. It was almost completely full, some 150 people. After the lecture I showed them the larger auditorium and the collection, or at least the half of it that had to be darkened quickly in the afternoon. Two former students of mine from Leipzig also attended the lecture; one of them had already visited me that afternoon. Airplanes flew over the city toward the east yesterday evening without letup. Probably it will start here

soon, too. So with the airplanes we have gone from the frying pan into the fire. Well, it is all pretty bad here. The only good thing is the provisions. One can eat meat meals in restaurants several times a week without coupons. Unfortunately, that will also end soon. If only I had another place to sleep! Last night was once again awful. This afternoon at six o'clock there is a meeting at the university, at which I hope to learn something about my institute's budget and personnel. At the institute, one room after another is gradually being put to rights.

Thursday, 1 May 1941

Today is a holiday. They are always terrible days when one is all alone in a city. But it is all right, since on Tuesday I got to know a colleague in mineralogy, Professor Köhler* of Vienna, with whom I can at least eat. Of course, on Tuesday I got to hear only nice, general talk, but nothing definite about my institute. Yesterday afternoon an intern was here who is interested in a position as assistant. Unfortunately he is also a zoologist, but cannot find a position at the moment. He made a very good impression, and I would be happy to get him. Regrettably I could tell him nothing definite, since I still do not know how many positions I will have. Yesterday the proofs of the first course catalogue of the Reich University of Posen arrived. There I discovered that I am now four-fold temporary director—that is, temporary director of all the institutes that are to be housed in this building but do not yet have directors.

Sunday, 4 May 1941

An awful day is almost over. Today my colleague returned home, and once again I am all alone at meals. If the weather were only different, warmer! Then it would not be so bad, for I am not afraid of being alone in itself. But you cannot do anything, work or read, for if you sit for an hour you freeze. Yesterday morning everything outside was white. For the last two days, almost uninterrupted driving snow. It all fits: time, place, and weather! Each as miserable as the next!

On Friday there was a meeting of the "faculty advisers," as they are so nicely termed, since the dean has not yet been appointed, with the rector and administrative director. We were informed at the same time that 23 people have registered so far in the Medical Department. Considering

* Alexander Köhler (1893–1955), mineralogist and petrographer, first in Vienna; 1942–45, professor at the Reich University of Posen; after 1950, mineralogist at the Vienna Technical College.

that this is only the first semester, this is quite a lot. I am convinced that many of the universities in Germany proper will have fewer beginners. I want to start my lecture on Tuesday, but I am afraid no one will come on that day, for the simple reason that the students have no idea when it starts. I did put up a poster in the main building, but when do students come there to read it? Well, perhaps some will find their way over after all, and that is enough for a start; the others will come later. Incidentally, I am supposed to get a chief assistant and a regular assistant, as well as a technical assistant, but I do not yet have it in writing. I am now reading Oswald, *The World of Neglected Dimensions*. I could already write a book entitled "The World of Neglected Professors." I have heard that a lovely dormitory has been completed for the students, but not for the professors. Nowadays they only come second. This afternoon I rummaged around in the library. One works and works to get the institute in shape, and perhaps it is all in vain. How long before a Russian bomb explodes here and destroys all our work? Well, at any rate, it would destroy us as well—that is a comfort.

Tuesday, 6 May 1941

This morning at ten o'clock I held my first lecture here. Seven students were present (three men and four women). Today I did not lecture for the entire hour; instead, after a short mention of the significance of this hour for me and for them, the students, I showed them the institute. Today, after nearly 14 days, there was finally sunshine again—alternating, however, with rain showers. Starting this week, ration coupons have been introduced at the restaurants here; in the past you could get everything, even meat meals, without coupons. I eat in the afternoon and evening at the zoo restaurants, which are very close by.

Thursday, 8 May 1941

This morning I had two hours of lectures, from ten to eleven System[atic] Anat[omy] I and from eleven to twelve General Histology. Tomorrow is the same. The number of students has increased somewhat, but is not nearly as large as the number of medical students registered at the university is supposed to be. Yesterday afternoon I received a visit from two colleagues from local hospitals. One of them, Dr. von Drigalski,* is chief physician in the Department of Internal Medicine; the other, Dr. Wi-

---

* Wolfgang von Drigalski.

denbauer,* is chief physician at the Children's Hospital. Both are lecturers, but not at the local university. I made an appointment to meet them next Wednesday evening at the Ratskeller.

Today at the university I learned that I will now receive a monthly salary of around 800 marks, after deducting all taxes, etc. In addition, I will receive another eight marks a day for running separate households. This is quite a bit more than in Leipzig. However, supplementary income through lecture and testing fees is pretty much eliminated.

Friday, 9 May 1941

Last night was again lively. Around 2:30—there was bright moonshine and I had just woken up—I suddenly heard an airplane thundering extraordinarily loudly. I thought, he's really flying low; naturally, I thought it was a German airplane that has often flown over the city recently. Then suddenly a mighty crash and a tinkling. I thought, the plane flew too low and crashed into something. At first I didn't even want to get out of bed, but then I saw out my window, in a northwesterly direction, the familiar yellowish spots lighting up the sky. I got up then, dressed myself quite calmly, and went downstairs. When I went out in the hall I saw the mess—shards of glass everywhere. I spent some time in the cellar with the gym teachers, who live here in the building, but all remained calm. Around 3:30 I climbed back into bed. But I didn't get much more sleep, since German flyers were still buzzing around. Not until this morning could one really see the extent of the damage. On the south side of the building almost all the windows are broken. In my "director's office," too, two windows on the south side are completely gone. Only on the west and north sides were almost no windows damaged. I was very lucky. First of all, of course, that the bomb did not hit the institute—approximately 150 meters south of the institute building, one or two houses on Herder Strasse were badly damaged and several people killed or wounded—and second of all that my windowpanes did not burst. For if they had, I would have had all the shards and splinters on my head, my bed was so close to the window. This morning, I could not read in the small auditorium because of the cold, but had to improvise an auditorium in one of the northern rooms with intact windowpanes. They were in fact English planes, with Polish pilots, of course. They say one was shot down. Thus, that which I

---

* Franz Widenbauer was director of the city and *Gau* children's clinics in Posen. He died in 1943.

never thought possible has happened once again: English planes fly from England to Posen and drop bombs on it, quite heavily in fact. The windowpanes in almost all the houses within a wide radius are broken. Thus, Posen's best characteristic, the absence of air raid warnings, is gone. And if there were another alarm here! But not a trace of sirens, no flak, nothing. The planes come out of nowhere. You hear them, and the bombs are already crashing down. A wonderful situation. At first I thought it was an attack by the Russians. If they also get started in the course of the summer, it could really get lively here. And after everything we're seeing here, there can no longer be any doubt that there will be war with Russia. The only question is when it will start. I hope the bad spring has delayed preparations somewhat.

Monday, 12 May 1941

Today there were 20 students at my lecture. That was a lot more than I had expected. I am very glad I can give lectures. Working with students is refreshing and encouraging; it always stimulates me, and under the present circumstances it is a particular comfort and encouragement to me.

Wednesday, 14 May 1941

Last night there was quite a fire in a factory on Glogauer Strasse, which I could observe quite well from the institute once I got up. Today I am lecturing in the small auditorium again, since the windows were repaired yesterday. It will probably take a long time in the other building. Across the street, the *Gau* air command is fortifying itself heavily against air raids. They are building walls uninterruptedly at night, under electric lighting, naturally using Polish labor. The day after tomorrow my Viennese colleague will be here again; then at least I will have some company at meals.

Sunday, 18 May 1941

My colleague Köhler arrived again on Friday and has a room at my institute. I now have some company on Sundays, which is very pleasant. The lonely Sundays I have experienced here have been awful. Yesterday afternoon we went out to Kuhndorf. There are very nice one-family houses there, and we decided we would like to live there. This morning we actually wanted to go out to Unterberg, but the train we had chosen from the schedule was canceled. So we went on an excursion, by streetcar and on foot, to Eichwald, a typical low-lying wood on the Warthe River. We met nothing but Poles from the suburbs there; thus, we saw how much of this miserable pack is still around. When you spend your time in the center of the city, you do not notice it as much. Today is the first pleasant spring day, warm and sunny.

Sunday evening, 24 May 1941

Today I want to travel to Leipzig, but I do not know what will come of it. Train traffic has been so much reduced that one hardly has any chance of getting on the two express trains that still go to Berlin. I want to try today, and maybe also tomorrow morning. This uncertainty spoils one's anticipation of the journey home. If it were up to me, I would not go at all at the moment. Arriving home is quite pleasant, but leaving again is all the more difficult, with the current situation what it is. But I must do all I can to get home, for Eva's sake. In Systematic Anatomy, 24 students are now registered. If we only knew what was going to happen here in the East. A huge deployment is in progress. Posen is practically one big military base; it is teeming with soldiers. Here in the basement of the institute building, there is a crematorium for bodies. It now serves the Gestapo exclusively. The Poles they shoot are brought here at night and cremated. If one could only incinerate the whole Polish pack! The Polish people must be exterminated, or there will be no peace here in the East. It is terrible that we are still dependent on Polish labor here at the institute.

Sunday, 25 May 1941

I arrived yesterday evening around ten o'clock [in Leipzig]. It is a miracle that I could board the train in Posen, it was so terribly overcrowded. The trip to Berlin was bad. I spent part of it standing, part sitting in the lavatory of a second-class car. Every seat in the car was filled with people and pieces of luggage. The train was delayed for an hour. At three o'clock I arrived in Berlin, and at 6:30 the trip continued. An hour and a half before the train left, I went to the platform where it was standing and got a seat. Except for an axle fire in Delitzsch, because of which the car involved was switched off, this trip went smoothly. It is magnificent here. The garden is wonderfully kept. Everything is growing and blossoming beautifully.

Whit Monday, 2 June 1941

Wonderful Pentecost weather, such as we have not had for years. Yesterday morning Eva and I went to the cemetery, as it was the anniversary of our son's death. He died two years ago. We are always happy to think that he did not have to live through these times. The Pentecost celebration was somewhat dampened by the fact that our housekeeper is leaving us. She is the second Bessarabian German we have had. Very good and capable. She and her parents are leaving on Wednesday for the Wartheland, where they will be taking over a Polish farm. I had already heard that many Poles had recently been evacuated from the countryside. The Poles are becoming quite impudent. They have started many fires, especially in mills, but I don't believe it does them any good. Their people is being decimated more and more because of such things. I think one should look at this Polish question without emotion, purely biologically. We must exterminate them, otherwise they will exterminate us. And that is why I am glad of every Pole who is no longer alive.

Friday, 6 June 1941

I arrived here at 11:30 in the evening the day before yesterday. Woke up at five in the morning, departed from Leipzig at seven; took turns with a lady sitting on my suitcase. Arrived at Anhalter Station in Berlin at 9:30. Then went to Friedrichstrasse Station, checked the suitcase, visited Herbert Bauer in Charlottenburg, and stayed until six o'clock. At 6:20, left for here. Only seat in the bathroom, like the first time, except that this time two other men and a woman shared this narrow space. But otherwise the trip was quite pleasant. A wonderful picture: the sun setting in a red ball of fire over the city of Frankfurt on the Oder. The ride through pine forests that stood out against the evening sky like silhouettes also offered lovely images. So during the trip, once again, I sat on the toilet seat and read from one of Seneca's works, entitled *On a Blissful Life!* I had to laugh to myself at the title of the book and the situation I found myself in. I arrived at the institute shortly before midnight. And then came another lovely surprise. I rang and rang and knocked at the door, but nothing stirred, no one opened the door. There I stood, all alone in the moonlight, wondering where I was going to spend the night. But one has to have a little luck and be able to take care of oneself. I had seen a light in the heating building right next door, where I knew Prof. Geisler,* the geog-

---

* Walter Geisler (1891–1945), professor of geography, was deeply involved in anthropological and physical-geographic problems in the border zones. He was especially interested in geographic research in the East. After working at the Herder Institute in Riga (1935–36), he was appointed to the Technical University of Aachen (1936–41), where he worked on economic and border problems in the West. He could devote himself to his actual area of interest, research on the East, as prorector of the Reich University of Posen (1941–45). In addition, he was head of the transregional

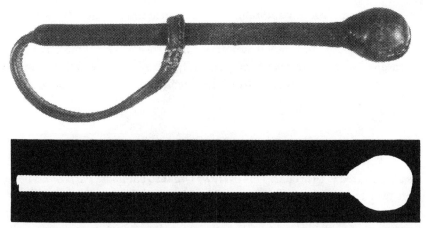

Hermann Voss walked through occupied Posen armed with both a pistol and a club. The x-ray picture reveals the truncheon's iron core.

rapher, lived. I rang the bell, and he soon opened the door. My colleague was still awake, and received me with great hospitality. I was able to lie down on the couch in his work room, and slept very well from one to seven o'clock. Yesterday, Herr v. H. [von Hirschheydt] told me that during the night, a man with serious knife wounds was found near the institute building. Yes, it has already become quite wild here in the East. It is not advisable to walk alone in the street unless you take a gun along. Therefore, I have brought my Mauser pistol from the world war with me. I hope it is still in working order. I will have to bring it to a weapons store and have it looked at. A flood of letters awaited me here at the institute. The red tape with the authorities is awful. So much paper is wasted unnecessarily, especially now, when paper is beginning to be very scarce.

Monday, 9 June 1941
Yesterday morning I accompanied my colleague Köhler on a very instructive geological excursion led by Prof. Thomson.* I learned a lot

---

working group on "Central Locations" of the Reich Association for Territorial Exploration (among other things, he was involved in the wartime research project "German East"), and worked on several research assignments on "central locations in the Eastern territories."

* Paul William Thomson (1891–1957), geologist, paleontologist, and phytopaleontologist. In 1928, he became lecturer in geology and paleontology at the University of Tartu (Dorpat, Estonia), and in 1932 guest lecturer in Königsberg, East Prussia. In 1939 he was visiting professor, and from 1941 to 1945 full professor and director of the Geological-Paleontological Institute of the Reich University of Posen. After about morains, etc.; in addition, I got a chance to really see the Warthe Valley for the first time. The landscape reminds me very much of my home in Mecklenburg, and thus is not at all alien to me. The climate is very pleasant. Generally dry warmth, but rarely the atrociously moist, humid air common in the Western part of the Reich, and also often experienced in Leipzig.

Sunday, 15 June 1941

Yesterday I viewed the cellar for corpses and the cremation oven that is also located in the cellar. This oven was built to eliminate parts of bodies left over from dissection exercises. Now it serves to incinerate executed Poles. The gray car with the gray men—that is, SS men from the Gestapo—comes almost daily with material for the oven. Because it was not in use yesterday, we could look into it. It contained the ashes of four Poles.* How little remains of a human being when everything organic has been burned! Somehow, looking into such an oven is very comforting. What did Marshal Ney say before he was executed? "Ou bientot un peu de poudre." The Poles are quite impudent at the moment, and thus our oven has a great deal to do. How nice it would be if we could drive the whole pack through such ovens! Then there would finally be peace in the East for the German people. Yesterday E. [Eva, his wife] wrote me; it looks as though Clara will be going to Munich. The two "men" at the institute there are thus under a great deal of pressure, since their positions are not secure. Well, it is good for them to know what it feels like for a change. In addition, I don't yet believe that C. is really leaving. Today I wrote to Prof. Schoen† in Göttingen and reminded him of my existence, in case they need an anatomist there. It won't do any good, but I want to take advantage of even the tiniest possibility of getting away from here.

1945 he worked at the State Geological Offices of Düsseldorf and Krefeld and at the University of Bonn.

* The cellar with the cremation oven at the anatomical institute was confiscated by the Gestapo in 1939; according to the testimony of Polish witnesses, the oven was often in use day and night and could hold four to six bodies, or, if they were quartered, up to ten bodies. The actual cremation process took some four hours. According to the records of the forensic and anatomical institutes, a total of 4,916 bodies of Poles and Jews murdered by the German police and judicial authorities were cremated between 1939 and 1945 in the cellar of the Reich University.

† Rudolf Schoen (1892–1979), professor of internal medicine in Göttingen.

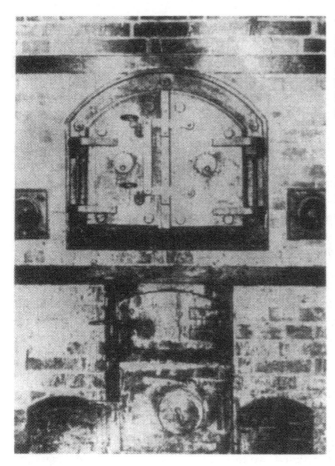

The oven at the Reich University's anatomical institute after being rebuilt in 1942.

Tuesday, 17 [June 1941]

Another announcement from the special court was posted that five Poles from Posen had been sentenced to death for murder and executed today. With all this work, our oven will probably go on the blink soon, since it is already a bit fragile; I sent a request yesterday that it be repaired, otherwise it will give up the ghost.* I do not understand why, given the

---

* The oven did in fact break down in the autumn of 1942. A description of the new oven can be found in the protocols of a viewing by the High Commission to Investigate Nazi Crimes in November 1945. This oven was erected in 1942 in place of the old one, which had burnt out. It was located in the basement of the building, and took up some 6 square meters of space. The dimensions of the oven were: length, 2.74 meters; width, 1.70 meters; height, 2 meters. Inside the oven were a cremation

present increase in attacks by Poles against German life and property, no stricter measures are taken. Why aren't a hundred Poles, or even more as far as I am concerned, killed for each murdered German? Today I received a letter from Herr Walther. He has left Holland and is now in Bromberg— that is, not very far from here. He wants to try to come here, but probably will not succeed. In this letter he is not as optimistic as in the past. Other people are also gradually beginning to realize that all sorts of things may lie ahead. The summer is passing, and it has not yet brought anything decisive. So far, we have been consistently victorious, just as we were in 1914–1918. And isn't America coming to England's aid, as it did before? So everything is the same, yet they expect it to end differently. I can't believe that, but I will be very glad if my expectations prove to be mistaken.

Thursday, 19 June 1941

Yesterday, two wagons full of Polish ashes were taken away. Outside my office, the robinias are blooming beautifully, just as in Leipzig. What I wouldn't give to be there still! In the last few days, a few more students have registered, so the number has grown to 31. The day after tomorrow, another week will be over. It is sad that one rejoices now over every day that passes. But that's just how we are.

Friday, 20 June 1941

Today I received an answer from my colleague Schoen in Göttingen. As always, I was too late. If I had inquired in time, I might have had a chance of being placed on the list. He writes: "Because you just received an appointment in Posen, we thought there was no point in suggesting your name." So this Posen is cutting off my other chances of appointment! That's all I need.

Sunday, 22 June 1941

Yesterday morning, in our coffee shop, we listened to the declaration of war on Russia. Everything is very calm here. No one seems worried,

---

chamber made of firebricks, and an iron grill through which the ashes of the burnt corpses fell into the ash holders. The inside of the cremation chamber was 2.30 meters long, .64 meters wide and .80 meters in height. Seven corpses could be cremated at the same time. To the left of the oven was a room with an area of 9 square meters and an iron door. It was used to store the ashes of the cremated bodies (GKBZH, i.e., High Commission to Investigate Nazi Crimes, *Ermittlungsakten des Greiser-Prozesses,* vol. 6, p. 6, cited in Olszewski, p. 205—see n. 5 for bibliographical details).

even though Posen is located within the range of Russian planes. I am curious what the coming days will bring; I am just glad I am not alone now, and that I have my colleague K. to discuss it with. Poor Eva, what anxiety she must be enduring! It is too bad one cannot listen to the radio now, except in the restaurant. Strangely enough, this time they did not announce when the fighting actually began. When will Russian planes appear over Posen? That is the main question now.

Thursday, 26 June 1941

So far, the nights have been quiet. Let us hope they remain so! The weather remains pleasant, but rather hot. But because it is dry heat, it does not cause one to suffer too much. On Monday, a bust of Bismarck was unveiled; it had been presented to the Reich University of Posen by the Technical College of Berlin. The rector of the T.C. presented it with a speech, and then the director Dr. Streit and his "young man," our rector, spoke.* I am surprised that this man, an SS man, doesn't mind playing such a miserable role. I would say "no, thank you" to constantly playing second fiddle to Herr Director.

Sunday, 29 June 1941

Today the first reports arrived on the battles in the East. We will defeat Russia, but what then? Here in Posen we have not yet received any visits from planes, and the most dangerous nights are now probably behind us. Whether that will remain so for long depends on developments in Russia. Frau Köhler came the day before yesterday. Very nice. I spend a lot of time with them, so I am no more lonely than usual. We also spend the evenings quite comfortably together—yesterday, for example, with a bottle of red wine, until around midnight. It is still not certain whether Eva will come in July. Her friend, our good Thiessing from Rostock, is there, but she is always on the go.

Yesterday evening, the Lecturers' Union met from 8 to 11. Rarely have I heard such nonsense. Yesterday afternoon I had a visit from a stu-

---

* The rector of the new university was 38-year-old Dr. Peter Johannes Carstens, a professor who, next to the administrative director Streit, was the reigning figure at the Reich University. A member of the Nazi party and the SA since 1930, he rose in the SS ranks after 1933 to become a colonel. In 1940 he was drafted into the *Waffen-SS, Leibstandarte* Adolf Hitler. His contemporaries described him as a brutal "master race" type. Carstens was a stockbreeding geneticist. He was elected rector of the university because agriculture was particularly important to the occupation and to the Reich University, due to the extensive resettlement programs (Goguel, p. 102f.).

dent who is a pastor and wants to study medicine; I spoke to him for some time. He invited me to come to the country with him on Saturday and Sunday to eat strawberries. He lives in Schlehen, a small village 20 kilometers from Posen that one can get to twice a day by bus. I was happy to accept the invitation, for I have often wanted to go out to the countryside here. Yesterday evening, the director announced an excursion to Gnesen on 26 July in which every lecturer must participate. The excursion will certainly be very interesting, but the date is bad; it is the day I wanted to leave, since the 27th is Eva's birthday.

Thursday, 3 July 1941

Today I received a card from Eva in which she announced she will be coming tomorrow evening. Let us hope she arrives safely. Traveling is very arduous at the moment. And hopefully she will bring good weather. Today it poured buckets the whole day without letup. Our troops' great success in Russia is the big news. Our excellent air force certainly protected us here in Posen from aerial attack. But in my opinion, the decisive thing in the war with Russia is not military success, but the destruction of Bolshevism by the Russian people themselves. Yesterday came news of the takeover of Riga. What is to become of the Baltic states now? And the Baltic Germans? Will they return home? That would leave a lot of room here—empty apartments in particular!

Monday, 7 July 1941

Eva arrived on Friday evening, shortly after eleven, after a relatively favorable trip—although she was on the road for almost 12 hours. We now live in Room 199 on the north side, as my previous room was too small. We are having a very pleasant time. While we men work, Eva and Frau Köhler go into town and shop. Today they bought various household objects for us "bachelors" (among other things a glass chamber pot!), and a large bucket of marmalade to take back with them. The weather has also improved again. And there are only two more Sundays before I go home.

Tuesday, 15 July 1941

On Saturday afternoon at two o'clock, we took the bus to Schlehen. Awful heat and overcrowding made the trip unpleasant. But we soon recovered in the vicarage over a cup of coffee and cake. The afternoon was spent viewing the garden and walking through the village and the fields. It was difficult to sleep at night because of the heat. On Sunday morning we took part in the service that Pastor Welke gave in the Schlehen church. After lunch we took a very pleasant trip by car through Klein Langenau, along Lussower Lake to Gross Langenau, and from there through Sassenheim to Tempelhof, an estate of over 4,000 acres, where we were received very kindly by Frau von Tempelhof and served real tea, etc. A walk through the beautiful park and the cattle stalls, which awakened lively memories of my youth, completed this visit. The return trip toward evening was very lovely. Everywhere, as far as the eye could see, fields of waving corn close to ripening. We returned Monday morning at seven o'clock, since I had to lecture at nine o'clock. Frau Köhler left yesterday evening, and on Friday Eva has to leave. . . .

Tuesday, 30 September 1941

Today I had a very interesting discussion with the chief prosecutor, Dr. Heise,* about obtaining corpses for the anatomical institute. Königsberg and Breslau also get corpses from here. So many people are executed here that there are enough for all three institutes.†

---

* Max Heise (1883–1956) was head of the prosecutor's office at the state court in Posen.

† On 31 October 1941, Voss wrote in the "Chronicle": "Today the institute received its first corpses: five executed Poles, one of them a woman." On 10 March 1942, Voss noted on the institute's first dissection exercise: "About 60 students took part in the dissection exercise. Nineteen corpses were dissected. Seven of them come from the Polish period, the rest had almost all been executed and injected a few hours after death with formol. In addition to the usual muscle and joint dissections, dissections of the breast, stomach, and sex organs were also made. The dissections of the organs of the executed persons were the loveliest I have ever seen in a dissecting room."

In fact, the students and teachers could have told more from these corpses than the simple fact that they were executed. This is proven by the results of a forensic examination, ordered by the prosecutor, of 48 bodies found after the liberation of Posen in the formalin-filled tubs of the *Collegium Anatomicum*. The report stated, among other things:

"The condition of the bodies (especially the marks of strangulation) showed—and the entry in the corpse register confirms this—that death occurred for 37 of the bodies through hanging by another. For 8 of the 11 bodies delivered from camps, death most probably resulted from insufficient nourishment, consumptive illness, and overexertion; the remaining 3 bodies showed such apparent traces of violence that one must assume mistreatment and torture as causes of death. On 8 of the bodies of the executed, injuries to the face and back in particular, but also to other parts of the body (bruised areas of the skin, hemorrhages, abraded skin, beating wounds) were found which suggest that these people were beaten and tortured before execution. Examinations of the teeth showed that for 5 of the bodies of those executed, the teeth, especially the front teeth, were missing. The condition of the gums and in part the remaining teeth showed that these teeth had been broken off after death. Since

Thursday, 2 October 1941

More medical professors are gradually arriving. The day before yesterday I had a visit from Prof. Masing, the former internist from Dorpat, and yesterday one from Dr. Rentz,* the future pharmacologist. Neither of them has an institute or a clinic yet. The day before yesterday the new forensic doctor arrived: Dr. Ponsold.† He is living here at the institute with his wife, but I have seen nothing of him yet. . . .

Posen, 17 October 1941

. . . The semester is now supposed to begin on 18 November. Yesterday I heard that a student company of air force doctors had been created. Twenty-eight students are already here.

---

no artificial teeth were found on any of the 48 corpses, it can be assumed that after death, gold teeth and gold crowns were broken off."

* Ernst Masing became professor of internal medicine at the Reich University on 1 January 1942; Eduard Rentz (1898–1962) became professor of pharmacology and toxicology on 1 December 1942.

† Albert Ponsold (1900–1983) came from the Baltics. In 1941 he became doctor of forensic medicine at the Reich University of Posen. He is still honored in Poznań as one of the few honest Germans in the occupation regime. This despite the fact that, according to the university class schedule, he taught the subject "human heredity and racial doctrine." Ponsold published memoirs (*Der Strom war die Newa: Aus dem Leben eines Gerichtsmediziners,* St. Michael, 1980) which describe only in passing the public, accepted character of the practice of murder in Posen: "At police headquarters in Posen, I happened to pass through a room in which Polish resistance fighters were being interrogated—two young men and a woman, apparently students. The officers sat around casually, one on the table, as if it was nothing important. When I saw a truck standing in front of the anatomical institute the next morning and asked what had been brought by, the driver pulled back the hood and revealed a horrifying sight: the three Poles beheaded, their heads between their feet" (p. 185f.).

In his memoirs, Ponsold describes himself as the only non-Nazi among the professors in his area. The files of the University of Halle and the Document Center in Berlin prove that, if there was a non-Nazi among the forensic doctors, it was not him. On the development of German forensic medicine between 1933 and 1945, see Friedrich Herber's book, *Gerichtsmedizin im Faschismus* (Leipzig, 1989).

In the meantime, the assessment of Ponsold in Poznań itself has been changing over the last decade: "Criminal psychological medical experiments took place at the Reich University at the Institute for Forensic Medicine and Criminology headed by Ponsold. Ponsold claimed that a tendency to crime was a racial category and only appeared in the so-called lower races." At any rate, this is what Piotrowski stated on page 173 of his 1984 book on the Reich University (see n. 5 for bibliographical details).

27 October 1941

The institute building has been heated since the day I arrived, but so little that one freezes to a block of ice when one sits too long in the rooms. I warm myself now and again by sandpapering the old Polish typewriter table. Our muscles are the best contributors of warmth, especially since we always have them with us. The dormitory for lecturers is simply not getting done. We will probably have to prepare ourselves to spend the winter in this ice palace. A wonderful prospect!

Thursday, 30 October 1941

Yesterday afternoon around six I visited the rector, Prof. Carstens, and received from him my certificate of appointment as a full professor. At 6:30, Xanderl and I visited Fräulein Müller, who had invited us over to say farewell. I have known Fräulein M. since my first day in Posen at the end of February. She is the secretary to the director, Dr. Streit. Another colleague of hers whom I also knew from the university, Fräulein Duwe, a Baltic German, was also there. Last Saturday we were both invited to visit the von Hirschheydt family. Tomorrow the anatomical institute will get its first bodies. Eleven Poles are being executed; I will take five of them, the others will be cremated.

Sunday, 2 November 1941

Yesterday we moved into the lecturers' dormitory. There I was given a large, pleasant room with two beds. We have finally attained what we had desired for so long. And yet it has become almost difficult to part from the familiar rooms at the institute, in which I experienced so much. Winter has already begun here, with snow and frost.

Thursday, 13 November 1941

. . . An east wind has prevailed since yesterday; it is blowing tiles and other things from the roofs. The air is filled with sandy dust. Yesterday afternoon, Director Papenfuss from the administration was here. I heard terrible things from him: a large institute for cancer research is to be forced upon our institute!* Well, let's wait and see what comes of that! . . .

---

* The so-called Cancer Research Institute in Posen was established in 1943 and 1944 with a budget of over 2.5 million reichsmarks. Deputy Reich Health Chief Blohme took part, as well as the German Research Society and the Kaiser Wilhelm Society. Various oral reports, for example that of the widow of Stegmann, the chief examiner for the Posen SS and police courts, indicate that toward the end of the war Posen

Wednesday, 26 November 1941

The second semester is in progress. There are some 50 students at my two lectures, and just as many in the dissecting room. The small auditorium is just large enough. My two "young people," med. stu. [Norbert] Hammer and [Alfred] Kalkbrenner, who have been appointed research assistants at my request, are doing quite well, so I do not have much difficulty with the dissecting room.

Saturday, 13 December 1941

. . . After next week, things here will be available only with ration coupons, as in Germany proper. On Tuesday afternoon, we joined the

---

must have become the site of brutal human experiments. The "Cancer Research Institute" was their focal point. Under the heading Bd. 304 abc in the archives of the High Commission for Prosecution of Hitlerist Crimes in Warsaw, there is a small group of files on an "institut w Pokzywno." These are the files collected by the Poznań prosecutor's office, which began investigations in 1946 on hard-to-identify buildings in Poznań-Pokzywno (Posen-Nesselstedt in German), a former Ursuline convent around which a high wall had been built. Additional barracks had been erected on its grounds, in particular a rough construction with a crematorium, a two-story cellar with tubs for bodies, and individual cell-like rooms. This house was equipped with a highly complex heating, and probably also cooling, system, which made it possible to keep the rooms far below freezing or unbearably hot. There were also plans for this building. It was labeled "Nesselstedt Animal Experiment Ward"; however, the individual rooms in this supposed animal experimentation ward contained two-meter-long beds, toilets, etc. Thus, the description was clearly camouflage.

To encourage further research, a few details from the files of the investigation: head of the construction site was a Dr. Gross of Vienna. Gross was an SS major, married to a doctor, who often traveled to Vienna. His deputy was a Dr. Raabe. Blohme, the Deputy Reich Health Chief, and Greiser, *Gauleiter* of the Warthegau, regularly inspected the site. The site leader was a Karl Büttner, the responsible planner in Posen a Herr Freust; his superior, the chief of planning, was named Döring. The architects were Walter Pretsch and possibly Richard Seifert. Shortly before the Red Army marched into Posen, the technical equipment and files of the institute were transferred to Thuringia, where two sister institutes already existed: Geraberg, near Weimar, and Ilmenau, near Erfurt. Gross once said to a worker, "This is to be the sister institute to Dachau." According to another worker, there was a similar institute in Poland, in Miedzychodzic.

Professor Schreiber of the former military medical academy in Berlin testified at Nuremberg: "In March 1945, Blohme visited me at the military medical academy in Berlin. Blohme had come from Posen and was very upset. He said that the rapid approach of the Red Army had forced him to flee the institute. He was afraid the Russians would recognize that an institute had been erected there for human experimentation. He made an effort to find someone to destroy all equipment and facilities." Schreiber stated further that he was unfortunately forced to make a similar institute in Sachsenburg available to Blohme, so he could continue his work there.

students to listen to the Reichstag session and the declaration of war on America. Now the world war has begun. I am not surprised, since I already predicted it in 1939. How is this ever to end? I do not believe they can defeat us. Our position is very different from what it was in the earlier world war; but how are we and Japan to defeat the United States? This war can end only through radical internal political change here or there. Let's hope it does not happen here, but to our enemies!

Thursday, 18 December 1941

Things are constantly occurring here to upset us. This afternoon I received word that the *Gau* air-raid emergency medical officer, Chief Physician Lieschke, commander of the student company that returned from Russia a few weeks ago, had died of typhoid fever. He visited me around three weeks ago. He may have infected me as well. If I can only get away tomorrow! I don't care what happens after that. As long as I get home. Yes, the "wild East" is nerve-racking. One day it will devour us. . . .

Wednesday, 31 December 1941

On this last day of the year, I always used to make a list of assets. But this year I don't feel like doing it at all. What will the new year bring? The future looks bleak to me because of the war with Russia. The Russians are constantly attacking. Will our forces hold out against this constant winter offensive by the Bolsheviks? How could the top people in the Reich have thought the Soviet army was as good as finished? Our side completely underestimated Russian military strength; that much, at least, is clear. But we lack the immense reserves the Russians have. In order to hold the eastern front, we must bring in troops from the occupied territories. This will soon spark large-scale uprisings. Fires will spring up all over Germany. Who is to extinguish them if our entire military force is tied down in the east? Perhaps it will be "finis Germaniae" as soon as next year. We wanted to make Russia into a colony; now probably the opposite will occur. Perhaps this is all too pessimistic. How happy I would be if it is, and if I am wrong about all these predictions. . . .

Posen, 15 April 1942

. . . The day I returned, the rector informed me that he wanted to appoint me dean of the Medical Department, and asked if I were agreeable. I answered yes. This means, thank God, no more of this ridiculous "supervisor" of the department, which I have been until now. But if I had not put up a fight, they would have let me play that part a lot longer. Today I already received a written appointment from the rector. . . .

Friday, 24 April 1942

Yesterday was my anniversary here in Posen. But I did not celebrate. I think a lot now about the first days and weeks here. It was a bad time, because my nerves were so shaken from the flu in spring of 1941. I am surprised that so many things I considered tragedies back then now seem completely unimportant and do not upset me at all. The number of students is approximately the same as last semester. I have to give many lectures and courses. Twenty-one hours a week. Thursday is the worst, with six hours; 8–9, system[atic] anatomy IV; 11–12, histology; 12–1, syst[ematic] anat[omy] I; 3–4:30, anatom[ical] working group; and in the evening, 8–9, construction of the human body (for students from all departments). But I am used to this from Leipzig, and am well-trained. Since 15 April I have had a technical assistant at the institute, Fräulein Bonitz. My institutional personnel now includes one chief dissector, two research assistants (instead of the two regular assistants), one technical assistant, one dissector, two institutional helpers, and one cleaning lady.* The last four are Poles. In addition, another air force doctor, Herr Gehrken, works at the institute, and another medical student already in her clinical semester is coming tomorrow; she is taking a semester off, lives here with her parents, and would like to do some scientific work. It is very nice that we can now stay at the institute and work in the evening. In winter it was not possible because of the cold in the rooms. When it begins to get dark, I wander over to the lecturers' dormitory, where I spend the rest of the evening very pleasantly, interestingly, and enjoyably with colleagues.

Sunday, 26 April 1942

Yesterday evening I went to the theater here for the first time, in order to get to know it at last. Herr Hammer, one of my "young people" at the institute, had gotten tickets for me. The piece, a modern operetta, was idiotic, but the theater and its interior rooms are very pretty. I just took a walk through the city park and visited the botanical gardens, which are really very nicely set up and in good condition. There I saw roses and lilac in bloom. It will be a long time before they have gotten that far on the outside. The weather is pleasant: sunshine from morning till night for days, but with a cold east wind. Last year, though, the weather at this time was much worse. Today I read in the Wehrmacht report that Rostock was

---

* The technical assistant, Renate Bönitz, married in 1942 and became Frau Berger. In 1944, Frau Ingeborg Naumann joined her. The research assistants were, according to the "Chronicle," the students Norbert Hammer, Alfred Kalkbrenner, Gerken, Lindemann, Kolloczek, Josef Meier, Seymer (Seimer?), and Finsterwalder.

badly hit by English planes the night before last. The Church of St. Niko-laus, the city theater, the registry office, and our old school were hit.

Monday, 27 April 1942

After lunch today, I sat upstairs for three-quarters of an hour right under the roof on our "bone whitener," soaking up the sun. To my right and left, Polish bones lay bleaching, occasionally giving off a slight snapping sound.* This evening our air raid warden was here, to give me the pleasant news that night watches must now be set up in the building. They are expecting air raids on Posen. That's great. But in the end it doesn't really matter where one croaks. . . .

Tuesday, 19 May 1942

On Sunday, Herr von H[irschheydt] told me he had gotten lice on Saturday from a louse-ridden Jewish corpse. He has been making plaster casts of Jewish heads for the Vienna anthropological museum. That was wonderful news, since the Jewish corpses delivered here have often died of typhoid fever. Because I was already in low spirits [English in original] that day, as the English say, this had quite an effect on me. I thereupon decided to go home for Pentecost to see my family again. You never know if it will be the last time. Yesterday I had to fight with the prorector about my trip. There is not actually supposed to be a Pentecost vacation. Rea-

---

* In July 1941, Professor Voss had made an agreement with the Gestapo under which not all the bodies would be cremated; some would instead be given to the anatomical institute for maceration and further dissection. Voss developed a booming trade in skeletons and skulls that he sold to Breslau, Leipzig, Vienna, Königsberg, and Hamburg; he received 15–30 RM per skull, or 150 RM per skeleton. In exchange, the Hummel firm in Leipzig sent Voss various animal skeletons, as shown in records kept by Alfred Kalkbrenner for the anatomical institute (see Goguel, p. 125). These skeletons of Polish resistance fighters are probably still being used today. On the technique of maceration, Voss wrote: "In order to obtain clean bones and skeletons, one must free them from all soft parts still adhering to them. This is first done mechanically, by cutting or scraping off the soft parts such as muscles, tendons, ligaments, etc. To remove the last traces of external soft parts and bone marrow within the bones, the bones are macerated. . . . Maceration of the bones can be accomplished in two ways: natural or decay maceration, and artificial or chemical maceration through the influence of solvent chemicals such as soda solution, potassium lye, antiformin, etc. . . . After thorough cleaning, the macerated bones are scoured with gasoline in the scouring apparatus, then bleached artificially by treatment with hydrogen peroxide or in the open air. Direct sunlight should be avoided, as otherwise cracks may appear in the bones. The bones of fresh corpses can be macerated best and most easily" (Hermann Voss, *Mikroskopisch-anatomische Präparationstechnik*, Leipzig, 1939, p. 26f.).

son: The Führer's last speech! I told him that, in that case, we shouldn't have a long university vacation either. Well, in any case, I managed to get permission to leave for eight days. The people at the top are all bastards; they are scared to death and have no courage. I will leave on Tuesday morning at four. I got a ticket at the station yesterday.

Monday, 8 June 1942

We just buried Herr von Hirschheydt.* It all happened as I predicted three weeks ago. When I arrived at the institute on the morning of 29 May, I was greeted with the news that Herr v. H. had become ill. I knew right away. It was good that Eva was here. I suffered through terrible hours. Our nerves are so on edge. These incidents don't seem to end. I used to like being at my institute. Now I hate it and will not remain there any longer than absolutely necessary. Tomorrow morning Eva is returning home. Then I will be alone again with all my worries. What a miserable life.

Thursday, 18 June 1942

The robinia, garlanded with clusters of blossoms, is peeking in at my office window at the institute once again. Unfortunately, the blossoms don't show up as well this year, because the weather is not as nice as it was last year at this time. For some time we have had an oceanic climate, which I have not yet experienced to this extent in Posen. Daily west winds, storms, and rain. Only one more hour of lecturing, and another difficult Thursday will be over. Some students from the country recently gave me 18 eggs and a piece of bacon. I sent the bacon to Leipzig; the eggs I ate myself. . . .

Saturday, 20 June 1942

Yesterday I had to head the first meeting of the Medical Department. I never dreamed a few years ago in Leipzig that I would once again have

---

* On the same day, Voss wrote in the "Chronicle" of the anatomical institute, "On 4 June, von Hirschheydt, the head dissector, died of typhoid fever. Some time previously, he had been asked by the Vienna Anthropological Museum to prepare plaster casts of Jewish bodies [apparently the Anthropology Department of the State Museum of Natural History in Vienna is meant. At the time, it was headed by Josef Wastel]. These Jewish bodies had been supplied from the Jewish camps, to be burned here in this building. They were often full of lice, and, as is now apparent, insufficiently disinfected. Herr v. H. caught lice from one of these bodies on 16 May; his illness began on 28 May. The anatomical institute has lost an unusually loyal and industrious employee, who was a great help to me during the early period and will be difficult to replace."

to play dean of a medical department. Besides myself, five members of the department were present: Monje, Masing, Ponsold, Grossmann, and Brandt.* The meeting lasted from five to seven o'clock. We decided to celebrate 6 May each year with a faculty meeting, and later, perhaps, with some other celebration. For that is the day medical education in Posen began, with my lecture. Tomorrow Köhler and I want to take part in an excursion to view a salt mine.

Monday, 22 June 1942

The war with Russia began a year ago today. It was a Sunday. I won't soon forget that day. The war with Russia is far from over. How shall it ever end? Yesterday we toured the salt mine Salzhof in Wapno. We left at 7:30 in the morning, first for Gnesen. There we had to change, and then it took about an hour more on the narrow-gauge railway, on the Nakel line, to Wapno. The salt mine is located right next to the station. After a short speech by the director we went down, clad in white coats, to the lowest level, 430 meters underground. The tour lasted about an hour and was really very interesting. It was very nice and warm down there, around 20 degrees [68°F]. Upstairs we then saw salt processing, which takes days. The salt processed here is so pure that it can be used as table salt, as is. After this tour through the plant, we had a bottle of beer contributed by the plant. We ate, and then went to the old gypsum quarry, in which gypsum used to be mined, for the salt is covered by a layer of gypsum that reaches almost to the surface. We collected various pieces of gypsum. I also took along a piece of salt and a salt crystal. At three o'clock we left, and were back here at six. A very pleasant day.

Tuesday, 30 June 1942

I left here on Friday afternoon at three o'clock and was in Leipzig by midnight. No streetcars were running, so I had to go on foot. I got home shortly before one o'clock. The way was pleasant: bright moonlight and the fragance of flowers on a summer night. On Saturday and Sunday we had bad weather: rain and cold. We had to turn on the electric oven for awhile. Left L. Monday at four, arrived here around midnight. In the "dormitory" I ran into colleagues who were just returning, around one,

* Manfred Monje (1901–81), professor of physiology in Posen beginning on 1 February 1942, succeeded Voss as dean and later became a professor at the University of Kiel. Hans Grossmann (1895–1973) was a professor of hygiene in Posen from 1 October 1941 on. Max Brandt (1890–1972) was a professor of pathology, and later a founding member of the Free University of Berlin.

from a meeting of the Union of Lecturers. We sat together until 1:30. In L. I received great news: The Medical Department hadn't even mentioned me on its nomination list. I never seriously expected to be Clara's successor there, but they could at least have put me on the list *honoris causa*. That is the thanks I get for 15 years of loyal service. But even this slap in the face by fate will not knock me down; it will simply make me stronger. Anyway, it is easier to bear than if I were still in Leipzig. Thank God, I am now even with Clara. I was in his debt for Posen, which was not at all pleasant to me. But that is now settled. If he had wanted to, he could have brought me to L. But he did not want to, because he wants to get rid of Herr Dabelow* in Munich, which he will doubtless succeed in doing. His friend de Crinis in the Ministry does anything he wants. He himself went to Munich against the will of the faculty. I now have to make the best of it. Who knows what use it all is. Here in Posen, my motto is victory or death. There can be nothing else. A slap in the face like this can often be quite a motivating force.

Sunday, 5 July 1942

Yesterday evening there was a medical students' party in the cafeteria. I had to make another speech. Then there was fish and potato salad, and afterwards all sorts of performances by the students. It was revealed to me in a lovely poem that I am called "Papa Voss" by the students. Nice and friendly in its way, but I can't stand this awful "Papa." It was much nicer in Rostock, when we students talked about "*Vatting* Barfurth." An anatomy guessing game was a very nice idea, with ten awards, consisting of bones that I contributed. The first prize was a very nice skull,† the tenth was two small sesamoid bones. Unfortunately, they kept trying to dance, which is now strictly forbidden. Because of this, I left by twelve. Wonderful Posen weather yesterday and today. Bright sunshine from morning till night, blue skies, and a light easterly wind. I am now sitting in the sun before the open westward-facing window of my office at around six o'clock, letting myself broil slowly. We now eat in the SS casino. The food

---

* Adolf Dabelow (born 1899), professor of anatomy in Leipzig from 1942, after 1945 in Mainz.

† In 1945, the porter of the *Collegium Anatomicum,* Jósef Jendykiewicz, described where Voss got his skulls: "The heads of the transported victims were thrown into a basket like turnips and brought in the elevator to the third floor for maceration. Here they were prepared and later used in our institute of anatomy, where some can still be found, or sent to various universities in Germany, or sold to students" (Olszewski, p. 42).

there is very good, and there is less of a crowd than in the usual pubs. Unfortunately, it is closed on Sundays, as we discovered this afternoon to our great distress. . . .

Litzmannstadt, Sunday, 18 July 1942, four in the afternoon
 Finally a break in this insane chaos. I am sitting in Litzmannstadt, Annenweilerweg 6, in the building housing the Insurance Doctors Association, on the second floor. There is a thunderstorm going on outside through which I can see this city's trademark, the numerous chimneys, hazily in the distance. The room I am sitting in, which I also sleep in with my colleague Brandt, is pleasant and cheerful. It even has running water, which is something special for this city, since it has neither water pipes nor a sewer system. Yesterday I saw a barrel truck that looked like a dung wagon driving through the streets, but it said "drinking water." This afternoon there is another tour, but I did not go along, which is understandable after everything we have already done here. I will describe it in order.
 On Thursday the 16th, we left Posen around 9 o'clock in the morning. All of the participants in this study trip to Litzmannstadt by the Nazi Lecturers' Union were accommodated very comfortably in a special express car attached to a passenger train. We traveled eastward through Wreschen-Konin to Kutno on the main Warsaw line, and from there southward. The trip was quite interesting, in part because of discussions with colleagues, in part because of the not so uneven landscape. However, it lasted quite a long time; we did not reach the Litzmannstadt station until four o'clock—incidentally, quite a wretched construction for such a large city. Then we took the electric streetcar, in two special cars, to the first hotel: the General Litzmann Guest House. There Mayor Ventzki* greeted us briefly, and quarters were assigned. After partaking of coffee, my colleague Brandt and I took the streetcar to our quarters, which are located rather far away. This gave us the opportunity to become acquainted with the city's wild appearance. In comparison with Posen, L. is no longer a German city, even if it still has some buildings and houses that one can immediately see were built by Germans; the Russian-Polish element predominates. In the evening, we attended a lecture by Ponsold on blood groups at the Center for Popular Education. Then we went by car to the home of a colleague, Dr. Schulz, a surgeon and student of Erwin Payr in

* As mayor of "Litzmannstadt," Werner Ventzki (born 1906) was responsible for the deportation of 55,000 Lodz Jews. After the war he served as a senior city councillor in West Berlin and represented the Ministry for Refugees.

Leipzig; my colleague Monje is staying with him. There we had very good wine, accompanied by all sorts of wild eastern stories that are said to have happened here in L. I was "home" by twelve, and chatted with my colleague Brandt until one.

In the morning I woke up early once again, so I only had a few hours of sleep that night. We had to be at City Hall by 8:30, where the mayor gave a very good, interesting speech on L. A tour of the city in two buses followed. Naturally, this tour included the famous and infamous ghetto of L., the organization of which had already been described to us by the mayor. In addition, in the southern part of the city we saw the battlefields of L. from the First World War; the hill of graves, a cemetery of honor, and the memorial hill that still does not have a memorial but is intended as such for the future. Lunch at the General Litzmann, then coffee and cake, which incidentally is still quite good here. At three, at the regional administrator's, the "academy" began; it consisted of five-six lectures and lasted until seven o'clock. I liked the lecture by my colleague Stavenhagen* the best. Dinner at eight o'clock at the General Litzmann, at the city's invitation. To bed around midnight, chatted until around one.

This morning at 8:30, a lecture by the president of the Chamber of Industry and Commerce; then we took a bus to a tour of the large Horak textile factory at 223 Breslauer Street. A true model factory, with a ventilation system and automatic extinguishers in the spinnery. It is a multilevel or complete factory; that is, it includes all processes necessary to the production of cloth, from the basic material (cotton, wool, flax, or rayon) to the finished product. The tour lasted until noon; then we went to the wonderful park belonging to the Horak family, said to be 25 acres, where we received a glass of beer at the tennis court. Incidentally, the tour was given by young Herr Horak himself. By the way, during this tour I discovered a wonderful model for loose and tight connective tissue, namely unprocessed rayon ready for spinning. Lunch at the General Litzmann at the invitation of the Chamber of Commerce. Then coffee and cake again.

Epilogue

The diary ends at this point. Voss would later find many more models for simplified description of human functions—something he is famous for.

* Kurt Stavenhagen was appointed a professor of philosophy at the Reich University on 1 October 1941.

The upper extremity is connected to the torso through an intermediate piece, the shoulder strap. On the torso, the shoulder strap forms a mobile socket for the free upper extremity, the arm, like the bed of a traveling crane.[10]

Muscle fiber is the elementary motor of the apparatus of movement. Fuel is supplied by the blood. Mechanical labor and creation of warmth are the tasks of this motor. It is dependent on the nervous system and the stimuli it produces; it is turned on and off by the nerves. The motor nerve fibers at the same time act as the ignition of this motor. If nerve paths are destroyed, the muscle motor is idle; it is paralyzed.[11]

At the elbow joint, this stem is interrupted by a joint, so that the interior of the moving shank is also accessible. Thus the arm is divided into two sections, an upper and lower arm. The lower arm is attached to pliers that are movable at the wrist—the hand.[12]

These various mechanical comparisons are reductions of complex human functions—as if the hand were a pliers or the mouth simply a chewing tool. This view of human beings—though not unique to German anatomists of the Nazi period—was developed at least in part with the help of Polish and Jewish bodies, ordered by Voss for the dissecting tables of the Reich University. They were not people, but apparatuses, motors; they had not been killed, their functions had been "interrupted." That is the background of the Vossian anatomy still being taught today.

Voss's diary shows that it was not an unbridled desire for scientific knowledge, but sheer hatred, that underlay his desire for extermination. Only as an afterthought did he use the many bodies for his own specific purposes as professor of anatomy—something also practiced by many of his colleagues. The examples of anatomists or anatomically inclined professors like Stieve, Hallervorden, Spatz, Rauch, Kremer, Hirt, Ostertag, and Wätjen[13] show the extent to which this type of research and these research conditions were considered normal; how scientists, without being convinced supporters of the regime, became beneficiaries of the optimal research conditions it provided—thus justifying an extermination policy whose scientific by-products proved useful to human progress, easing the consciences of the actual perpetrators.

The human experiments performed by one of Voss's mentors, Hermann Stieve, stand out in this context of scientific collaboration. Stieve was considered the gynecologists' anatomist. He was born in 1886 and died in 1952 a recognized professor at East Berlin's Humboldt University.

In 1921, he participated as a volunteer in the repression of the Central German workers' rebellion; Voss describes in his diary the commotion that arose when Stieve's gun, still hidden for counterrevolutionary purposes, was accidentally discovered in 1936 at the anatomical institute in Leipzig. From 1935 on, Stieve taught and conducted research at Berlin's Charité Hospital, where he became an advocate of human experiments—an activity that his obituary in East Germany confirmed more than it concealed:

> For Stieve, the times brought with them an opportunity to pursue questions involving the male and female sexual glands, which had already interested him during his earliest investigations as assistant to Rückert. As early as 1918, he reported that in experiments performed in 1913, caged hens no longer laid eggs, while in experiments a year later in the same place they had become accustomed to imprisonment. The reason for this varying behavior became clear to Stieve only later. It consisted in the fact that in 1913 a fox and several cats occupied the same stall, though also in cages; their presence, perceptible through smell, apparently greatly frightened the hens.[14]

What the "times brought with them" was Stieve's opportunity to conduct human experiments of the most repulsive kind, enabling him to reach sweeping conclusions on the psychosomatic conditions of the female cycle. What Stieve investigated before the First World War on caged hens, he continued to work on in the '40s in cooperation with the Ravensbrück concentration camp and the execution site at Plötzensee:

> In 1942 I had the opportunity to examine a woman in whom such exceptional bleeding had begun. The woman was twenty years old. Her first period had occurred at fifteen and taken place regularly from then on without complaint every 28 days; the woman had rarely had sexual intercourse, and pregnancy had always been prevented. As a result of great nervous excitement, she had not menstruated for 92 days; upon hearing news that agitated her greatly, blood flowed heavily from the vagina, and the woman believed menstruation had begun. However, this was not the case. . . . Later (1943), I had the opportunity to investigate a large number of such cases. . . . I later had many opportunities to observe the effect of highly agitating events on female sexual organs.[15]

Stieve determined that "this was not the case" by examining the—executed—woman. The "news that agitated her greatly," comparable to the smell of the fox in the henhouse, was the announcement of her own execution. This was then postponed long enough to allow Stieve to make a gynecological examination of the bleeding in the living prisoner, enabling him to prove afterward on the dead woman that the bleeding was a result of fright without ovulation; that the woman's psychological situation affected her reproductive capabilities, not only emotionally, but through provable anatomical changes in the respective organs.

The experiments on imprisoned and executed women, hinted at in Stieve's obituary and in his publications, have not been investigated to this day. Meanwhile, however, the "Influence of Fear and Psychological Excitement on the Construction and Functioning of Female Sexual Organs," as Stieve titled one essay, has been accurately, not at all pseudo-scientifically, researched and internationally accepted—based on the studies undertaken at the Institute of Anatomy and Biological Anatomy of the University of Berlin.

While Voss at first ordered fresh bodies "only" for educational purposes, to resell the bones, and to make anatomical plaster casts, he soon began to perform his own experiments at execution sites; Voss's assistant, Robert Herrlinger,* not only received his professorial qualifications in this way but also made a name for himself as "anatomist of the spleen"—an organ he had already examined in his medical dissertation,[16] though at that time he had used white rats. In 1947–48, he described "some examinations" of "eight male corpses."[17] They had been healthy men between 18 and 48 years of age, who were "available" to Herrlinger and Voss "for blood tests and laparotomy forty to eighty seconds after death." That is,

---

* On Herrlinger's career in Posen, the "Chronicle" states: "27 September 1942. The assistant at the anatomical institute in Jena, Dr. med. et phil[.] Robert Herrlinger, has been hired as assistant starting 1 September, and as chief assistant beginning 1 October. At the moment, Dr. H. is a physician on the Russian front. I will apply to have him granted leave to conduct classes in the coming winter semester, which is to last from 1 December to 31 March." This application was not successful until a year later:

"28 November 1943. Dr. Herrlinger has been furloughed from the Wehrmacht at my recommendation to the Reich Chief of Health, and has been at the institute since the beginning of October."

"13 May 1943. . . . On 6 May, Dr. Herrlinger passed his academic orals before the faculty, and has received the title of Dr. med. habil. He was excused from the Eastern front for a few days because of this."

"26 November 1944. . . . In the past week, from 20–25 November, Dr. Herrlinger and I took part, along with our students, in trench-digging near Guntershausen, where we worked on the construction of an antitank trench. Lectures and exercises were canceled this week."

Voss's last entry in the "Chronicle" informs us:

"18 December 1944. Dr. Herrlinger was appointed lecturer."

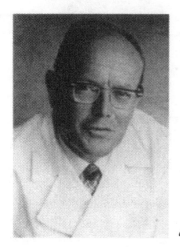
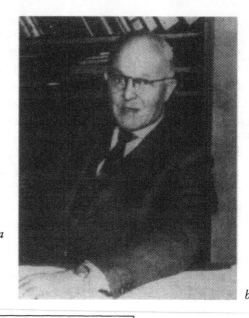

a

b

Bekanntmachung.

Der Strafsenat des Oberlandesgerichts in Posen hat

am 13. Oktober 1942

        Stanislaus Mazurek   beide aus Leslau
        Janina Lech

am 27. Oktober 1942

        Wanda Daszkowska   aus Leslau
        Henryka Wojdyllo   aus Wolne Kreis Hermannsbad

wegen Auflehnung gegen das Reich

            zum Tode verurteilt.

Die Urteile sind vollstreckt worden.

(Übersetzung:) Strafsenat des Oberlandesgerichts in Posen skazal na śmierć za zbuntowanie się przeciwko Rzeszy

dnia 13 października 1942

        Mazurek Stanisław   oboje z Leslau
        Lech Janina

dnia 27 października 1942

        Daszkowska Wanda z Leslau
        Wojdyllo Henryka z Wolne, pow. Hermannsbad.

Wyroki zostały wykonane.

Posen, den 28. November 1942.

Der Reichsstatthalter (Generalstaatsanwalt)

im Reichsgau Wartheland

d

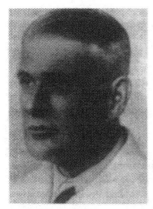

Research at the guillotine: (*a*) Robert Herrlinger; (*b*) Hermann Voss; (*c*) Hermann Stieve; (*d*) poster announcing execution of Polish resistance fighters; (*e*) an execution site in occupied Posen.

c

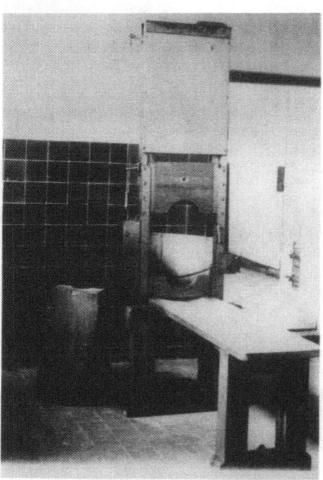

e

the two anatomists waited with their pipettes and dissecting tools right next to the Posen Gestapo's guillotine. To Herrlinger, who described a split neck as an "operating area" in his essay, the guillotine must have seemed merely a somewhat coarse operating tool and the executioner nothing more than an assistant. "The arterial blood was taken first, from the still-pulsating carotids." This occurred "in the usual fashion, using numerical pipettes."

These were certainly optimal conditions for research on still pulsating, beheaded bodies. Yet there were also disadvantages: "Sometimes, however, because of immediate evacuation of chyme from the oesophagus, an accurate examination of the carotid blood became impossible. . . . During pipetting of the carotid blood, the abdominal cavity was opened, the spleen removed as carefully as possible, and the numerical pipette filled by sucking off the drop of blood appearing at the stump of the vena lienalis near the hilus. This blood sample was taken on an average of 120–180 seconds post mortem."

In this way, Herrlinger answered "the question that had long existed on the morphological composition of the blood of the spleen in people with stroke." To convince any doubters, he also mentioned that those "examined" had experienced similar living and nutritional conditions; that is, they had obviously been imprisoned for a long time.

This essay was published in Jena in 1947–48 with the permission of the Soviet military government; that is, without the slightest fear or sense of wrongdoing on the author's part. After all, the tradition of anatomical work "in the shadow of the guillotine" was an old one.[18] This publication, however (and herein lies its exceptional nature), later did, in fact, affect the author's career: in the 1950s, Hans Wollheim, an internist who had been a victim of racial persecution, and Josef Ströder, a very conservative professor of pediatrics, did everything they could to prevent Herrlinger from becoming a professor of anatomy in Würzburg. He had to be satisfied with a post as medical historian in Kiel.[19] He died there, in 1968, at the age of 53; according to Fridolf Kudlien, he, unlike Voss, clearly suffered pangs of conscience resulting from his deeds in Posen, which were publicized by Wollheim and Ströder within the scientific community. When the Polish author Teresa Wróblewska addressed a written inquiry to Voss in Greifswald in 1978, asking what he had to say about his diary today, he responded: "I am 83 years old and want nothing but peace."[20]

Hermann Voss is recognized as an educator. From 1942 to 1945, his main concern was efficiently instructing the medical students who had been furloughed from military service in order to complete their studies

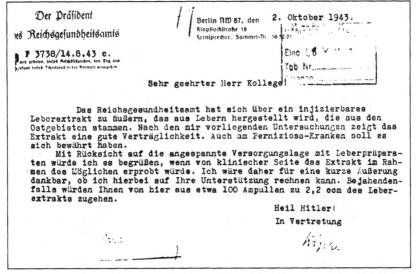

This document shows how openly the Reich Health Office invited the deans of medical departments to participate in crimes. The extract discussed here is made from livers "from the eastern territories"—clearly a euphemism for the fact that the medicine was made from human livers. The handwritten note at the bottom left says, "Seen on 10/15/43, Voss."

"The Reich Health Office must evaluate an injectable liver extract made from livers from the eastern territories. According to the studies available to me, the extract is well-tolerated. It is also said to have worked well in tests on patients suffering from malignancies.

"Considering the difficulty of supplying liver preparations, I would be happy if the extract could be tested clinically as far as possible. Therefore I would appreciate a brief statement on whether I can rely on your support. If this is the case, I would have approximately 100 ampules at 2.2 ccm delivered to you.

Heil Hitler!"

quickly. Thinking and questioning were to be avoided. In this situation, he and his assistant, Herrlinger, laid the groundwork for their future manual. When it was published in 1946, paper was scarce; there was an urgent need for rapid, achievement-oriented training, especially in the newly created GDR, where a new generation aimed to break the bourgeois educational monopoly. This demanded an egalitarian simplification of knowledge. Meanwhile, paradoxically, developments in West Germany took a parallel turn: more narrowly focused studies and limitations on students' freedom required a simplified, easily teachable compendium. Books, too, have their histories.

Notes

1. The annotator has given copies of the diary to the institutes of medical history in West Berlin, Kiel, and Leipzig, as well as the Stiftung für Sozialgeschichte (Foundation for Social History) in Hamburg.

2. H. Voss and R. Herrlinger, *Anatomia cztowieka Repetytorium* (Warsaw, 1974).

3. S. Rózycki, "Państwowy Uniwersytet Niemiecki w Poznaniu" (The German Reich University in Poznań), *Nowiny Lekarskie* 3–4 (1945): 1–8.

4. Proces Artura Greisera przed Najwyzszym Trybunalem Narodowym (Trial of Arthur Greiser before the Supreme People's Court) (Warsaw, 1946). The files of this trial can be found in the archives of the High Commission for the Prosecution of Hitlerist Crimes in Warsaw.

Material on the anatomical institute in Posen can be found in the records on bodies cremated at the *Collegium Anatomicum* (592 z/II) and the records on receipt of bodies by the institute in Poznań (592/I–IIz, 593/I–IIz).

5. Karol Marian Pospieszalski and Edward Serwański, "Materialy do sprawy eksterminacji w tzw. Kraju Warty" (Materials on the extermination in the so-called Wartheland), *Przegląd Zachodni* 1–2 (1955): 298–354.

See also Karol Marian Pospieszalski, "Z pamiętnika profesora 'Reichsuniversität Posen'" (From the diaries of a professor at the Reich University of Posen), *Przegląd Zachodni* 1–2 (1955): 275–98; Halszka Szoldrska, *Walka z kulturą polską: Uniwersytet Poznański podczas okupacji* (The battle with Polish culture: The University of Poznań during the occupation) (Poznań, 1948); Marian Olszewski, *Straty i martyrologia ludności polskiej w Poznaniu, 1939–1945* (Losses and suffering of the Polish population of Poznań, 1939–1945) (Poznań, 1973); Stanislaw Kaguna, "Morderstwa faszystowskich najeźdźców w Poznaniu w okresie drugiej wojny światowej" (Murderous deeds of the Fascist intruders in Poznań during the Second World War), Archiwum Medycyny Sądowej, *Psychiatrii Sądowej i Kryminalistyki* 2 (1961): 57–67; Bernhard Piotrowski, *W służbie rasizmu i beprawia: "Uniwersytet Rzeszy" w Poznaniu, 1941–1945* (In the service of racism and injustice: The "Reich University" of Posen, 1941–1945) (Poznań, 1984).

6. Rudi Goguel, "Über die Mitwirkung deutscher Wissenschaftler am Okkupationsregime in Polen im zweiten Weltkrieg, untersucht an drei Institutionen der deutschen Ostforschung" (diss., Humboldt University, Berlin, 1964), p. 124.

7. The "Chronicle" consists of 17 pages, handwritten by Hermann Voss. They are preserved at the *Collegium Anatomicum* in Poznań.

8. Hermann Voss, "Die experimentelle Herstellung von parthenogenetischen Froschlarven durch Anstich des Eies mit einer Glasnadel" (Med. diss., Rostock, 1919).

9. Kurt Herschel was the medical illustrator at the anatomical institute in Leipzig; Hans-Georg Schäffner was the head dissector—according to Voss, "a true master of his discipline."

10. H. Voss and R. Herrlinger, *Taschenbuch der Anatomie*, 2d ed., vol. 1 (Jena, 1948), p. 29.

11. Ibid., 10th ed. (Stuttgart, 1961), p. 23.

12. Ibid., p. 29.

13. On Julius Hallervorden, Hugo Spatz, Hans-Joachim Rauch, Berthold Ostertag, and Julius Wätjen, see Götz Aly, Chap. 4 in this book. On Johann Paul Kremer, a professor of anatomy active at Auschwitz, see, e.g., Jan Sehn, "Fall des Arztes J. P.

Kremer von Auschwitz," in *Unmenschliche Medizin: Anthologie*, vol. 2, pt. 2 (Warsaw, 1969), pp. 1–49; in Polish, first published in *Przegląd Lekarski Oswięcim* (1962).

14. B. Romeis, "Hermann Stieve," *Anatomischer Anzeiger* 99 (1953): 420f.

15. Hermann Stieve, "Eine Schreckblutung im Klimakterium," *Anatomischer Anzeiger* 98 (1952): 361–68.

16. Robert Herrlinger, "Die Milzgefäße der weißen Ratten" (Med. diss., Heidelberg, 1938).

17. Robert Herrlinger, "Das Blut in der Milzvene des Menschen," *Anatomischer Anzeiger: Zentralblatt für die gesamte wissenschaftliche Anatomie* 96 (1947–48): 226–34; the following quotations are from this work. Among Herrlinger's other scientific achievements in Posen are the essays "Neue funktionell-histologische Untersuchungen an der menschlichen Milz," *Zeitschrift für Anatomie und Entwicklungsgeschichte* 114 (1949–50): 340–65; "Die Sinus und das venöse Abflußsystem in der menschlichen Milz," *Folia haemat.* 70 (1950): 132–39; "Anatomie der Milz," *Anatomische Nachrichten* 1 (1949): 89–90; "Neuere Erkenntnisse über den anatomischen Bau der Milz," in *Handbuch der gesamten Hämatologie*, 2d ed., pt. 1, ed. Ludwig Heilmeyer and Anton Hittmair (Munich, Berlin, and Vienna, 1957), pp. 407–12.

18. See, e.g., Alfred E. Hoche, "Im Schatten der Guillotine," *Jahresringe* (1941): 226ff.

19. On Herrlinger's career, see "Bibliographie Robert Herrlinger (1914–1968)," in *Mitteilungen aus dem Institut für Geschichte der Medizin und Pharmazie an der Universität Kiel*, Special Issue, intro. and comp. Edith Feiner (June 1970). This also lists his obituaries.

20. Teresa Wróblewska, *Uniwersytety Rzeszy w Poznaniu, Pradze, i Strassburgu jako model hitlerowskiej szkoly wyższej na terytoriach okupowanych* (The Reich universities at Posen, Prague, and Strasbourg as models of Nazi universities in the occupied territories) (Toruń, 1984), p. 154.

CHAPTER FOUR

Pure and Tainted Progress

by Götz Aly

Psychiatric Reformers of the Weimar Republic

Professor Nitsche, with whom I had frequent contact, was a thoroughly good man, always concerned with his patients' welfare. He did everything possible to exhaust every opportunity to achieve a cure. He believed euthanasia would heighten doctors' sense of responsibility.[1]

In Bresler's 1913 compilation *Mental Hospitals in Words and Pictures,* the chief physician of the Dresden Municipal Mental Hospital, Paul Hermann Nitsche, described the progressive conditions prevailing there. Establishment of this institution could with justice "be described as a milestone in the development of the German hospital system." In 1908, "the department that cared for the mentally ill [in Dresden] was separated" and placed under independent administration. This new department was headed from the start by the author of the report, Dr. Nitsche. Some years earlier, in 1903, a large number of chronically ill patients had been "relocated" in order to "relieve the institution." Therapy consisted of the usual methods of the period: baths, rest cures on covered terraces, isolation. Those who responded well to therapy were discharged, or at least placed in their family's care under Nitsche's supervision. Those who remained chronically ill were transferred from Nitsche's Department II to Department III, where they worked as much as possible: hauling coal, binding books, caning, pasting paper bags, braiding rope, and rolling twine. Nit-

Capers Rubin assisted with part of the translation of this chapter.

Für Unterricht und Forschung
wichtiger Fall!

Prof. Pohlisch bittet, von Verlegung
Abstand zu nehmen.

File label from the Bonn University psychiatric clinic. The label says: "Important case for teaching and research! Prof. Pohlisch requests that no transfer occur." Pohlisch was a consultant for T-4.

sche called this form of forced labor "occupational therapy."[2] Nitsche's friend, the psychiatrist Carl Schneider, characterized the "period around 1900" as a period in health care in which people "generally spoke a great deal about kindness, love, compassion, gentleness."[3]

During the First World War, conditions for the mentally ill underwent an abrupt change. In his testimony before the Frankfurt prosecutor, the department head responsible for "clemency" in the Führer's Office, Hans Hefelmann, summed up the beginning of the "euthanasia operation" in 1939, as well as Paul Nitsche's role in it:

Asylum directors pointed out that there had been an alarming mortality rate during the First World War. It had been much higher than the number of extremely severe, incurable cases that would have been considered for euthanasia. (As far as I remember, Nitsche had figures on mortality rates during the First World War that proved this.) During that time, many doctors and nurses had been called up for military service. Food and pharmaceuticals had become scarce, leading to a great increase in the mortality rate, because what was available had to be distributed equally among the curable and the incurable. One doctor's suggestion that curable cases be given better treatment than incurable ones was rejected by the others. The doctors also suggested a nurse-patient ratio of one to approximately three or four in serious cases and eight to ten in other cases; thus, in spite of the departures of nursing staff for military service, if euthanasia were administered to the most serious cases, it would ensure a peacetime level of therapeutic care for less severe cases by making available a relatively large number of nurses within the institution.... In this discussion, the doctors stressed that the numerous deaths, confirmed by all parties, that had occurred after even greater suffering during the First World War would provide the justification for the recommended euthanasia measures.... They took what they saw as a favorable opportunity to demand that more be done in terms of therapy than had previously been the case. As far as I recall, schizophrenia was mentioned in particular. This request by the psychiatrists may have been the reason that Brandt, through Brack, later had a special department organized in T-4 under Professor Schneider especially to deal with concomitant improvements in therapy.[4]

In fact, tens of thousands of institutionalized patients starved to death during the First World War. In Prussia alone, the figure was estimated at 45,000; in Saxony, 7,840.[5] A 1920 book by Karl Binding, a respected liberal legal scholar, and Alfred Hoch, an equally distinguished professor of psychiatry, called *Destruction of Worthless Life,* represented not only a rationalized outburst of hatred against the underclasses on the part of middle-class professors who felt existentially threatened but also a justification after the fact. While hunger had affected all asylum inmates equally during the First World War, twenty years later, in their view, the death of the least useful among the "useless eaters" could ensure sufficient food and nursing personnel for those who might still be made economically viable through therapy.

Paul Hermann Nitsche was a reformer, and it was as such that he started down the road that would lead to his execution in Dresden on 25 March 1948, at the age of 71, for his leading role in the euthanasia murders. In his chapter, written in 1929, on "General Therapy and Prophylaxis" in Oswald Bumke's *Handbook of Mental Illnesses,*[6] he developed ideas for more humane as well as more efficient psychiatry. Medicine, he wrote, had to strive to "find a causal therapy for every illness," even if psychiatry, with its "preponderantly symptom-oriented" methods of treatment, was still far from that goal. Nitsche discussed at length the principles propounded by Hermann Simon, director of the former provincial sanatorium at Gütersloh, for reforming therapy; then he turned to the issue of staff conduct in a modern institution of the kind he desired. In institutional life, he argued, there existed a danger of "conflict between nurse and patient": "The nursing staff must be warned expressly against the dangers of incorrect attitudes; they must be made aware that a lack of skill and kindliness can brutalize psychiatric nursing. The patient should always feel that the intention is kind and benevolent. 'It's not what you say, but how you say it'; it is certainly possible to be firm without being harsh."[7]

According to Nitsche, this approach created a generally suggestive atmosphere and was essential if active therapy were to be effective. Like

Simon, and already in the style of his later T-4 activity, Nitsche showed himself to be an action-oriented physician: "Thus, efforts must focus on actively including as many patients as possible in therapy, for each refractory individual [each individual not amenable to the therapy] spoils the institutional routine, the use of suggestion."[8]

For Nitsche, psychotherapeutic educational influence came first, even as he laid the groundwork for a therapeutically selective utopia of extermination. Thus, the psychiatry he propagated broke with involuntary treatment, physical restraints, and torture: "Banishing any type of compulsion from the usual apparatus of therapy is rightly considered the basic premise of modern psychiatric treatment. Mechanical constraint, an everyday event prior to the introduction of 'no-restraint,' is inhuman and undignified, brutalizes the spirit of doctors and nursing personnel, and damages patients physically and mentally."[9]

Wet wraps, for example, still a normal disciplinary tool at the time, were "a means of compulsion that totally confines the patient" and were to be "unconditionally forbidden." In this manual, Nitsche rejected bed treatment as well as continuous therapeutic drug treatment, which had caused far too many deaths. Nitsche saw "institutionalization as by no means the best method of treating the mentally ill." In defiance of the practices of his day, he advocated a concept of "open care" outside of institutions (precisely what social psychiatric services offer today), which he was able to include in Saxony's public welfare law in 1925:

> As much as possible, everyone active in branches of public health care should be instructed on the treatment of the mentally ill, so that they can make referrals for patients of whom they become aware in the course of their activities. It is particularly important to refer persons who exhibit symptoms of some psychic anomaly. In many cases, the doctor can offer counseling and assistance without institutionalizing his patients or even taking them away from their jobs. This often means a great deal to patients and their families, not only psychotherapeutically, but also economically.[10]

Valentin Faltlhauser, a physician who would later be an adviser to the T-4 operation and was involved in extermination at Kaufbeuren in Bavaria, became particularly prominent in the twenties as a theoretical and practicing activist for open care and outpatient counseling. In Erlangen-Nuremberg, Faltlhauser was able to arrange that patients discharged from the institution into public care (or the families caring for them) receive support payments of from two-fifths to three-fifths of the daily institutional costs.

> The state thus saves on public assistance costs, because it does not need to pay the considerably higher institutional costs (approximately 2/5-3/5 higher); the institution and the district (province) save on institutional beds. It will also be easier for patients to reacclimate, to gain a foothold in the outside world even under difficult conditions. However, in addition to the more or less official sources of support underwritten by public welfare agencies, means of rapid assistance must also be available.[11]

This system linked state-mandated care with a therapeutic and charitable apparatus. Nitsche further incorporated supplementary self-help organizations also discussed at length by Faltlhauser, "associations for the relief of the mentally ill of the sort that have existed for decades in various countries": "Their goal was, and is, to provide material and economic support to mentally ill patients living on their own, as well as the families of institutional charges. They grant financial assistance, find work, provide counseling and support, and educate the populace about the mental health care system."[12]

Hermann Simon, the Gütersloh director who was highly praised by Nitsche, was also interested in making clear distinctions between incurable and curable mental patients, and in social reintegration of the curable to the greatest extent possible. He was considered the founder of work therapy, an honor he vehemently rejected; his method, he said, went far beyond a single therapy. It aimed at total institutional reform that would allow patients to benefit from living in an institution. In his book *More Active Treatment of Patients in Mental Institutions,*[13] he summarized the reform model he had begun to develop around 1905 (and as director of Gütersloh from 1919 to 1934). Among contemporary specialists, Simon's results were considered spectacular, and numerous visitors came to Gütersloh to witness the effects of "more active treatment." Simon explained the comparative phrase "more active" as follows:

> Initial failure does not spell the end of therapeutic efforts, but only of one stage, which is followed by new stages until finally a way is found that leads to progress. The justification for this "more active therapy" is an awareness that, among asylum inmates, there are very few with whom it is not possible to work successfully—even if success is modest and often consists merely in preventing them from sinking more deeply

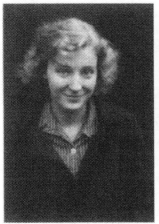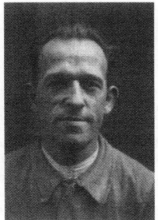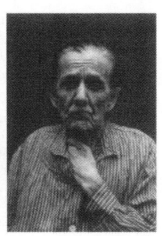

Some of the victims.

into a more degraded condition than that to which their illness would lead in any case.[14]

In 1942, a commission of experts from T-4, the central office for euthanasia, that toured and evaluated German institutions was highly impressed by the therapeutic activism carried over from Simon's term in office. T-4 doctor Herbert Becker wrote of Gütersloh:

> The director is Dr. Hartwich, the head physician. It is probably the most beautiful institution in Westphalia, and is structured entirely along Simon's principles. The main building, in a most beautiful park, was created using the institution's own labor. Because of the work therapy, the conduct of which is perhaps overly military, even the most restless reception wards maintain a peaceful atmosphere that is beneficial and contrasts strikingly with other institutions. Flowers, vases, and tablecloths are intact, even around the most agitated patients. Outside, everything is cultivated and forested by the patients themselves. Because of the work, the patients are less agitated and require less personnel. The personnel ratio is only 1:9. Dr. Hartwich could document that many interested visitors from abroad continued to seek out the institution even in wartime. He introduced serology and medication therapy to the hospital, which had previously used pure work therapy. An outstanding laboratory with a technical assistant is available. The Hohlfelder process [mass x-ray examinations by the x-ray battalion (*Röntgensturmbann*) of the SS] was conducted at the institution and indicated a 5 percent rate

of tuberculosis. Insulin and cardiazol therapy is carried out. The asylum has its own electrical and water systems. In the laundry, a great deal of washing by hand. All in all an institution that merits extensive study and support. Suggestion for use: asylum.[15]

The reformers of the 1920s considered "general prevention of mental illness" to be part of sensible therapy and care. Simon and Nitsche thought this could be achieved through active forms of treatment, but also through mass sterilization; even when exact genetic lines were unknown, this was advisable because of the "enormous importance . . . of this prophylactic question, simply on the basis of probability." Every inch the scientist, Nitsche wrote: "Those we advise and the general public must draw and act upon the practical conclusions."[16]*

Structural Reform and Euthanasia

Planning

As he awaited execution in 1946, Nitsche stated that the "office" he had led "oversaw the individual institutions [involved in euthanasia],"

---

* During the Weimar period, the demand for mass sterilization was not the eugenic battle cry only of notorious Nazis. Advocated by numerous intellectuals and proletarian victims of the future National Socialist regime, it signified that scientists had descended from their ivory towers and taken on social responsibility.

The German Bundestag's 1975 psychiatric commission report (*Bericht über die Lage der Psychiatrie in der Bundesrepublik Deutschland: Zur psychiatrischen und psychotherapeutischen/psychosomatischen Versorgung der Bevölkerung (Psychiatrie-Enquête)*, Drucksache des Deutschen Bundestages, 7. Wahlperiode, 7/4200 [Anhang 7/4201], p. 382ff.) reflected this mood when it vehemently advocated sterilization of those "not capable of consent" (to the procedure), but who, on the grounds of "equality before the law," "integration," and the "right to rehabilitation," should have free access to sexuality—except that they were to be sterilized beforehand, with the consent of their legal guardians and "the involvement of expert and independent authorities." The reform-minded authors of this report then accused the Bundestag of avoiding its legal responsibilities in order "to avoid anything which could in any way recall forced sterilization of the National Socialist variety." The renunciation of coercion, they said, had been "undisputed . . . since the collapse [of the Third Reich]."

The closing chapter of *Zwangssterilisiert, Verleugnet, Vergessen: Zur Geschichte der nationalsozialistischen Rassenhygiene am Beispiel Bremen* (Bremen, 1984), by Norbert Schmacke and Hans-Georg Güse, demonstrates strikingly how far from the truth this was. Using the files of the Bremen health authorities, the book reveals the and—so he said—"completed all the preparatory work for uniform organization of the mental health care system planned for after the war."[17] Planning and collecting data had long been among Nitsche's specialties. As a young man, he recorded the achievements of his Dresden institution with pride and precision: The nurse-patient ratio in Department I was 1: 2.5; in Department II, 1:6.5; in Work Department III, 1:7.9. In Dresden, medical zeal did not end with the patient's death: "In 1910, a total of 367 autopsies was carried out."[18] When the Reich Office of Statistics stopped compiling institutional statistics in 1932, Nitsche encouraged the German psychiatrists' organization to respond: "In spite of the value of statistics on mental illness, shortages prevent the Reich from revising them until further notice. Therefore, the German Psychiatric Association has decided to continue collecting them." Nitsche revised these statistics and made a name for himself as a private psychiatric statistician until 1936, when the Reich Ministry of Health made his voluntary services redundant by returning statistical supervision of mental hospitals to the state.[19] A 1975 West German psychiatric investigative commission praised this initiative. Although not expressly named, Nitsche, who in the period under discussion was already preparing to process patients for euthanasia, received a very strange memorial in the commission's report:

Data Collection, Data Utilization, Data Protection
Among the great difficulties this commission faced at the beginning of its work was the lack of reliable, useful data. . . . From 1877 on, the German health authorities kept "Reich asylum statistics," later called "mental illness statistics." In 1932, the Psychiatric Association took over this task, in hopes of making the statistics more complete and more precise. The *Mental Illness Statistics of the Society of German Neurologists and Psychiatrists* (Psychiatric Department) for 1936 were published in 1938. This was the last complete overview of its kind, and was described as "complete for the first time." It was organized according to categories of mental illness under the so-called Würzburg diagnostic system, and also included two categories indicating the type of hospital and its sponsors.

---

continuity of personnel and content connecting Nazism and the postwar discussion of eugenic sterilization. With the way paved by "progressive" functionalization of the body and voluntary mass sterilization under the rubric of self-determination, the shame felt at the link with Nazi practices is coming to an end.

The Reich Commissioner for Mental Hospitals

As early as 1940, the planned euthanasia law provided for a central state office that would take control of the fragmented German institutional system. This office was known as the Reich Commissioner for Mental Hospitals.[20] Paragraph three of the proposed law created the legal basis for this office, which was to be responsible to the Ministry of the Interior. As far as can be reconstructed from surviving notes on the discussion of the draft, §4 defined the powers of the Reich Commissioner, which were extensive. The Reich Commissioner was to appoint the "implementing doctors"—in other words, the hangmen who were to carry out the "mercy killings" that had yet to be legalized.[21] At an experts' hearing, Max de Crinis, a psychiatrist and neurologist from Berlin, suggested that patients be discharged from institutions only with the Reich Commissioner's approval.[22] The centrality of the office of the Reich Commissioner to the euthanasia law is reflected in an opinion submitted in June 1940 by Dr. Irmfried Eberl, a Brandenburg physician involved in extermination, on the draft law on "extermination of those incapable of living":

On §2, §3, §4
Every inmate of an asylum who has been institutionalized for more than three . . . years and for whom discharge is not imminent must be reported to the Reich Commissioner on a prescribed form. The Reich Commissioner will assign a member of an expert committee appointed by him to examine the patient based on this form and write a short recommendation on the results of his examination. The report form and recommendation will then be given separately to the other committee members, who will decide whether the patient in question is covered by the law or not. The decisions by individual experts will then be forwarded to the Reich Commissioner, who will make a final decision. The office of the Reich Commissioner will administer its own asylums, which will admit patients covered by the law. There, the lives of people to whom the law applies will be terminated. Patients must be observed for at least seven days in the Reich Commissioner's asylum before their lives may be ended. The head of this institution may appeal the committee's opinion to the office of the Reich Commissioner. It must then appoint another expert committee, which will make a final decision in the presence of the head of this institution. For greater efficiency, the meetings of this second expert committee will take place at the Reich Commissioner's asylum, so that all the experts can personally examine and observe the patient in question. The costs of the stay in the Reich Commis-

sioner's asylum are to be assumed by the responsible public welfare association.[23]

The testimony of the future managing director of T-4, Dietrich Allers, that the laws on mercy killing and on establishment of the office of the Reich Commissioner were discussed simultaneously is both plausible and correct. The regulation involving the Reich Commissioner was approved on 23 October 1941 and published four days later in the Reich legal bulletin "in slightly modified form," as Allers testified.[24] Two months after the suspension of Operation T-4, which had carried out nonlegal mass murders, the Nazi regime published the first part of a body of laws on institutionalized euthanasia (see Chap. 2, p. 46ff.).* After a general introduction, the law established that the Reich Minister of the Interior would appoint the Reich Commissioner, who would be responsible for all institutions "concerned, even in part, with the accommodation and treatment of the mentally ill, feeble-minded, epileptics, and psychopaths." Paragraph 2 addressed "wartime economic measures," a euphemism for mass murder used by the Reich administration as well as by the German Conference of Mayors (*Gemeindetag*), health insurance companies, and churches. It thereby elevated the most important term of Nazi linguistic camouflage from a "secret Reich matter" to the status of a published law; though formally only a decree, it was printed on the first page of the Reich legal bulletin. It legalized the formerly covert Reich Association of Mental Hospitals, the organization that had already killed over 70,000 people. The wording of the paragraph that permitted and indeed announced this "necessary measure" went as follows:

> The Reich Commissioner for Mental Hospitals has economic tasks to carry out regarding mental institutions. He is subordinate to the Reich Minister of the Interior and is authorized to take necessary measures in coordination with the head of the Reich Association of Mental Hospitals.[25]

From this time on, the Reich Ministry of the Interior assumed centralized control of the destruction of unusable Germans on the basis of a published law, rather than a vague authorization from the Führer. Until then, the Ministry of the Interior had functioned as an auxiliary to the Reich Association as well as to the Führer's Office that backed it. From

---

* This practice better suits the mood of general euphoria in the late summer of 1941 than does the explanation that religious resistance, the strength of which is constantly asserted, forced the Nazi government to abandon euthanasia.

then on, the relationship was reversed. The *Ministerialblatt der Inneren Verwaltung* (Ministerial bulletin of domestic administration) soon published the name of the new officeholder: "On the basis of Paragraph One of the decree of October 23, 1941 (Reich Legal Bulletin 1, p. 653), I have appointed the Ass't Sec'y in the Reich Ministry of the Interior, Dr. Herbert Linden, Reich Commissioner for Mental Hospitals."[26]

The extent to which Linden actually received the full powers reflected in the legal discussions of October 1941 is still unclear. However, the official in charge of T-4 personnel, Arnold Oels, later testified: "We did not have the impression that we were part of a Party office, but rather of a branch of the Reich Ministry of the Interior."[27] Furthermore, Linden was appointed chief consultant. This was the office a man like Nitsche would call on in difficult cases, and whose decisions he had to respect. Herbert Linden was a central, though ambiguous, figure in the euthanasia program; Allers characterized him as "a very closed man,"[28] while a Viennese mother who encountered him in his Berlin office called him "small and inconspicuous, but enormously kind."[29] Hans-Joachim Becker, of the central T-4 clearinghouse, who was related to Linden's wife Hanna, described finding his cousin's husband processing report forms during an evening visit. "I asked him why he had to work even in the evening, and he answered, 'I have to do this for "your association" as well.'" Linden processed and annotated the forms "one after the other." When Becker asked why he, an official of the Reich Ministry of the Interior, had anything to do with these reports, he responded, "My name has to be on them, too."[30]

Although Linden's work initially concentrated on planning for available institutional space and future use of the buildings, everyone involved was waiting for the second part of the euthanasia law. Numerous comments in reports by the planning commission indicate the extent to which euthanasia figured in their calculations. They assumed that orderly, reformed psychiatric hospitals would require the extermination of a large number of patients.

In Bavaria, for example, a planning commission arrived at a figure of 30,000 mentally ill asylum inmates who were still alive following the mass murders, with an existing target of 14,000 available beds. This problem "can only be solved with the help of the Operation or a euthanasia law."* It was not possible to hold to the previous years' target figures,

---

* The distinction between the (unlawful) "Operation" and the "euthanasia law" indicates that, despite their later defensive statements, the participants did in fact distinguish between what was legal and illegal, and that they never considered the "Führer's authorization" to be a quasi-law. This distinction, made in October 1942, also

since they had been proposed "on the assumption that the Operation would continue." Asylums could only be used for other purposes "if the Operation continues."[31]

In Danzig, West Prussia, the same planner issued an opposite warning. In 1943, the region was still approximately 60 percent short of the necessary number of beds: "Here, as in other states, the low number of patients following the Operation can never serve as a basis for planning for the future."[32] Conditions in Pomerania were similar: "Closing facilities, which is possible because of a temporarily low patient census (the Operation), unfortunately does not lower morbidity in the population." There were 7,000 beds in Pomerania before the war, with only 4,800 necessary according to the new target figures; but "this number [was] very low and could only be maintained in hopes that the law would have certain effects."[33]

The planning department was set up in the spring of 1941 under the direction of T-4. It was headed by Dr. Herbert Becker, a former school and sports physician from Leipzig, who had belonged to the "circle around Professor Nitsche." He led the planning department until it ceased functioning in the winter of 1943–44, probably for reasons other than general wartime cutbacks.[34] Starting in October 1941, this department reported to the new Reich Commissioner. A report of a discussion on the issue between Linden, Heyde, Nitsche, and Allers notes:

> The work of the Reich Commissioner should be organized such that Professor Nitsche, along with the gentlemen of the planning commission, are to inform Assistant Secretary Linden of the prior work of the planning commission. Assistant Secretary Linden will then contact state and provincial authorities. Finally, decisions will be made on future use of the various asylums in consultation with Herr Jennerwein [cover name for Brack].
>
> From a purely technical point of view, the work will proceed such that the planning commission will remain in the building on Tiergarten-strasse, while only one gentleman, who is still to be chosen, and a secretary will move to the Ministry of the Interior.[35]

This man was Ludwig Trieb, administrative director of the Günzburg Asylum before and after the war. Günzburg was considered a model

---

shows that at that time, the institutional murderers were not certain whether their activity would ultimately acquire a legal basis or whether another "Operation" would take place.

institution because of its highly efficient administrative structure. In March 1941, Trieb, along with T-4 doctor Aquilin Ulrich, the Bavarian Assistant Secretary Max Gaum (who introduced his superior to the euthanasia organization in Bavaria), and a photographer named Wagner, toured the Bavarian institutions. "The commission was charged with recording the financial condition of the asylums."[36] Trieb later stated that this had nothing to do with the criminal aspect of the action; they were interested in "purely financial issues"—as though it were not criminal to consider these patients "purely financial issues!"

Nitsche must have had a reason for writing to Blankenburg to request that Allers and Trieb be included in a discussion of the euthanasia question.[37] In his analysis of the Rummelsburg Workhouse in Berlin, for example, Trieb suggested that since its "Working Group I" employed people "supposedly incapable of work," the group "could be reduced correspondingly"; the "remainder" would then have to "improve their work performance."[38] And in a 30-page analysis of the Bethel institutions he determined, to his surprise and satisfaction, that nonworking patients there received perceptibly worse care than working ones, and women worse care than men: "Bethel has long been doing what public institutions will merely be discussing excitedly and at length for a long time to come."[39]

Trieb would later testify about his activities:

In Berlin I spoke with Assistant Secretary Dr. Linden at the Reich Ministry of the Interior. The office was on Schadowstrasse. He basically informed me that he was the Reich Commissioner for Mental Hospitals. I was to visit and survey the various asylums in Austria with the same commission with which I had gone to Bavaria. . . . Shortly before Christmas of 1941 I returned from a trip to Austria. As always, I reported to Dr. Linden. During this stay in Berlin, I was invited to a Christmas party at 4 Tiergartenstrasse, where I met Herr Allers, among others. Dr. Linden was also there. . . . In the winter of 1941–42 and afterward, the remaining unregistered Reich areas were registered, or more precisely, stock was taken. I was assigned to a new doctor, Dr. Herbert Becker, from Leipzig. . . . After the stocktaking was done, I drew up an index. It included every institution, even the smallest. . . . Once the index was completed, current statistics on occupancy were entered in it every month in columns, based on the records. After the government office on Schadowstrasse was bombed, the evaluation took place in an office at 4 Tiergartenstrasse. My involvement actually first began at this time.[40]

In contrast to Becker, Trieb was active until 1945; as late as 1943–44, he led the "barracks operation," and during the final months of the war he directed the "operation to build bunk beds in asylums."[41] He also drew up plans for Linden, his superior, on "occupational therapy in mental hospitals during wartime"; according to these plans, economic officials, with the consent of physicians, were to "guide and oversee the correct use of workers"—in other words, to organize forced labor by the patients.[42]

According to the 8 August 1943 plan of organization of the Central Office, the planning division was part of Main Department II, Technical Execution. Becoming Subdivision IIg Planning (Asylums) Dr. Becker—Trieb, it joined the Transportation System, the Central Index, and the offices in charge of dismantling extermination centers no longer in use.[43] Though planning focused on peacetime, Herbert Becker tried to achieve certain minimal aims under wartime conditions. In proposals formulated for a discussion between Linden and Conti at the beginning of 1943, he combined the goal of more active, aggressive scientific therapy with simplification of the institutional bureaucracy:

> 1. The mental health system requires a central headquarters that will direct scientific activity, with the capacity to obtain information on occupancy of even the smallest asylums, in order to ensure that beds are available in case of emergency, such as during wartime.
>
> 2. For this reason, an index, to be updated monthly, will be created following a planning trip. . . .
>
> 4. All institutions near cultural centers are to be maintained, in order to ensure the availability of new psychiatric personnel.
>
> 5. Work therapy will be expanded, and along with the often extremely outmoded, old-fashioned, and overstaffed bureaucracies, will be modernized.
>
> 6. Each *Gau* is to set up an institution that provides leadership in these two areas. Other regional institutions can learn from these asylums. Setting these up would be a rewarding task for Chief Inspector Trieb, who has experience with work therapy and modern administrative methods (model: the Günzburg asylum). . . .
>
> 8. The Reich Commissioner can pressure industry to furnish the asylums with electroshock apparatus.[44]

In 1943, against this background, Trieb compiled a guide entitled "How to Manage Asylums so as to Achieve Higher Occupancy in Case of

A T-4 index card for registering mental institutions. Developed by Ludwig Trieb.

Emergency." He claimed that the guide, which has not yet been rediscovered, was sometimes requested even after the war "in order correctly to plan construction and reconstruction of asylums."[45]*

The guidelines for mental hospitals issued by the Reich Commissioner foresaw fifteen hundred psychiatric beds per million inhabitants by the end of 1941. That would be 60 percent fewer hospital beds than in 1939. Twenty-five percent of the patients had been murdered; in order to implement their program, therefore, the planners had both to shorten the length of hospitalization considerably and to set their sights on new killings. In January 1942, the figure of fifteen hundred was raised to two thousand psychiatric beds per million inhabitants.[46] This may have been done to rescue beds from the claims of other Nazi institutions suffering from space shortages; in that case, the increased target figure could be interpreted as rapid adaptation to a changing wartime situation. Or it might have occurred because the therapeutic activists among these institutional murderers wished to avoid arbitrarily reducing the number of potential victims, which would also diminish their own importance and the number of directorial positions open to them. Perhaps, however—and this seems most probable—the Reich Commissioner was reacting to pressure from department heads in the various states and provinces. Linden attempted to keep his centralized directives flexible, in order to accommodate the practitioners' desire for change:

> In order to advance the work of the Reich Commissioner, a meeting will be convened in Berlin during the second half of January 1942. The number of participants will be as large as possible; we think it important, for the sake of smooth planning in the future, to invite participation by state governments on behalf of the urban asylums, and regional administrators on behalf of public and private institutions, rather than merely heads of health departments. At this meeting, the Reich Commissioner will present his guidelines and program. . . . Afterward, the states will be given a deadline by which to indicate their wishes. . . . Our files will be revised in light of these requests. After our report is made,

---

* After the war, Trieb remained administrative director of the Günzburg district hospital. He continued to be an active member of the Society of German Hospitals and the Professional Association of Administrative Directors of German Hospitals until very late in life, and participated in planning Bavarian psychiatric clinics. He also published, of course; for example, essays on "genuine efficiency in hospitals" (*Krankenhausumschau* 33 [1964]: 291ff.).

there will be a second meeting, separately with each state, and the final plan will be discussed.[47]

Those in charge of asylums for the state governments were involved in reshaping the institutional system, along with the insurance companies that bore the costs. From the start, Herbert Linden's program to minimize social costs was broad-based. As a "financial expert and institutional specialist," Trieb coordinated the "incoming request lists from the various *Gaus*."

Statistics on institutional beds "put to other uses" indicate that "inferior" inmates had to make room for those still categorized as more valuable. By the summer of 1942, over 6,300 "mothers and children" had been assigned to homes after chronically ill patients were killed. Almost 5,000 beds were reassigned for use as reserve hospital space for the expected large-scale bombardment of northwestern Germany; and 4,600 new beds were prepared to institutionalize "antisocial tuberculous patients," a figure that, according to the report, "fell far short of the demand." Some 800 beds were added to foster care institutions. Here, too, this was only the beginning: "The figure falls far short of demand, which is increasing as processing of juveniles improves."

This analysis by the T-4 statistical department summarized the sociopolitical connections between the annihilation of chronically ill, useless "fellow Germans" (*Volksgenossen*), on the one hand, and the advantages it brought for the "dignified aged" and "large families," on the other:

> Beds available in small homes are only included in individual cases in the figures presented above. These have become available through the removal of mentally ill juveniles and middle-aged persons; they are now free to accommodate old age homes. The head of the medical department of the Württemberg Ministry of the Interior has pointed out that, by creating a larger volume of vacancies for old people, he has made housing previously occupied by single people available to young couples. This is most apparent in the heavily populated industrial areas of Württemberg and Saxony, and can also be observed in the Reich *Gaus* of the *Ostmark* [Austria], such as the Upper Danube and Tyrol, where the heavy workload of the mountain farmers creates great demand for dignified accommodations for workworn, elderly family members.[48]

While the T-4 planning experts were quite secure when dealing with the difference between "usable" and "unusable," "worthy" and "unworthy" lives, and whether patients could be employed as "marginal labor," they were apparently unable to take account of actual social conditions in their planning. They held stubbornly to their target figures. As late as October 1943, Becker reported to his chief "on the eventual number of peacetime beds in Germany": "Our latest calculation was two thousand psychiatric beds per one million inhabitants; that is, for a population figure of 87,308,930 persons we would require 174,618 beds for the mentally ill. If the ideal institution averaged 700 beds, 250 such institutions would be necessary in Greater Germany."[49]

The figure of 700 beds in an ideal institution was very low, almost revolutionary, for the time; however, at least according to those documents that have survived, the planners never considered that the highly industrialized regions of central Germany might produce more mental illness than, say, East Prussia. When reports took note of social distinctions, they did so only with the greatest reluctance. For example, Saxony was described as a "heavily populated industrial area" with "proportionately high admissions figures" and a "great demand for beds," which had to be taken into account despite the "effects" of the Operation and the "particularly high mortality rate that might exist in Saxon institutions."[50] The plans for Bremen stated: "Dr. Wex attributed the higher instance [of mental illness] in Bremen to 'dockworkers' illnesses' (syphilis, alcohol) and Nordic inbreeding."[51] The same "illness" was acknowledged in Hamburg, which exceeded its quota of psychiatric hospital beds by almost 100 percent, in comparison with Bremen's mere 25 percent oversupply.[52]

It is difficult to determine whether this mechanistic orientation ever became a problem for the T-4 planners. However, a paper entitled *Zur Planung!* (On planning!), by Robert Müller, a close collaborator of Nitsche's in T-4, was obviously written in protest. In it, he demands that only "*one* factor" be decisive—prewar admissions figures, an indicator Müller was the only one to note in his planning proposals.[53]

The extermination plans were based on precise investigations by commissions throughout the German Reich; in 1942, they covered not only large institutions but even the smallest old age homes, poorhouses, and workhouses. In these cases, planning was always linked with very practical evaluations and proposals for extermination. The following examples are from Saxony, where the planning commission, led by a doctor named Gerhard Wischer, visited 82 homes and institutions:

Report on the Mittweida Reformatory and Home
. . . It is headed by Director Wendelin, who has a very positive attitude. The home regularly reports any severe cases of feeble-mindedness that

occasionally appear among juveniles, or transfers them to neighboring institutions.

Report on the Schottenberg Home in Buchholz-Saxony
. . . The home makes quite a good impression. The large number of retarded and mentally ill inmates (45 percent) is striking. It was suggested to the director of the home and the resident physician that a number of disruptive mentally ill inmates be transferred to asylums. Both completely agreed with this, and intend to transfer 20 inmates to asylums in the near future.

Report on the Nursing Home Kauschwitz near Plauen
The institution is run by the city of Plauen; originally it had 100 beds. It admitted chronic psychiatric cases from the Psychiatric Department of the Plauen Hospital (Dr. Gaupp). A hospital for chronically ill patients from the Departments of Internal Medicine and Surgery of the Plauen Hospital has been established at the institution (44 beds). An additional 44 beds accommodate senile dementias. At the time, there were only eight psychiatric cases in the home, of which two were to be sent to Arnsdorf in the next few days. Dr. Gaupp did not intend to take any more psychiatric cases at all in the future, so that K. will become purely an old age home. . . .

Old Age Home in the Rural District of Auerbach (Vogtl.)
. . . This old age home is located in the rural district of Auerbach. It is currently directed by Inspector Kirchhoff. The district magistrate of Auerbach, Dr. Becker, has already purged the home of most of its feeble-minded and mentally ill inmates, and in the future only the aged will be accepted. For this reason, no new report forms will be filled out. The heads of the home made a very good and sensible impression. . . .

The Wettinstift Old Age, Retiree, and Children's Home in Coswig, Dresden District
. . . Because the inhabitants of this old age home are kept occupied, they do not feel useless and are protected from monotony, etc. Even minor achievements by the inmates, who cultivate all their own crops and butcher animals (in the home's own slaughterhouse), make it possible to keep food costs down (adults 1.90, infants .80, preschool children 1.20, and school-age children 1.40). The home operates without any subsidies.

Report on the City Home in Döbeln-Saxony
. . . There is a strikingly high incidence of feeble-mindedness and even schizophrenia and idiots who are uncontrollable among the elderly

nursing cases. There was even a healthy child of approximately 10 years of age in the home, supposedly only temporarily. I would mention, for example, an old lady of 74 who was in a cold cell, supposedly because she was unable to behave calmly "due to depravity." She was severely ill with arteriosclerotic delirium; the woman was entirely withdrawn and no longer responsive. With the help of the Döbeln district physician (Dr. Brendel), I arranged to transfer this woman and a particularly disruptive idiot to a hospital.[54]

Patients with diverse illnesses were no longer to be treated in the same institutions. Diagnoses and reasons for institutionalization were carefully distinguished. The planners suggested turning numerous institutions into homes for the old and infirm, in order bureaucratically to separate problems resulting from poverty in old age, arteriosclerosis, and abandonment from psychiatric problems. Other institutions would be turned into pure reformatories or—if their location was particularly attractive—convalescent homes for soldiers or German mothers. The loss of institutions during the early period of euthanasia greatly reduced spatial options. The planners ascertained the precise economic and therapeutic capacities of each institution, as well as the state of the property, and made suggestions for future use. The end product included picture portfolios of each institution—for example, over 300 photographs of Bethel—and an index, updated monthly, with short notes on the year of construction, the owner, layout, size, commercial undertakings, railroad stations, and railroad connections (see fig. 4.3). Because of the progress of the war, these data could no longer help promote the original goal of relatively comprehensive, optimized psychiatric care throughout the Reich. However, starting in the spring of 1943, they became important in laying the groundwork for the phase of institutional murder—the phase in which, in response to large-scale air raids on German cities, a new, rapidly growing wave of exterminations ensured the availability of emergency medical care.[55]

Because of the course the war took, conflicts over the future of the new institutions were never settled. The planning commission under Becker and Trieb had clearly distinguished between actively therapeutic psychiatric hospitals near cities and cheap holding asylums "for hopeless cases." The T-4 psychiatrists had another vision, however, more horrible in its sterility, to offer Becker, the sports physician, and Trieb, the economist. Robert Müller formulated this concept in a 1942 report of an inspection tour by psychiatrists (rather than administrative specialists) through asylums in Baden:

The Rastatt home (now a prisoner of war hospital) raises a basic question. The planning commission wants this institution restored to its original purpose as a home only for hopeless cases no longer requiring therapy. I would like to think that such homes will no longer exist in the future. In implementing the contemplated euthanasia law, we cannot allow asylums to attain the reputation of institutions of death—in other words, asylums in which death awaits those transferred there. One of the basic conditions for implementing euthanasia is that it be as inconspicuous as possible. This means, first of all, an inconspicuous milieu. And this is undoubtedly best provided by the institutions that have been asylums until now. There we can accommodate incurable, chronic, or far advanced cases for which euthanasia will be or has been decided upon, in the usual wards or houses for the disruptive or infirm. These establishments and the general conditions for euthanasia cases must be indistinguishable from traditional nursing institutions. Euthanasia directives and their implementation must remain completely integrated into normal asylum routine. Thus, with few exceptions, euthanasia deaths will be all but indistinguishable from natural deaths. That is what we strive for. . . . Thus, we hope for the future not asylums for serious cases but instead hospitals with active therapy and scientific activity— and facilities for euthanasia.[56]

The Development of the "Operation" into the Reich Office for Mental Hospitals

Calculating costs for patients transferred to intermediate institutions and later killed elsewhere proved endlessly complicated. In the spring of 1941, T-4 hired two new administrative specialists: administrative lawyer Dietrich Allers and administrative expert Hans Joachim Becker from the Hessian state welfare agency.* Becker became the actual director of the new Central Clearinghouse for Mental Hospitals (Zentrale Verrechnungs-

---

* There were three Beckers involved in T-4. Hans Joachim Becker came to T-4 in 1941 to direct the Central Clearinghouse. In 1943, he also became office manager at the Hartheim extermination center. He had acquired the necessary professional experience at the regional office in Hesse. Dr. Herbert Becker probably also came to T-4 in 1941 to direct its planning department. In internal correspondence, the two Beckers were distinguished as "Becker" and "Dr. Becker." In addition, August Becker, Ph.D., played a role. He belonged to the Main Office of Reich Security and was employed as a gas specialist for T-4 and later in the gassing operations in Poland and the Soviet Union.

stelle der Heil- und Pflegeanstalten; ZVSt). "The clearinghouse was essentially the financial intermediary between the cost carriers and the so-called intermediate institutions and euthanasia facilities, the names and existence of which were to be kept secret."[57] This new procedure elegantly resolved bureaucratic frictions.

The procedure did not, however, close the gap in the camouflage, as was originally intended. On the contrary: "The invoices we were to issue indicated that a large number of mental patients had died within a very short space of time. From these invoices, even the most simple-minded person would have noticed what was going on here, that it was a planned operation. To top it off, in most cases incidental costs of around 20 RM were added."[58]

Initially, the new office was attached to T-4, though it had its own separate address. In September 1941, even as the office of the Reich Commissioner was taking legal form, the clearinghouse became a separate public institution, the office of the Director of the Central Clearinghouse for Mental Hospitals. Allers, who continued to manage T-4, was named director. Routine operations were conducted by Hans Joachim Becker.

He conducted them so well that the organization soon began to turn a profit, which Becker passed on to T-4's economic department to enable the organization to finance itself. This earned him the nickname "Million Becker." These funds were probably also the source of a generous donation by T-4 to the Society of German Neurologists and Psychiatrists in 1941. Professor Ernst Rüdin thanked T-4 for this 10,000-mark contribution.[59]

T-4 money was obtained not only from the assets of murder victims but also from the gold in their teeth, a practice begun long before its better-known use in connection with the extermination of the Jews. Its most important source of income, however, was the fact "that no costs were incurred during the euthanasia cases' final days; however, we charged for the cost of care up to the day of death."[60] H. J. Becker billed even beyond the actual day of death, with the help of falsified death certificates.

Of course, these methods could not be taken too far without triggering renewed disputes with state welfare agencies. Where no resistance was to be expected, however, namely in the case of murdered Jewish asylum inmates and the Jewish health insurance that had been forced upon them, the billing experts enriched T-4 relentlessly. They added several months onto the lives of murdered Jews who had supposedly been deported to a fictitious "Cholm, Post Lublin": "Thus, this operation brought particularly high profits." According to Becker's estimates, the "large bill" he

1. Name: ~~[redacted]~~	Vorname: ~~[redacted]~~	bei Frauen auch Geburtsname:

2. Geburtsort: *Danzig* 3. Geburtsdatum: ~~[redacted]~~ *1898*

4. Kostenträger: *[handwritten]* 5. Staatsangeh.: *[handwritten]* 6. Rasse: *[handwritten]*

7. Anschrift der nächsten Angehörigen: —

8. Anschrift des gesetzlichen Vertreters: /

9. Wie oft in Anstalten (Kliniken)?	3	16. Diagnose: *[handwritten]*
10. Wie lange im ganzen? (in Jahren)	16	Zustandsbild in Stichworten *[handwritten]*
11. Besteht Vormundschaft?	0	*[handwritten]*
12. Erhält Patient regelmäßig Besuch?	0	*[handwritten]*
13. In Familienpflege?	0	
14. Wert der Arbeitsleistung?	0	*[handwritten]*
15. Art der Arbeit?	0	Grad der Ausprägung: [3]

	Sa +	Rein Ø	Bemerkungen:
17. Nicht erbliches Leiden?		0	
18. Erbliches Leiden?	+		
19. Belastung? (Soweit bekannt)		0	Womit? /
20. Idiotisch? Dement? Kontaktunfähig?*	+		
21. Körperlich hilflos?		0	
22. Therapie aussichtslos?	+		
23. Auch Arbeitstherapie aussichtslos?	+		
24. Asozial? Gemeinschaftsfeindlich?*		0	Auch prämorbid? [0]
25. § 51 Abs. 1, Abs. 2, § 42b, § 42c?*		0	§ 51 Abs. 1 oder 2 alt?* [0]
26. Besteht körperliches, unheilbares Leiden?		0	Welches?

* Zutreffendes unterstreichen.

A new, "objectified" T-4 registration form from 1943. Entries on form: (1) name, first name, maiden name; (2) place of birth; (3) date of birth; (4) insurance agency; (5) citizenship; (6) race; (7) address of closest relatives; (8) address of legal representative; (9) how often has patient been in institutions (clinics)? (10) how long in all? (in years); (11) is there a guardian? (12) does the patient receive regular visits? (13) is patient in home care? (14) value of labor? (15) type of work? (16) diagnosis—notes on condition; (17) nonhereditary illness? (18) hereditary illness? (19) problems? (to extent known): what kinds? (20) idiotic? dementia? incapable of contact? (21) physically helpless? (22) no chance of successful therapy? (23) no chance of successful work therapy? (24) asocial? antisocial? premorbid? (25) Para. 51 sec. 1, sec. 2, Para. 42b, Para. 42c? Para. 51, sec. 1 or old sec. 2? (26) is there physical, incurable illness? what kind?

wrote earned "approximately two to three hundred thousand reichsmarks."[61]

The Central Clearinghouse had still broader goals; it hoped to use financial leverage to reform and standardize the entire German institutional system, making it possible to introduce "uniform regulations throughout the Reich following the war." The varying legal conditions of institutionalization and treatment were to be reconciled and a uniform cost system created. T-4's system of patient transfers and its centralized, anonymous billing system paved the way for standardization.

H. J. Becker recovered money from hundreds of cost carriers—municipalities, welfare agencies, health insurance and pension funds—and paid the costs of intermediate facilities and extermination centers. Above all, however, he simply reconciled differing regional rates without becoming involved in conflicts with individual cost carriers: "It [is] the nature of my office to pay the effective rates to admitting institutions and collect the effective hospital rates from cost carriers."[62] Different supply systems and payment modalities could thus be standardized quite simply. Varying costs for different methods of care and treatment were reconciled without any changes being required of the cost carrier. It was possible to allow an incurable patient to starve, while using the money thus saved to lavish upon another patient the full arsenal of treatments then available to psychiatry. At least theoretically, this system also allowed T-4 to bill the same amount for outpatient treatment as for institutionalization.

> When, for example, a mental patient from Tapiau in East Prussia was transferred to Altscherbitz in the province of Saxony, the welfare agency responsible for Tapiau had to pay the mental patient's expenses to the Altscherbitz institution. Since, in the province of Saxony, the cost of hospitalization was one Reichmark per head per day higher than in East Prussia, the two welfare organizations came into conflict. After creation of the Central Clearinghouse, the East Prussian state welfare agency would pay the clearinghouse the old rate for transferred patients; the clearinghouse then paid the new institution its higher rate. Since this was reversed in other cases, i.e., the new rate was lower than the old one, a balance was generally maintained.[63]

Paragraph seven of the Ordinance to Simplify the Welfare Law of 7 October 1939 had already established a partial legal basis for these practices. The paragraph, a typical Nazi enabling clause, permitted the Reich Ministry of the Interior to determine "final responsibility for welfare payments, where it deviates from the ordinance on welfare responsibility." [64] At first, this vague, nonspecific regulation, which may have been issued in connection with the beginning of the euthanasia program, was not implemented. In early 1944, Allers suggested "uniform regulation of the entire body of mental health law throughout the Reich" and elimination of the "unimaginably large number" of individual regulations. Admissions procedures and costs were to be standardized. The new central office would not only make the Reich Commissioner for Mental Hospitals superfluous but would allow all department heads, bureaucrats, and regional office workers responsible for the institutional system "to be abolished." In addition, "charitable institutions" could be "slowly phased out," and "the operation of private asylums [could be] prevented by changing Reich business regulations." Through these small legal steps, "the entire mental health care system" would eventually be collected "under one roof." [65] Allers's paper also addressed the question whether institutions could be expropriated, with or without compensation, for the benefit of the Reich and in order to promote centralization.

Two days earlier, H. J. Becker had put together a proposal containing an even clearer statement: In recent years, the state had "shown great initiative in the care of the mentally ill." It had "introduced measures" that had led to a "completely new orientation of the mental health care system." The "practical work"—this formulation refers to the thousands of murders—had succeeded in spite of all existing legal difficulties, and "the task had been accomplished." Only an "administrative foundation" could make this work "truly fruitful," however. This should be implemented from above, with the help of a Central Office for the Care of the Mentally Ill. Becker wanted to create a new high-level office, the Director of the Reich Office for Mental Hospitals. [66] Those immediately responsible to the director would be the planning department and the institutional supervisors. Two self-contained subdivisions of this office would take care of so-called practical work.

The second projected department of the planned Reich office would be called the Arbeitsgemeinschaft der Heil- und Pflegeanstalten (AHA; the Association of Mental Hospitals). Becker only hinted at its activities; however, he sketched the consensus among "favorably inclined" German psychiatrists briefly and accurately:

> The predominant activity of this department is medical work. From a purely practical standpoint, it is responsible for evaluating report forms and carrying out the measures following from them. Through intensive collaboration with asylums, it will assure that everything possible is

done in cases worthy of treatment and research. It is the job of the AHA to ensure that personnel receive continuing education in the care of the mentally ill through meetings with medical directors. Further, it is to carry out all research in this area.[67]

The other main department of the new Reich office would be the office of which Becker was already the acting head; that is, the Central Clearinghouse for Mental Hospitals. This department would record all asylum inmates in a central index and reimburse institutions for the costs of care, while collecting these costs from insurance carriers. Billing, however, would no longer be done by name, but only according to the number of days in care. This would create a central clearinghouse in which only the overall balance mattered, not individual transfers. Becker also considered whether regional cost carriers ought to be billed at all, or whether the revenue redistribution should simply be "made possible through corresponding cuts in tax remittances to cities and districts." The new office would allow a 15-fold reduction in necessary administrative personnel: "For its activities, the clearinghouse . . . will require an estimated 30 employees, predominantly female. As discussed, these activities consist almost exclusively in indexing, cataloguing, and statistical and registration work. A bookkeeping system organized along commercial lines will be able to manage with two or three workers."[68]

Like the planning department of T-4, H. J. Becker did not have a strategy of integrating murder into normal institutional routine; instead, he had a clear plan for different institutions that could be made economically viable through variable costs of care.

A = Special Hospitals
(All types of treatment applied in cases worthy of treatment)
B = Mental Hospitals
(Predominantly admitting and transit institutions, and for treatment of non-long-term cases)
C = Nursing Institutions and Homes
(Specifically for nursing or custodial cases, whereby the nursing homes are intended more for the aged infirm).[69]

For Becker, this implied complete control over the patients in C institutions, a conclusion that apparently remained unchallenged within T-4. If patients were incurable, their fate was not a matter for doctors but for economists and bookkeepers. H. J. Becker saw the issue as one of state economics as well as of business management; he even calculated economic losses due to friction resulting from "unproductive excitement" over the death of a "useless person." Becker and Allers's team applied industrial psychology in a breathtaking optimization of trouble-free death, which they continued until the military collapse of the Nazi regime. The more difficult external and internal conditions became, the more they refined their "Instructions for Institutions Admitting the Mentally Ill from Other Areas of the Reich," which has survived in different forms (quoted here in the version of 28 April 1944). It illustrates the power of the Central Clearinghouse and its murderous flexibility.

I. (a) *Discharges and Long-term Leave Leading to Discharge:*
The decree of the Reich Minister of the Interior of 11 May 1943—Az. IV g8958/43–5100—applies to patients from areas threatened by air raids. It permits discharges only when it can be guaranteed that the patient will probably not be reinstitutionalized for a significant period after discharge. The institution may act according to its own judgment. My office's involvement is unnecessary. If there should be difficulties in special cases, correspondence as well as the patient's files are to be given to me so that I may make a decision if necessary. . . .

II. *Notification of Relatives:*
(a) It is necessary for at least one relative to receive brief notification that *admission* has taken place. The address of the closest relative will be easy to ascertain from the files. I consider it expedient to inform them simultaneously that visits can only be permitted in exceptional cases due to the great distance and strained transportation situation.
(b) *Concerned* relatives must be notified by mail of significant *deterioration* in the condition of the patient. This information can be omitted for relatives who, according to the files, care little or not at all about the patient.
(c) In *case of death,* a telegram is to be sent immediately to the closest relatives. The telegram must state that the patient will be buried in the usual way in the institution's cemetery (or the local cemetery) unless other arrangements are made immediately. In order to enable relatives to participate, the funeral generally should occur not less than four days following the day of death.
(d) Should letters or other messages arrive for a patient after his *decease,* I request that a short notice regarding the patient's death be sent back, and that notations such as "addressee deceased" be avoided as far as possible. . . .

IV. *Notification of Change:*
I must be immediately notified of any change in the number of patients. The forms I have made available are to be used for this. Two copies of the form are to be submitted. Names and dates must be filled out with extreme care, as they will be the basis for billing. I ask that forms be requested early.

In group transfers, the forms are not to be used. It is sufficient to submit a list to me.

I will notify cost carriers. No report should be made to them by the institution.

V. *Handling of the Estate of Deceased Patients:*
The property of deceased patients should be sent to the relatives. This applies to underclothes and clothing as well as objects of value, insofar as these are mementos or other objects of minor value. They will be shipped at the recipient's expense. I request that packaging be used that is already available, where possible. Where objects of *real* value are included in the estate, I am to be consulted as to whether they should be claimed to partially cover costs. . . .

VI. *Miscellaneous:*
(a) *Funeral Costs:* . . .
In general, the institution should not submit written requests for funeral expenses to relatives. An exception is to be made—as stressed in III(b)—when relatives pay the funeral costs to the institution immediately after burial. Should relatives inquire as to how funeral costs are handled at the institution, they should be referred to me.

(b) *Transport of Bodies:*
If relatives insist on transporting the body despite the difficult transportation situation, they must bear all resulting costs.

(c) *Costs of Visits:*
Under certain circumstances, I can approve a contribution to the additional expenditures made by needy relatives who have incurred considerable additional expense to visit a patient in seriously deteriorating condition or to participate in a funeral at the institutional cemetery. I request that, in cases which seem appropriate, the relatives be informed and referred to me.[70]

Starting in the winter of 1943–44, Allers and H. J. Becker were the most influential people at number 4 Tiergartenstrasse and in the newly established central office at Hartheim Castle, where the bulk of the extermination and planning bureaucracy was moved in August 1943. At the end of 1943, Allers had Nitsche's planning doctor, Herbert Becker, fired. Becker complained self-pityingly to his mentor: "All the planning will probably be done from Berlin by Allers and Fräulein Schwab, on the side, as it were."[71] Though Herbert Becker regretted "all the work, time, and expense," the time for amateur medical planners was over. His plan, which failed to distinguish between rich and poor, paying patients and government pensioners, was replaced by a three-tier care and extermination plan with room for special cases such as Bethel. This institution was safe from the Reich's standardizing grasp, not only or primarily because of Friedrich Bodelschwingh, the director, who opposed the euthanasia program, but because of its patient composition—which horrified Herbert Becker, though he did not analyze its class structure: "Sixty-five percent of its patients are private!!!"[72] T-4's business department, its Central Clearinghouse, and its executive management had reduced the doctors to subordinate suppliers of information, returning them to therapy and healing. They were still permitted to decide marginal cases, but nothing more. An old man like Nitsche was weak enough for this role.

As late as February 1945, Hans Joachim Becker issued a form with which doctors were to report sick forced laborers who "would probably remain in the institution more than four weeks." In the final days of the Third Reich, a forced laborer who might not be able to work for more than four weeks had lost the right to live. The decision was no longer made by a physician but by the Central Clearinghouse on the basis of a few lines in a "report of findings."[73]

Murder of Children and the "New German Children's Hospital"

The "Children's Operation" carried out by the Reich Committee for the Scientific Processing of Serious Genetic Diseases (18 August 1939–April 1945) was more than simply one facet of Nazi mass murder. After the war, the adjective "scientific" in the Reich Committee's long-winded name was dismissed all too readily as camouflage.

In 1944, Hans Heinze, a psychiatrist implicated in both extermination organizations, recommended the "Reich Committee's experiences" to T-4 as a "model" that could "steer things in the right direction."[74] Unlike the rapid elimination of adult mental patients, implemented with the help of hurried expert opinions and gas chambers, the Children's Operation, which began slowly, was intended as a progressive Nazi health policy. After cases were thoroughly reviewed by three experts, handicapped children were killed individually by specially authorized and trained doctors.[75] Science, research ambitions, and reformist zeal combined in the Reich Committee to form an explosive mixture of progress and extermination.

In the spring of 1942, Reich Committee expert Ernst Wentzler registered the Association of German Children's Hospitals with a district court in Berlin. It was sponsored by Reich Health Leader Leonardo Conti. Representatives of the Führer's Office (Viktor Brack), the Nazi party's Main Office of Public Health, and the Health Office of the Nazi party social services agency were present at its establishment. Wentzler, who had initiated it, was elected chairman; Brack became his deputy.[76] The association's goal was to double pediatric beds per 10,000 inhabitants from 3.9 to 8, a target that required a program to build 300 children's hospitals. Small, manageable hospitals with approximately 100 beds were the goal; "mammoth institutions, . . . generally unmanageable and soulless because of their size," would be a thing of the past. It was time "to make fundamental changes in the accommodation of sick children in pediatric hospitals," in three ways: (1) from a psychological and pedagogical perspective, (2) medically, and (3) in regard to finance and construction.[77]

The association formulated a transition from children's hospitals managed on public financial principles to the German children's hospital "of the future" conducted on a commercial basis. Today, years after West Germany's social-liberal coalition passed a new hospital financing law in 1978, many hospitals still function on this basis. "Hospital management is conducted according to private-sector economic principles. The advantages of public health institutions ought to be combined with those of private hospitals. In general, a hospital is to be organized so that no contributions become necessary from the hospital's sponsor. Nevertheless, institutional management must serve the public good in all respects."[78]

"When at all possible," however, this "new German children's hospital" was to have no more than 200 beds "so there is constant human contact between the medical director, the parents, and the children entrusted to him."[79] The monopoly on treatment enjoyed by doctors in private practice would not be stubbornly defended; instead, the hospital was to be a "polyclinic . . . in friendly collaboration with independent practitioners."

> Psychological and pedagogical care of the children is to be taken consciously into account during construction and organization, and applied particularly as a therapeutic factor in the treatment of the children.

(Colors in the rooms, units of 12 to 16 beds, consultation with pre-school and school teachers, etc.). . . .

For this work to be successfully organized, centrally regulated clinical collaboration will be arranged and practiced by all institutional directors and nearby specialists in other medical areas. The rule will be that the specialist actually comes to the child, and not vice versa, as has generally been the case.

Above all, the chief pediatrician is to be responsible for the whole child, so that, despite his acknowledged importance, the consulting specialist's role will be merely supplementary and generally a one-time-only occurrence. . . .

A state-accredited school for infant and pediatric nurses is planned for "German children's hospitals" with a particular number of beds and isolation units. . . .

Preventive health care is to be emphasized—mother and child counseling, prevention of rickets and infectious diseases, particularly tuberculosis, diphtheria, and scarlet fever, and regular pediatric dental care.[80]

The location of the office (44 Zeltingerstrasse, Berlin-Frohnau) was Wentzler's private pediatric clinic, where handicapped children were also murdered. With the participation of the architecture professor Walter Krüger and the respected Freiburg professor of pediatrics Carl Nöggerath, a new model building for the Wentzler clinic was to be erected on a "parklike site with pines and deciduous trees" in the Berlin district of Frohnau. The war was not considered a disadvantage, since wartime limits on construction made particularly intensive planning possible; this, in turn, would make its realization "that much better and more flawless."[81]

At the same time that Wentzler was pursuing this reformist program, he made the decision to murder thousands of handicapped children. The Association of German Children's Hospitals was not a "secret Reich matter." Nevertheless, it was based on euthanasia of children, and it was hardly accidental that the 200,000 Reichmarks it donated to finance its planned model children's hospital was capital confiscated from a Catholic order considered "hostile to the state."[82] Expropriation from "enemies of the state" and destruction of unusable people were both preconditions and complementary elements of the new, cheery, reformed German children's hospital.

On 18 August 1939, an unpublished decree by the Reich Ministry of the Interior introduced "mandatory reporting of deformed, etc. new-

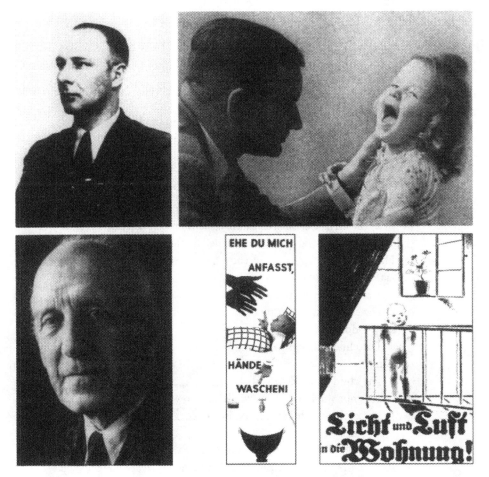

The planners of the New German Children's Hospital: (*top left*) Viktor Brack; (*top right*) Ernst Wentzler; (*bottom left*) Carl Noeggerath. (*right*): health measures in an educational brochure by the euthanasia doctor Wentzler.

borns." Reports were to be sent to the Reich Committee for the Scientific Processing of Serious Genetic Diseases, Berlin W9, P.O. Box 101. The committee was responsible to the Office of the Führer of the Nazi party. To be reported were: idiocy, Mongolism, microcephalus, hydrocephalus, deformations of all kinds, such as spina bifida, and paralyses, including Little's disease. The expanded 1940 text of the report form read as follows:

Report of a case of _____
in the child _____
1. Information on the disease or illness
(a) Most apparent symptoms _____
(b) Is the illness stable or progressive?
2. Information on the birth of the child _____
(a) . . . does the same or similar illness appear in the family?
(b) Other major illnesses _____

If the report was made by a midwife, the following group of questions on development was to be completed "to the extent possible" by the district health official:

(a) Does the physician believe improvement or cure can be expected?
(b) Will the child's life span be shortened by the condition?
(c) Has the child _____ already been medically or institutionally evaluated?
(d) Has physical development been normal until now?
(e) 1. The child sat up during the _____ month—sits—does not yet sit—does not sit on its own.
   2. The child learned to talk in the _____ month—does not yet talk.
   3. The child learned to walk in the _____ month—walks—still does not walk—does not walk on its own.
   4. The child was toilet trained in the _____ month—is still not toilet trained . . .
(f) Was the child always or sometimes noticeably calm or restless?
(g) Does the physical development of the child correspond to its age— to what extent does it not?
(h) Have any marked symptoms, in particular convulsions, been observed?*

* In the 1960s, this questionnaire was still being used in Bavaria in its original written form. The form was based on the secret decree on child euthanasia of 18 August 1939, as well as the Bavarian ministerial decree (*bayerischer Ministerialerlaß*) of 18 April 1950, III8–5292a5. The files used by the author also contain an 11 December 1945 directive from the regional administrative head in Munich (no. T 5000/48) stating that "under the ministerial decree 5346 b 1 of 30 November 1945, mandatory reporting of deformed etc. newborns using the form created in 1939 will continue until further notice." Moreover, the files also contain a decree (*Erlaß*) of 30 June 1958 (no. II/12–5009 c 17), "Betr.: Erhebung über Mißbildung bei Neugeborenen" (Re: Inquiry on deformities in newborns), which stated: "Dr. Saller of the Institute of Anthropology and Human Genetics of the University of Munich, Richard

Midwives, family doctors, pediatricians, and district health officials filled out the report forms—at first only for newborns and children up to three years of age, later for children up to sixteen years of age.

The information requested under (e) on the questionnaire matches child development "milestones" still in use throughout Germany today. Consistently enough, Wentzler, the Reich Committee expert, created a "developmental table" in 1966; Wilhelm Bayer and Hannah Uflacker, physicians who had been involved in the extermination program, propagated this scientifically flavored poison in hundreds of thousands of editions of popular household guides to infant care.

In 1949, the indictment against Reich Committee expert Richard von Hegener provided some details of how this decree was implemented:

> Members of Office II of the Reich Office emptied the mailbox daily. Von Hegener's job was to check over the reports that arrived daily with great care and separate out cases that would probably be treated. All cases that, in his view, absolutely had to be exterminated were copied initially in triplicate. V. Hegener then forwarded the copies to the so-called consultant committee of the Reich Committee for the Scientific Processing of Serious Genetic Diseases, which consisted of three doctors appointed by Hitler's personal physician, Dr. Brandt. This committee had to go through the file of the child to be exterminated and return it to the committee with a recommendation. If the recommendations were approved, they were presented to Hitler's attending physician, Dr. Brandt; with his signature, he essentially indicated that nothing more stood in the way of killing the child in accordance with the circular. After Dr. Brandt approved the extermination, the files went back to Hegener, who, in a confidential letter, informed the district physician responsible for the child's place of residence that the child with the said disease whom he had reported for treatment was to be transferred to one of the Reich Committee for the Scientific Processing of Serious Genetic Diseases' "pediatrics departments" at the _____ institution.

According to von Hegener, by the time he stopped working, when the

---

Wagnerstr. 10, has requested support from the State Ministry of the Interior for an inquiry on the incidence of deformities in newborns. Health officials are instructed to support Dr. Saller in his project, and in particular to allow representatives of the Institute to examine files on hereditary illness and midwife reports of deformities." Geneticist Karl Saller was one of a very few German professors who refused to participate in the Third Reich's medical crimes (Oberbayerisches Staatsarchiv München, Gesundheitsamt Weilheim, "Meldepflicht missgebildeter usw. Neugeborener").

Third Reich collapsed, approximately 100,000 such reports had been submitted to the Children's Operation, of which, according to him, approximately 5,200 were sent for treatment (killing).

According to von Hegener's statement, a "pediatrics department" of this sort existed in every *Gau* of what was formerly known as the Greater German Reich, generally in mental hospitals, but some also in children's hospitals. At the end of the war, there were approximately 20 to 25 such "pediatrics departments."

In summary, von Hegener's role in the so-called Children's Operation consisted primarily of:

1. Screening all daily incoming reports from health offices, approximately 50 per day, and registering same,
2. Reproducing same and forwarding them to the experts,
3. Obtaining authorizations and correspondence with health officials to admit children into "pediatrics departments," instructions to treat (exterminate) same,
4. Obtaining reports of findings,
5. Taking charge of and calculating the costs of care, etc.[83]

This description of von Hegener's activity is essentially accurate. Of the 100,000 reports, Reich Committee officials directed approximately 20,000 to three permanent consultants: Professor Hans Heinze (director of the Brandenburg-Görden Asylum), Professor Werner Catel (director of the Leipzig University Children's Hospital), and Dr. Ernst Wentzler (pediatrician in Berlin and director of a small private clinic).

Where research and diagnosis were concerned, the extermination departments of the Reich Committee quickly expanded beyond their original purpose. These pediatrics departments soon became more than merely killing sites. In the cases of Lüneburg, Brandenburg-Görden, Stadtroda, Loben, Vienna, and Berlin-Wittenau, we know that all children who came to the attention of psychiatrists or physicians were admitted, diagnosed, and transferred; only in exceptional cases were they killed. The following classification scheme comes from the pediatrics department in Loben (Lubliniec) in Upper Silesia, headed by Ernst Buchalik and Elisabeth Hecker:

Following admission to the clinic, throat cultures were taken from the children and they were examined for diphtheria. During the entire period, there was never an epidemic among the children. The hospital had an average of 60 children ranging in age from 8 months to 18 years.

They remained in the hospital for six to eight weeks at most. After examination, they were separated and transferred:

    1. children between the ages of 4 and 8, boys and girls, who were found normal were sent to Orzesze, where there was a children's home with a school;

    2. retarded children who could learn a trade, boys and girls from 5 to 18, were sent to Lesznica (Bergstatt);

    3. psychopathic children, boys and girls ages 14 to 18, were sent to the Klosterbrück institution;

    4. boys ages 14 to 18 referred by the court were sent to the reformatory in Grotkow (Grottkau);

    5. girls from 14 to 18 referred by the court were sent to the reformatory in Lubliniec;

    6. retarded children, idiots, epileptics, mongoloids, those with hydrocephalus, paralysis cases, etc., were sent to department B in Lubliniec.[84]

The hospital reported only children listed under item six to the Reich Committee. Department B was the extermination department. On Heinze's initiative, those who carried out this highly developed diagnostic selection were repaid with a better address; the selection centers became known as "juvenile psychiatric hospitals."

In his "Suggestions for Future Reorganization of Juvenile Psychiatric Institutions,"[85] which were to be given to Karl Brandt as a supplement to the 1943 reform memorandum, Heinze called for "differentiated planning" in accordance with the categories used in Loben. To begin with, a "department for admission and observation directed by child psychiatrists"—as in Loben and elsewhere—was to observe patients and "strive for separate accommodation in separate institutions." A "definite educational and treatment plan" was to be established; only there could the "tasks set for the Reich Committee be carried out without problems." Educable and ineducable retarded children were to be separated; children damaged primarily by the environment would be distinguished from "inherently aberrant children." Children with nervous and mental disorders obviously would be accommodated in another special department.

Heinze also wanted the institutional *Hilfsschulen* (special schools for retarded children) to be reorganized.* Theoretical intelligence was to

* The term *Sonderschule* [translator's note: special school, in the sense of *absondern*, to segregate, as well as *Sonder,* special] replaced *Hilfsschule* [translator's note: spe-

be strictly separated from practical intelligence, simply to keep from over-taxing certain children and "to find a way to enable them to occupy a modest position in working life . . . given sufficient practical ability."

These classifications and assignments required a diagnostic system. In Brandenburg-Görden, Heinze relied particularly upon psychological tests.[86] The euthanasia recommendations by Heinze's interdisciplinary team of doctors, psychologists, and remedial educators were brimming with conscientiousness and supposedly objective analytic language. Classifications were detailed; the chances of survival for those who did not satisfy the criteria were minimal. The classification system was refined under the conditions of the euthanasia program, as child psychiatry in general experienced an upswing as a result of these murderous activities; it has been retained uncritically in the postwar era.

Based on tests administered by a resident psychologist, who used the most up-to-date methods of the day, Heinze and his ward doctor Hans Fischer evaluated a 15-year-old boy committed to a reformatory for stealing:

At age 14.85, Walter performed at age level 8.60 on the Binet-Simon intelligence test, thus indicating an intelligence lag of 6.25 years. During

cial school, in the sense of *helfen*, to help], which was oriented toward fostering children individually. The *Sonderschule* aims to segregate. The term is more modern. The literature states that the Ministry of Education's Permanent Conference introduced the term into German educational law in 1960. In point of historical fact, however, the term, like the apparently neutral term "handicapped" (*behindert*), comes from the Reich Mandatory Education Law of 6 July 1938. Paragraph six governs "mandatory education of intellectually and physically handicapped children" (RGBl [1938, I], p. 799). (Until then, the German language had had no general expression for these disabilities—only the words "cripple" for the physically handicapped and "idiot" or "feeble-minded" for the mentally handicapped.) They "are required to attend the *Sonderschulen* appropriate for them or the special education especially suited to them." And further, "Whether this requirement exists in individual cases, and which *Sonderschule* the child must attend or which special education the child must participate in, is to be decided by the officials in charge of the schools." Paragraph seven of the law regulates "accommodation of school-age children in institutional and family care." Whether such children were to be compelled to attend such institutions was decided by "school officials together with responsible welfare officials." Only in this case were the children's guardians *supposed* to be heard before compulsory measures were ordered and carried out. The term *Sonderschule* thus stems from a linguistic milieu which also produced the *"Sonderaktion"* (special operation), *"Sonderbehandlung"* (special treatment), or the *"Sonderauftrag"* (special assignment), and which Joseph Wulf has documented and analyzed (Joseph Wulf, *Aus dem Lexikon der Mörder: "Sonderbehandlung" und verwandte Worte in nationalsozialistischen Dokumenten*, Gütersloh, 1963).

An intelligence test used as the scientific justification for the clinical execution of a boy from Berlin at Brandenburg-Görden. The child's age ("LA") was 11.5 years; the institution's psychologist estimated his mental age ("IA") as corresponding to that of a normal 5.8 year old.

the testing, he was responsive and somewhat anxious, and made an effort to respond correctly. His school and general knowledge was not at all commensurate with his age. He was unable to state his date of birth or the date of testing. He was not capable of spontaneously writing simple sentences. In preparing a personal record, he was unable to make himself comprehensible orthographically or with regard to content. In arithmetic, he could only perform operations in the first two basic forms of calculation with numbers from one to ten. He could read only simple syllables, and only by spelling them out. His verbal expressive ability was primitive and frequently ungrammatical. He proved hardly capable of learning in school exercises. Even after repeated explanations, he could not understand the process of division. . . . His performance in technical areas was just as poor. He had difficulty understanding the technique of braiding, and could work only with assistance. In pasting with colored paper, his work was very sloppy and primitive. He was approximately the equivalent of a five-year-old boy. He showed little skill at the simplest practical tasks. He dusted carelessly. Here, too, he was barely able to learn. After a three-week stay here, he could not make his bed in a sufficiently orderly manner, despite repeated instruction. . . . He was hardly able to occupy himself sensibly in his free time. In general, he sat or stood about idly. Along with physical infantilism, infantile psychological trends clearly appeared. From the beginning, he spent his time with the much younger school children. He never asked to be allowed to stay up in the evening with those his own age. His favorite occupation was stringing glass beads like a small child. There was no sign of serious vocational interest.[87]

Objectified and scientifically sterilized in this manner, scientific and bureaucratic interests in extermination fused into a unified whole.

Documentary Digression

Psychiatric Advances, 1943 and 1975

On 23 July 1943, de Crinis and Nitsche discussed resumption of the centrally administered murder of the chronically ill with Karl Brandt, head of the military and civilian health systems.[88] The murders were to be part of the preparation for emergency medical aid to bombed-out cities, which was also centrally managed. As a legacy of their now-irrelevant years of reformist activity, Nitsche and de Crinis read a memorandum at this meeting—"Gedanken und Anregungen betr. die künftige Entwicklung der Psychiatrie" (Ideas and suggestions on the future of psychiatry).[89] They had formulated this document with Professors Ernst Rüdin, Carl Schneider, and Hans Heinze, on the basis of various drafts.

In 1943, German psychiatry had to cede the scope for reform it had acquired through euthanasia to the headquarters charged with waging total war. Although recent attempts at research on and intensive therapy for mental illness (including individual, intentional murders as a last resort) had already given way to an immediate program of undifferentiated mass murder, the euthanasia reformers hoped to salvage at least their constructive ideas before the uncertain end of the war.

I am not comparing the various points in their report with corresponding points in the 1975 West German psychiatric report in order to denounce the latter as "fascist." Instead, the comparison is meant to show that the Nazi murderers, equipped as they were with professorships, were neither common murderers nor racists committing crimes of passion; their deeds were anything but clumsy bungling. Their "psychiatry of the future," designed in 1943 and based on organized euthanasia, was modern. It gained significance after 1945 under different political conditions.

The "historical introduction" to the 1975 report states, "In spite of the struggle for better care and treatment of the mentally ill, after the First World War an important trend in the opposite direction emerged with the discussion on 'sanctioning destruction of worthless lives.'"[90] In fact, the reverse is true. The connection between "better care and treatment" and the simultaneous goal of extermination is obvious. Like the authors of the psychiatric report, the criminals in 1940 opposed "conditions unworthy of human beings," "simple custody," deficient "interest in therapy." Mental institutions were renamed clinics and hospitals beginning in 1942, against a background of therapeutic optimism and "transfers" of long-term patients. The term "nursing" or "maintenance" (*Pflege*) was expurgated from the care of the chronically ill. Today, to a rapidly increasing degree, persons excluded from treatment (the Nazis would have used the term "disqualified"—*ausgeschieden*) by authorities on rehabilitation because they require constant care are materially and socially downgraded by Germany's public welfare system. (Klaus Dörner, a prominent German psychiatrist, speaks of "social euthanasia.") Concerned care and security for the chronically ill are not discussed in either the 1943 or the 1975 report. Post-Nazi reforms should be evaluated according to whether they seek improvements for all (for example, everyone subjected to psychiatry), or attempt to help some by quietly omitting others.

In order to facilitate comparison of the 1943 report with the 1975 report, I have interwoven the two. Each of eleven sections from the 1943 "Ideas and Suggestions on the Future of Psychiatry" is followed by a section (set off in brackets) from the 1975 report of the psychiatric investigative commission released by the West German Bundestag.

> 1943: In the last two decades, the state of psychiatry in Germany has undergone a fundamental transformation. First a move developed toward goal-oriented educational psychotherapy and active psychotherapy. In this context, patient occupations underwent considerable development and expansion; particular indicators were elaborated. In well-run clinics and institutions, these efforts have already brought about a conspicuous change in the psychoses of acute and chronic patients, insofar as the symptoms of illness have substantially diminished. Among other things, the heretofore highly unsatisfactory conditions on

wards for agitated patients have undergone extraordinary improvement; in such institutions, "padded cells" in the old sense no longer exist at all.

[1975: The development of pharmacotherapy, psychotherapy, and rehabilitation methods; new models of care; and therapeutically more effective forms of social treatment have made it possible to treat many mental illnesses successfully and to influence diseases previously considered incurable. Even where the effects of treatment are limited, satisfactory rehabilitation can often be achieved. This means that many mentally ill and handicapped persons can be given the opportunity to regain their place in society, and long-term stays in hospitals avoided. Diagnosis and therapy have become more exact, in large part due to increased consideration of social conditions and the effects of psychological disturbances. (p. 4)]

1943: Other new methods of treatment have also been gradually added—in particular insulin, electroshock, and hormone and dietary therapies. Considerable success has already been achieved in curing and encouraging remission in endogenous psychoses. Melancholia, in particular, has been reduced, and many arteriosclerotic personalities have shown improvement in overall physical and psychological condition. It is to be expected that the progress of research and improvements in therapeutic methods will improve the rate of cure. In any case, it can be said that psychiatry today is a healing discipline in the truest sense of the word.

In light of these developments, the diagnostic and therapeutic goals of psychiatry have increasingly required studies of internal processes, as well as development of a psychiatric metabolic pathology, constitutional morphology, and hormone research.

Above all, however, the psychiatrist in the National Socialist state has fundamental responsibilities concerning methodical registration of and research on the genetic health of the German people, as well as prevention of hereditary illnesses. Psychiatry must not only take an active role in this, but must educate the medical profession in general. The increased importance of the psychiatrist's pathological and anatomical work, especially in light of genetic research and practice, should be emphasized in this context. . . .

The close relationship between neurology and psychiatry is becoming ever more apparent. In light of the facts, we can no longer deny that these branches of medicine very much complement each other, and that psychiatrists require a strong neurological background to the same extent that neurologists need good psychiatric training. This should be stressed especially in the interests of accomplishing medicine's tasks in the area of eugenics.

[*1975:* The expert commission thus strongly advocates the view that psychiatric hospital care is *a fundamental component of general medicine.* The special relationship between psychiatry and neurology is particularly noteworthy in this regard. (p. 205)

From a psychiatric point of view, the central issue in the planned legal arrangement is the *sterilization of mentally handicapped people* who are—to a greater or lesser extent—*incapable of consent.* The drafts fundamentally reject the admissibility of a legal guardian making this decision even for this category of persons . . . although many good reasons may exist for such sterilization in emergency cases; the national association Lebenshilfe für geistig Behinderte (Counseling for the mentally handicapped) has emphatically supported recognition of these reasons.*
(p. 383)]

1943: In the years just before the war, German psychiatry energetically addressed the problems of child psychiatry. Regarding these efforts, see . . . the summary of a recent lecture by F. Stumpfl—known to be a psychiatrist with a strong genetic perspective and research orientation. . . .

Considering the tasks facing psychiatry today, the leadership of the state and those responsible for health care require a productive psychiatric profession and productive hospitals and institutions in order to achieve their national and health-policy goals. It is important to educate these specialists properly, and above all to bring capable young people into the profession. . . .

[*1975:* It is particularly important to encourage specialization in child and juvenile psychiatry. Between the introduction of the specialization in child and juvenile psychiatry in 1969 and 1 January 1972, only 124 doctors in the Federal Republic of Germany, not including West Berlin, had been certified as such. (p. 392)]

---

* The former T-4 expert Professor Werner Villinger was co-founder and chairman (until his death in 1961) of the scientific board of "Counseling for the Mentally Handicapped." This is documented in an important book by Udo Sierck and Nati Radtke, *Die Wohltätermafia: Vom Erbgesundheitsgericht zur Humangenetischen Beratung* (Hamburg, 1984; privately printed).

1943: Everything must be done to combat the frequent denigration of the psychiatric profession, and to emphasize, in contrast, the importance and the scientific as well as practical value of psychiatry. The involvement of these specialists in maintaining genetic health, using measures that naturally often meet with distaste and lack of understanding from the masses, is likely to detract from the regard in which the nation holds psychiatry. However, the more often capable specialists make the public aware of the successes of modern therapy, the more often victims of chronic mental infirmity are cured or at least made capable of returning to work and independent life, thus helping reduce the labor shortage that can be expected in the coming decades, the more the public will consent to genetic measures. It will realize that the medical profession, which is primarily responsible for carrying out these measures, is simultaneously engaged in the large-scale work of healing and prevention; nothing eliminates mistrust of doctors more naturally than visibly successful treatment. For example, good therapists can now expect successful cures and rapid curtailment of suffering in an illness as tormenting and protracted as melancholia; thus, everything must be done to introduce new treatment methods into all clinics and institutions.

[*1975:* The mentally ill and handicapped often face rejection from society in the form of both attitudes and behavior. It is not only the afflicted who perceive this, but also employees of institutions where these people are treated and cared for. . . . Health education and instruction will have to struggle to make available to a broad public information on prevention, therapy, and rehabilitation methods in the area of care of the mentally ill and handicapped. (p. 79ff.)]

1943: Euthanasia measures will meet with more general understanding and approval when it is assured and made public that in every case of psychological illness, all possibilities are explored for curing or improving patients so they can be provided with economically viable employment, either in their own vocations or in another form. That the latter is possible, and indeed without an unreasonable expenditure of resources and nursing personnel, has been shown by the last two decades of psychiatric treatment and research, and in particular by many years of experience employing inmates in agriculture.

It should be stressed here that previous mention of a serious crisis regarding the new generation of psychiatrists was in no way exaggerated. Capable young doctors are already taking flight from psychiatry;

that is, there has been an exodus of trained personnel into other areas of medical activity.

[*1975:* Varied groups of mentally ill, handicapped, and socially isolated patients are collected in large psychiatric hospitals; it is a fact that many of them do not need hospitalization. These often long-term inhabitants of existing psychiatric hospitals should be transferred to other treatment facilities appropriate to their needs. . . .

Aside from a minority of mentally handicapped persons clearly in need of hospitalization, the psychiatric hospital is basically not suited to treat or care for this category of people. (p. 205ff.)]

1943: Regarding the future shape of psychiatric work, the following must be taken into account: It has already been established that all asylums in the Greater German Reich that treat and care for the mentally abnormal are to be registered by a central office and closely monitored. The results of these findings are kept in an index that is continually updated through a requirement that institutions report all changes in patient census and organization.

This creates a reliable basis for future regulation of the institutional system, in the context of which the *following fundamental changes* are to be made:

[*1975:* Collection and evaluation of all relevant data is indispensable in order to ensure adequate planning. (p. 17)]

1943: 1. Uniform organization of the German mental health care system.

2. Basic assurance of psychiatric direction or overall psychiatric supervision of all institutions for the mentally abnormal.

3. Abolition of all private and denominational institutions for the mentally abnormal.

[*1975:* 1. The expert commission recommends an *institution organized at the level of the eleven federal states.* This institution must be set up through agreements between the states. (p. 30)]

1943: 4. All institutions for the psychologically abnormal are to be opened for research through organizational connections with the German Institute for Psychiatric Research, university hospitals, and other research institutes.

5. Acknowledgment and, to the greatest possible extent, application

of the basic principle that asylums should be close to seats of scientific education; in other words, near university hospitals and larger cities with lively medical and scientific communities, in which resident physicians can and must take part.

This principle will be decisive in determining whether existing asylums are to be retained for psychiatric purposes after the war. Such well-situated institutions should not be dismantled or put to other use; if the latter took place during the war, these institutions should revert to psychiatry.

6. Regarding selection of institutions under point 5, as well as possible new construction, it must also be recalled that, depending on their location, institutions can be used for industrial or agricultural work to an extent sufficient to reap economic benefits from occupational therapy.

7. In the interests of treatment, the institutions are to be equipped with all diagnostic and therapeutic equipment.

[*1975:* The clinic of the *Max Planck Institute of Psychiatry* in Munich [formerly the German Institute for Psychiatric Research] is active in applied research, in addition to the basic research undertaken by its Theoretical Institute. (p. 379)

It is particularly important and urgent that we *involve psychiatric hospitals* in medical education. Although many psychiatric hospitals are unfavorably situated in relation to university towns, all psychiatric hospitals should be assigned to a university hospital and should participate in teaching psychiatry, psychotherapy and psychosomatics. (p. 328)]

1943: 8. In order to ensure successful treatment and employment, outpatient clinics are to be set up at institutions to ensure continuing treatment of patients who have been discharged.

9. Where possible, it is recommended that psychiatric clinics and institutions be attached to hospitals for physical illness, since modern psychiatry must maintain a close relationship with somatic medicine, and especially with internal medicine.

(For example, some time ago a general hospital was built in Troppau-Sudetengau on the grounds of an existing asylum and was linked to it financially. In the judgment of the doctors who work there, this has proven extraordinarily useful.)

10. Institutional psychiatrists are to be involved in the racial aspects of juvenile welfare, in criminal-biological treatment in certain districts, and in similar areas of activity.

11. The education of resident physicians should make them competent in every respect for the tasks required of them, and should therefore include racial hygiene and genetics, internal medicine and neurology.

[1975: It has become apparent that the mentally ill in need of preventive care, particularly those requiring intensive aftercare, easily fall through the cracks in existing outpatient services. This results in relapses, chronicity, and setbacks in rehabilitation. Many inpatient readmissions could be avoided if outpatient care were extended and coordinated with inpatient care. (p. 10)

A fundamental guiding principle, particularly with regard to planning and construction of new psychiatric treatment centers, is the forging of close links to general medicine. There are many ways to pursue this goal, such as attaching psychiatric departments to general hospitals (the British model) or integrating a general hospital into an existing psychiatric hospital or one under construction (the Scandinavian model). (p. 218)]

1943: 12. Pathological anatomy must be cultivated in the spirit of the resolution taken by the Society of German Neurologists and Psychiatrists.

13. Continuing scientific training of institutional physicians is to be strongly encouraged.

14. The goals of child psychiatry are to be encouraged in all respects.

15. Institutions are to be directed by physicians. Only scientifically trained, experienced physicians are to be appointed clinical directors. In addition to his scientific qualifications, a clinical director must become familiar with the institution's organizational needs through a preparatory period as acting clinical director, and must prove capable of employing patients in work therapy.

[1975: Medical assistance, especially psychotherapeutic, psychological, and social assistance, and, in certain areas, educational assistance, must supplement one another; they form an integrated whole in the treatment of the mentally ill. (p. 205)

This traditional special position no longer corresponds to the possibilities and demands of modern psychiatry. (p. 204)]

1943: 16. The social position of institutional physicians and nursing staff is to be appropriately structured.

17. The responsible authorities must ensure dissemination of a true image of psychiatry and its work, rather than the often largely inaccu-

rate assessment common at present, and prevent condemnation of these specialists. It appears particularly necessary to provide regular instruction on psychiatric issues to heads of *Gau* offices for public health at their regular conferences. A start in this direction should be made through directed educational activity.

[*1975*: Such educational work will be particularly necessary, however, in areas in which overdue political decisions are not made with the necessary speed. This must be expected in great measure when the necessity of community-based care for the mentally ill and handicapped is not acknowledged, or where resulting local obligations are not taken up vigorously. (p. 81)]

Research on Victims

The interconnections between destruction and modernization, between extermination and research, were the basis of the euthanasia murders. Those involved saw themselves as reformers, as standard-bearers of progress, who would deal a death blow to the oppressive institutional milieu. Through intensive early treatment, a preliminary group of outpatient care facilities, and etiological research, they believed they could utilize the death of thousands to promote the public good.

A March 1939 decision was appended to the 1943 report:

In the interests of public welfare, the Society of German Neurologists and Psychiatrists considers it necessary for autopsies to be performed in all cases of patient deaths in public asylums. Given the importance of these measures for the clarification and understanding of hereditary illnesses, we call for the introduction of a legal requirement that these institutions perform autopsies.

The aim should be to have one institution in each administrative district in which one doctor primarily carries out difficult pathological-anatomical examinations. This is possible using simple methods. Collaboration with a larger institution (a university hospital or research institution) is recommended. Starting in this way, an anatomical institute should be developed for the administrative district if possible.[91]

Carl Schneider

"The more active, critical therapists enter the field, the more conclusively the bleak period of inactivity in psychiatry will come to an end."[92]

Schneider, who wrote this in 1943, inspired such a team of young assistants. He belonged to the Sicherheitsdienst (SD; Security Service) and directed the racial policy office of the Baden *Gau;* yet, in 1937–38, after a tremendous struggle, Schneider himself succeeded in driving inflexible, unscientific Nazi doctors out of the Heidelberg University psychiatric clinic, which he directed.[93] Without outwardly conforming, Schneider personally combined the interests of science and the state, justifying each with the other. In a 1944 "Report on the Condition, Opportunities, and Goals of Research on Idiots and Epileptics in the Context of the Operation," he stated:

> From the beginning of the entire operation, the medical participants knew that the opportunity for researching, combating, and, above all, curing and preventing mental illness should not be allowed to slip by. Even before I began to participate actively in the work, I had the opportunity to attend a discussion with the Chief of Reich Lecturers, at which the problems this occasioned were considered. At the time, it was the unanimous opinion of the scientists present (almost exclusively full professors in different fields) that such an occasion ought not to be missed.[94]

In this research, the "causes of nonhereditary forms of imbecility were to be clarified"; once they were known, "ways and means will be found to intervene preventively, even during pregnancy or the immediate postpartum period." It was hoped that, in the near future, a considerable number of people who otherwise would have been handicapped would simply not be born. (In 1940 the Reich Committee, to which Schneider also belonged,[95] had already switched to intrauterine extermination—i.e., eugenically determined abortion.)[96]

In postwar interrogations, Hans Hefelmann also referred to the link between extermination and intensive therapy and research:

> Right at the beginning of the asylum operation during the Second World War, a general consensus was reached that the institutional manpower, medications, and therapeutic opportunities recovered through euthanasia should benefit the 80 percent of institutional inmates that would probably remain. To this end, a psychiatric expert, Professor Schneider of Heidelberg, consented to be appointed to the Reich Association to further expand therapy and research. This circumstance underlined the moral justification for carrying out the euthanasia measures. In the course of Professor Schneider's appointment, we visited the therapeutic section of the Eglfing-Haar Asylum, which at the time was directed by

Professor Braunmühl. Professor Braunmühl had achieved outstanding therapeutic success with electroshock and insulin therapies that were ahead of their time. Professor Schneider's research department was to spread them to other institutions as well.[97]

Anton Edler von Braunmühl is known in psychiatric history as *the* theorist of shock therapy* of the postwar period.[98] In 1945, he successfully convinced the Americans that he had been a member of the resistance.[99] In May 1942, Braunmühl wrote a (now lost) "Plan for the Orga-

---

* See in particular the impressive essay by Angelika Ebbinghaus, "Kostensenkung, 'Aktive Therapie,' und Vernichtung," in *Heilen und Vernichten im Mustergau Hamburg,* ed. A. Ebbinghaus, K. H. Roth, and H. Kaupen-Haas (Hamburg, 1984), p. 136ff. Using Hamburg as an example, Ebbinghaus describes the development of psychiatric therapies up to the shock therapies of the 1930s. "Even in the past, doctors had often abused the bodies of the mentally ill. Patients were whipped, strapped into revolving chairs, or thrown into cold water, and had to endure other, similar cruelties inflicted upon them with therapeutic intent. In the 1930s, psychiatrists discovered that the brain could be treated in cases of psychic suffering and disturbances. A contemporary psychiatrist correctly identified this development: the transition from body shock to brain shock therapy." Loss of consciousness induced by hypoglycemia during insulin "shock" made the patient "more obedient and easier to control." "Cardiazol convulsion therapy" was based on an antagonism between schizophrenia and epilepsy that was never actually proven. "The convulsions produced artificially by cardiazol almost always released a type of devastated feeling and great anxiety in the patient. These aggressive, brain- and personality-destroying treatments served primarily to quiet patients and make them submit to institutional life."

Ebbinghaus further reports that as early as 1936, 80 out of 320 beds at the Hamburg University Psychiatric Clinic were "reserved exclusively for patients undergoing insulin therapy." "The patients' fear of this very 'active' therapy was enormous. No practicing doctor could fail to notice it." The therapists themselves reported "panic-like anxiety attacks" and also, right from the beginning, deaths. According to Ebbinghaus's information, from 1936 on, admissions figures from the Hamburg University Psychiatric Clinic rose sharply and the duration of stay was radically curtailed. Statistics from the department involved indicate a clear connection between the use of "therapy" and "therapeutically" induced deaths, which can be traced to the newly introduced shock procedure.

Year	Number of Inpatients	Number of Inpatient Deaths
1936	1,333	85
1937	1,990	142
1938	2,196	154
1939	2,516	188
1940	2,113	235
1941	2,391	290

nization of New Treatment Methods for Certain Psychoses at the Present Time" for T-4.[100] It concerned the introduction of electroshock treatment, now that insulin for artificial induction of "therapeutic comas" had become scarce and was forbidden for psychiatric purposes. The provision of asylums with electroshock equipment, which this paper advocated, was later pursued by T-4, the Reich Commissioner, and the Führer's Office as particularly "important to the war effort." In 1943 and 1944, practically all public asylums received electroshock equipment through Richard von Hegener (simultaneously a consultant to the Reich Commissioner and procurement adviser to T-4).[101] Whereas Braunmühl's career got off the ground after the war, Schneider hanged himself in American custody.

Born in 1891, the son of a pastor, Schneider grew up near Leipzig, where he, like many of his future colleagues, attended the university. After a year as Förster's assistant in Breslau and a year at the German Institute for Psychiatric Research in Munich, he transferred to Arnsdorf as government medical officer for Saxony. From 1930 to 1933, he was the first medical director of the Bodelschwingh institutions in Bethel.[102] As Schneider later wrote, this appointment was "accomplished by the state"; as a rule, charitable institutions were headed by church officials, and when the state pressured them to hire doctors at all, they did so "based essentially upon membership in the church."[103]

In 1933, Schneider was named professor of psychiatry and neurology at the University of Heidelberg. Precisely how he came to participate in the euthanasia program is not clear. His membership in the SD, his experiences with the Lutheran Church, and his connections in Leipzig may have been influential; but above all, perhaps, his scientific abilities and interests brought him into the program. Schneider became an expert for T-4 as of 1 April 1940; his chief physician, Konrad Zucker, joined him three weeks later.[104] But not until January 1941 did they succeed in adopting a "Psychiatric Research Plan"—"in accordance with the discussion on 23 January 1941."[105]

This meeting was conducted by Professor Walther Schulze,[106] who headed the Health Department of the Bavarian Ministry of the Interior. From the beginning, Schulze actively promoted euthanasia, while also serving as head of the Reich Lecturers' Association. The location of the meeting was probably the German Institute for Psychiatric Research (the Kaiser Wilhelm Institute). The plan concentrated on schizophrenia, feeble-mindedness, and epilepsy. Mass examinations would assist in researching, among other things, blood composition, physical chemistry of

Name d.Pat.: _X Y_   Diagnose: _Schizophrenie_

.3..Elektroschock am _12.10.43._ Tageszeit. _9.5_ Wetter: _trüb_

Krampfdosis: a) _15 mA/1sec mA._ Spannungs=   a) _+.3.²_
(a. etwaige   b) _20.:/1mA._   schwankungen b) _.12.%._
Abortiv-Krämpfe) c) ....   c) ....
              d) ....   d) ....
              e) ....   e) ....

Beobachtungen beim Ablauf des Anfalls:
      zu a) _abortiv_
      zu b) _Krampfdosis_
      zu c) ....
      zu d) ....
      zu e) ....

1. Dauer der Latenzzeit. _2." _ Sekunden.
2. Traten dann auf ? :   a) "Hampelmann": _+_
                     b) Kieferöffnung: _+_
                     c) Initialschrei: _+++_

3. Dauer vom Ende d.Latenz=
    zeit bis zum Ende der
    Streck-s t a r r e _12."_ Sekunden.
4. ~~Traten bei bzw.nach~~
    der Streckstarre auf   a) Giraffenhaltung: _0_
                     b) Muskelwogen. _0_
                     c) Gänsehautphänomen. _++_

5. Dauer der
    s y m.Zuckungen _21."_ Sekunden
6. Dauer der
    S c h l e u d e r-Z.: _13."_ Sekunden
7. Dauer d.Atemstillst.: _4."_ Sekunden Grad der Cyanose. _++_

Mithin Gesamt-Dauer. _52."_ Sekunden.
==

    Art und Menge des Speichels: _Häufig, wenig._
    Trat Einnässen auf. _0_ .... Trat Einkoten auf: _0_ ....
    Trat Samenabgang auf: _+_ .... Trat Luxation auf: _0_ ....
    Rückenschmerzen nach dem Anfall. _0_
    Kopfschmerzen nach dem Anfall. _+_
    Bemerkungen : _keine_

Prov. Obermedizinalrat,
Direktor Dr. Mennecke
Landesheilanstalt Eichberg (Rheingau)

!28139

Therapeutic research connected with the euthanasia program. This was a
standardized form for electroshock observations at the Heidelberg University
psychiatric clinic.

the brain, chromosomes, metabolic pathology, constitutional type, and the chemistry of aging. After "full clinical examinations," each series of experiments was to conclude with autopsies of the examined patients. That the patients were to be killed after the experiments was not explicitly stated. To prevent the mass experiments from failing due to the lack of skill of the mainly young, inexperienced "implementing physicians" at the extermination centers, Nitsche circulated the following instructions in May 1941: "I request that, at the meeting at Hadamar, directors be informed that a 4–5 percent formalin solution must be used to preserve the brains, that the solution must be changed every three days, and that the brains are to be suspended from the main artery so that they do not rest on the convex surface."[107]

In September 1941, as this research was being planned, the *Zeitschrift für die gesamte Neurologie und Psychiatrie* (Magazine of neurology and psychiatry) published a lavishly illustrated, practical "Introduction to the Physical Examination of the Brain and Skull of a Corpse" ("submitted 28 March"). A. Dohmen, Werner Heyde's assistant in Würzburg, wrote these guidelines for the busy reader. In the article, he briefly and simply described and illustrated techniques for "measuring the body size" of corpses, "sawing open the skull," "removing the brain from the skull cavity," and professional "weighing."[108]

In 1941, Carl Schneider wrote a report for the sixth annual meeting of the Society of German Neurologists and Psychiatrists in Würzburg. The meeting, which was supposed to take place 5–7 October 1941, was then canceled. The final remarks in the draft of his report on "modern treatment procedures in the therapy of endogenous psychoses" have survived. Schneider attributed new significance to therapy and healing in a way that radicalized and simplified the views of earlier psychiatrists: "We find ourselves at a decisive turning point in psychiatry in general. Psychiatry has finally cast aside therapeutic nihilism, which the historian may regard as the belated remains of ancient spiritual and demonic beliefs, and has accepted therapeutic experience as the only means of exorcising psychoses."[109]

Schneider's concept of biology attempted to combine social, psychological, physical, and constitutional phenomena. The pseudoscientific ideas propagated by geneticists were consciously expanded in Schneider's work. Psychiatrists agreed upon forced sterilization of the sick and racially undesirable, in which medical judgment and action combined. They did not agree, however, on the length of time doctors should treat patients whose ailments resisted their curative efforts. In 1941, Schneider formulated the semiofficial state psychiatric position:

> Soon even so-called incurable mental illness will be amenable to therapeutic efforts; patients will be saved from chronic illness and lifelong institutionalization, so that after sterilization they will remain active members of the community despite their illnesses.
>
> To many fellow Germans who are intelligent but nonetheless unacquainted with the state of affairs, such a psychiatric program appears unnecessary and untimely. . . . Indeed, agencies on which psychiatric institutions depend for funding and further development are presently run by officials who think it unnecessary to do anything more for psychiatric institutions and psychiatry, because they will soon be redundant. [This refers to his archenemy, SS colonel Fritz Bernotat, responsible for the Hessen Nassau district organization, with whom Schneider had a running feud because of his neglect of the Eichberg Asylum] . . .
>
> All current measures to relieve economic pressure on our people resulting from expenditures for useless institutional inmates, and all eugenic measures in the broadest sense, are long-term measures. It will take centuries to lower the incidence of endogenous psychoses in the populace to a level normal for a population with completely healthy psychological genes that experiences the normal rate of mutation toward psychoses. Only then will insane asylums really be empty, and only then will it be possible to keep them empty. During this long period, it will be both humane and economically expedient to use intensive treatment as far as possible to prevent both chronic mental illness and the need to institutionalize numerous patients suffering from endogenous psychoses. But it is still possible to relieve our people of a great number of congenital, hereditary, or acquired chronic mental infirmities in other ways.[110]

The document reveals both the scientific optimism and the openness of the discussion at the time. "Current measures to relieve economic pressure on our people" was a common euphemism for murdering the sick, as were the formulations "all eugenic measures in the broadest sense" and "other ways" in which the Volk was to be relieved. In the draft of his speech, Schneider went so far as to use the word "euthanasia" publicly in another part of this report. These were the types of sentences that were to have been presented at the 1941 meeting of the Society of German Neurologists and Psychiatrists. At the same time, Schneider intended to admit publicly a fact that had already become a commonplace among leading Nazi eugenicists: mass sterilization would only be effective in centuries, if at all. What remained for the practicing psychiatrist who was responsible for the health of the nation as a whole was the choice between extermination and active, increasingly aggressive "therapy." As a consequence of this development, "treatment" became a code word for murdering patients.

Until the medical death sentence, however, a patient remained the object of therapeutic efforts, not as a person with a unique life history who had fallen ill, but as a functionally disturbed member of the *Volksgemeinschaft* (national community). Treatment administered to the sick individual was to serve the *Volksgemeinschaft*. Measures were justified only because they ultimately served the healthy majority. Likewise, it was considered legitimate that upright, hardworking citizens should wish to be rid of the "social burden" of the ill. Where a collective, rather than an individual patient, was the object of curative efforts, mass murder could be considered a quasisurgical operation on the body of the nation. In Schneider's words:

> If psychiatry sacrifices the opportunity for successful progress along this path through premature loss of the necessary research tools, it would be like depriving a state's armed forces of the tools necessary to invent and test promising new weapons, in the belief that we could avoid wars through other relationships among nations, entirely mistaken as to the amount of time it would take to reach such a distant goal. No, only if enough money is spent on real treatment now, as psychiatry approaches its great turning point, will we achieve the goal of relieving the nation of the burden of incurable psychoses in every conceivable way.[111]

Treatment of sick people was declared a war, and the laws of war are different from those of peace:

> These organizational measures were also conditioned by the fact that, in terms of the national psychology, euthanasia can only be carried out properly when it is certain that the patient was adequately treated not only in medical, but also in social terms; that is, that he could be classified appropriately through work.[112]

Work therapy had made clear the extent of the damage wrought by custodial institutions. Modern therapy and euthanasia saved money, which Schneider hoped would be used for further psychiatric research. He had planned and partially executed extensive research projects, with the help of the Reich Association of Mental Hospitals:

> The road to ultimate relief lies, not in withholding the funds that current measures allow us to save, but in appropriately spending a portion of them on psychiatric research. In addition, however, there must at last be moral recognition of the work to be done by the psychiatrist for the good of the entire nation. . . . Men whose knowledge of the biology of the psyche and the dangers slumbering within it enables them to protect the nation from these dangers are as indispensable as bacteriology, bacteriological institutes, and researchers became, once the bases for treating numerous diseases were discovered.
>
> As long as people have psychological functions, there will have to be a science within medicine concerned with the links between physical illness and psychological processes, and the alleviation of all kinds of disturbances in this area. Indeed, such a science will become all the more indispensable, the more seriously we intend to transform the slogan of the totality of life into a real understanding of the biology of this totality in health and illness. This science may be called psychiatry or something else; it may eventually be defined as something other than medicine, given the changing classification of the sciences. Increasingly, psychiatry will be one of the basic tools to describe, recognize, and control this psychophysical totality.[113]

Schneider perceived responsibilities extending beyond medicine. In his opinion, psychiatry would be the cornerstone in the edifice of enlightenment, instructing mankind on its own spiritual nature and thereby shedding light on a still largely unknown sphere.

> At last it is time for a discipline that cures human beings to intervene in humanity's intellectual history. A researcher will one day do for psychiatry what Copernicus did for astronomy: exorcise the superstition of religious ideas and dogma from the essence of the soul, thus opening the door to a more profound, richer life for our people, in harmony with its own powers and talents.[114]*

* In keeping with this kind of rationalism, Schneider's subordinate Zucker wrote his postdoctoral thesis on the "psychology of superstition" and requested of Victor Brack that "some of the offices of the Gestapo share their records . . . on those elements in larger cities that are involved in fortune telling and horoscopes, etc., for more or less illegitimate commercial purposes" (Letter from Zucker to Brack, 2 July 1941, BA-MA, H 20, 465). Zucker received the records he requested from the state

Although a general ban on conferences—imposed as the tide of battle turned against Germany—prevented Schneider from delivering his closing remarks to the German neurologists and psychiatrists, he was nevertheless able to begin his research. After years of financial battles with the German Research Association and the university administration, he believed the time had come for a major, long-term project underwritten by a third party. Psychiatry would no longer play second fiddle to scientific medicine; research on mental illness and the well-founded recommendations that would result would make psychiatry the psychohygiene of the national community, the queen of medical knowledge par excellence. Schneider applied for five doctors, five laboratory assistants, and five secretaries; since his research group would of course be interdisciplinary, he also applied for a psychologist and several philologists, to ensure "extensive preliminary work on scientific history and problem studies."* According to Schneider, "All things considered, . . . paying this staff, along with the actual work of the entire enterprise," would "cost approximately a million reichsmarks annually." Schneider further calculated that his long-term "comparative developmental research" would require "total expenditures of RM 15,000,000" over 15 years. In any case, the size of the sum was "disconcerting to the uninitiated."[115]

For the period following the 15-year research phase, Schneider fore-

---

police in Karlsruhe. One year later he completed the thesis, and again asked for help from a higher official. Brack wrote to the chief of the security police:

"Professor Zucker, an academic employee of the operation directed by me and known to you, has written a book on the 'psychology of superstition.' In a letter dated 11 December 1941, you informed him that there were no reservations as to publication of the work. In a letter dated 22 December 1941, Professor Zucker requested that you confirm your interest in publication of the book, in order to obtain the paper necessary for printing. Professor Zucker has not yet received an answer" (Letter from Brack to the chief of the Sicherheitspolizei, 9 April 1942, BA-MA, H 20, 465).

The security service approved the paper on 2 July 1942, "because the book is intended to inform and is free of any occult tinge." Delayed by the development of the war, the book was published in Heidelberg in 1948. The foreword suggests why the chief of the security police paid so much attention to this book: "For those who wish to know when a superstitious inclination remains harmless under all circumstances, and when it can suddenly burst all restraints at the right moment like a swelling subterranean fire and become a rapidly spreading blaze" (Konrad Zucker, *Psychologie des Aberglaubens*, Heidelberg, 1948).

* Zucker's second postwar book, *Vom Wandel des seelischen Erlebens: Eine Seelengeschichte des Abendlandes* (Heidelberg, 1950), probably contains the findings in this area of euthanasia research.

saw "conversion to an institute for biological anthropology." Heinze would move from Brandenburg-Görden to Wiesloch after the war.[116] In the meantime, he was running a T-4 research department in Görden separate from the one in Heidelberg. There, however, he was responsible to Schneider. Alongside his intensive efforts to carry out these research programs at Görden and Wiesloch, Schneider considered editing a new textbook on psychiatry, one that would "obviously [be] a special edition."[117] In the fall of 1942, he urged "inauguration of a series of scientific journals by the Reich Association, in order to record research and make its results accessible to the public."[118]

Schneider adapted his ambitious plans to wartime conditions. His outline of the 15,000,000-RM project included an appendix, "Emergency Measures and Deviations from Normalcy Resulting from the War."[119] According to this plan for Wiesloch, "The psychiatric hospital currently has three doctors, Dr. Hans-Joachim Rauch, Dr. Fritz Schmieder, and Dr. Carl-Friedrich Wendt. Dr. Rauch has been released for special assignment."[120] A short time before, after a dinner at the Bracks', Schneider had requested that the Führer's Office declare Rauch indispensable.[121] He was successful: "The Wehrmacht physician," Schneider later wrote, "agrees to their [the assistants'] employment on the special assignment, and has agreed to allow them to remain at the hospital for the duration of the special assignment."[122] Thus they were released, not to conduct their normal activities, but on special assignment to conduct research connected with the murder of the mentally ill and handicapped. During that period they were only marginally attached to the Heidelberg University Psychiatric Clinic. Their employer was a "new office" that, at least externally, "was officially part of the Heidelberg research department of the Reich Association of Mental Hospitals."[123] The Heidelberg research assistants received a supplementary monthly payment of 150 reichsmarks from T-4.[124]

In addition to the doctors mentioned above, participants included Dr. Johannes Suckow of Leipzig-Dösen and Dr. Ernst-Adolf Schmorl, who had been delegated by Heinze from Görden to Heidelberg. Research began in the spring of 1942 in the constricted conditions of the Heidelberg University Psychiatric Clinic. However, a separate research department in nearby Wiesloch was planned. After "80 patients had been deported from Wiesloch" to make room for the new department, and following complicated contractual negotiations and reconstruction, "it went into full operation in December 1942."[125] It comprised two sections. In retrospect, Schneider later reported:

Each section was occupied by approximately 20 patients, predominantly feeble-minded persons and idiots, but also some epileptics. Clinical and work therapy-related observations and genetic research were in full swing; most of the patients could also be treated from a constitutional-morphological perspective. Neither metabolic examinations nor the filming of unusual disturbances had begun, so examinations could not be comprehensive. Also, of course, not all of the genetic material could be collected. The findings were placed in safekeeping; only Dr. Schmorl's studies on seizures could be utilized (distinguishing between spontaneous and induced seizures in the same patients).

In the anatomical department, the majority of the brains sent us from the Eichberg institution were examined. New and surprising findings constantly emerged, as well as disturbances which had never before been described. Only the continuation of these investigations can ensure further information; thus we urgently request a greater number of brains of idiots and severely feeble-minded patients.[126]

From the beginning, Wiesloch failed to provide accommodations for everyone employed in the research department. "Histology [Rauch] and photography [Schmieder] had to remain in Heidelberg." A few weeks after the opening of the research department, Schneider announced the first requests that patients be murdered. "We plan to make our first applications to the Reich Committee. . . . I can only hope they also support us. It would be best if they were transferred to Eichberg, with precise instructions that the brains be given to us."[127]

Just as Schneider treated sick people as objects in his research, he treated objects as though they were almost human. In the same letter in which he announced the killing of children, without using the words "child" or "killing," he complained with great annoyance about the equipment of the Wiesloch laboratory. "I cannot work without chemicals, and if I cannot set up the chemical laboratory properly . . . then I must declare that the whole undertaking threatens to lapse into incurable infirmity."[128]

Schneider's research program focused upon the following:

Heidelberg, 21 January 1943
Psych.-neurology clinic of the University of Heidelberg
To:
    Reich Association of Mental Hospitals in Berlin.
    Regarding the research department in Wiesloch, I would like to inform you that work is under way, with the exception of the metabolic

investigations. At present, aside from extremely intensive collection of material on idiocy, the following scientific problems are being considered:

By Dr. *Suckow*, 1. the development of motility through experiments on idiots;

2. special factors in insulin and shock therapy in various mental illnesses.

By Dr. *Schmorl*, 1. experiments on the differences between induced and spontaneous seizures in humans;

2. hydrogen experiments on patients with convulsive disorders, including idiots.

By Dr. *Schmieder*, 1. constitutional types in exogenous convulsive disorders, including head injuries suffered in combat;

2. prevention of vertebral fractures in cases of convulsive shock.

By Dr. *Rauch*, brain histopathology in idiots.

By Dr. *Wendt*,* a collection of material on functional endocrine disturbances in developmentally induced physical dysplasias, particularly in the context of experiments with idiots.

It has become apparent that Dr. Wendt's work is greatly impeded by a shortage of laboratory assistants. Herr Diehl cannot manage the metabolic investigations alone. We therefore need to hire another laboratory assistant immediately, as has already been approved for the histological laboratory. I therefore apply for approval of a second laboratory assistant for the metabolic laboratory, so that the collection of material on idiocy, and especially other laboratory work, can proceed more rapidly.

Heil Hitler!

Dr. Schneider.[129]

Schneider and his assistants linked their "experiments on idiots" with the "brain histopathology in idiots." They reckoned from the outset with their victims' death. The phrase "collection of material on idiocy" referred to people both living and dead.

The close connection between research and extermination in this scheme was described by Nitsche on 18 September 1941: doctors, he said, should begin "thoroughly investigating available cases of congenital

* Hans-Joachim Rauch, Carl-Friedrich Wendt, and Fritz Schmieder became respected professors after the war in Heidelberg and Gailingen. Some years ago, prosecutors in Heidelberg began to investigate them for alleged complicity in murder, but the investigation was dropped several years later. Justice officials have known about the documents cited here since 1960.

feeble-mindedness and epilepsy before disinfection." [130] The word "disinfection," as used by these doctors, meant killing. Two days later, he expressed himself even more clearly: "Until now, cases of congenital feeble-mindedness and epilepsy have simply been transferred from nearby feeder institutions to Görden, the intermediate asylum, from which they are then forwarded to one of our institutions, following the necessary examinations." [131] "Our institutions" were the extermination centers, which continued to exist even after euthanasia was supposedly suspended in August 1941. Werner Blankenburg, the official in the Führer's Office charged with these matters, had obviously agreed to this exception to the "suspension"; he had also agreed that exterminating doctors should rapidly acquire anatomical knowledge. In September of 1941, a doctor from each extermination center was to be assigned to "an institute of pathology and anatomy, most likely Professor Wätjen's in Halle." [132] Research on patients before and after death was not possible before 1939, according to Schneider; since the "idiots obviously did not die immediately, the linkage between anatomical data and clinical conditions remained open." The systematic extermination of research patients made it possible, "to a far greater extent than in other scientific discussions and psychiatric work, at last to solve the most important and practical problems affecting public health, since, thanks to the operation, rapid anatomical and histological clarifications could follow." [133]

On 31 March 1943, "following the misfortune of Stalingrad," after four and a half months, Schneider had to disband the Wiesloch department. He became severely ill with an abscessed auditory canal and could not return to research until August. So as "not to allow things to come to a complete standstill," he reserved three or four beds at the university psychiatric clinic: "That would mean that approximately ten to twelve idiots could be examined monthly." [134] Even though the department at Wiesloch had been disbanded, the "Reich Association's research department" in fact continued to exist. Nitsche had suggested that "after the dissolution of our research department there—in other words, from 1 April on—the four doctors, Dr. Suckow, Dr. Rauch, Dr. Schmieder, and Dr. Wendt, should receive a consideration for their help in research matters, the amount of which must be determined." [135]

The doctors mentioned were indeed called up for military service, but they remained at the Heidelberg hospital as military doctors. They conducted research for T-4 alongside their own work; as Schneider put it in 1944, "Given current procedures, the studies naturally take a relatively long time, as the gentlemen can only devote a few hours to these tasks." [136]

The victims, however, were still in the hands of the researchers: "After the dissolution of the department at Wiesloch, most of the patients were transferred to other institutions. However, the researchers were informed of all transfers. The Ministry of the Interior ensured, and received corresponding orders, that whenever a patient died the brain would be sent to us. Thus it is hoped that at least some of the Wiesloch studies can be utilized for research. Here, too, wartime conditions have interfered."[137]

Schneider continued his research, despite mounting difficulties. In August 1944, he requested that his monthly salary supplement be discontinued, as he was able to conduct research only on a small scale, taking "approximately one or two idiots from Eichberg per month." Indeed, "it [was] probably no longer possible to obtain metabolic data," but "clinical, morphological, and x-ray examinations" could still be conducted. He explained that even though the research department of the Reich Association had to be "formally" disbanded due to the "totalization of the war," he still wished to continue research at his clinic.[138] Contrary to expectations, he was assigned Julius Deussen, a specialist educated at the German Institute for Psychiatric Research, to assist with human experiments. Deussen could "devote himself entirely to the work," and motivated Schneider to develop new plans: "With Herr Deussen now completely free to concentrate on this work, psychological observations and full examinations of the children could be essentially perfected if we could erect a small barracks in the hospital garden. Even if it contained only two or three rooms, we could include a bedroom, a recreation room, and a room for experiments on the children."[139]

In the meantime, Schneider had fallen back on doctoral candidates: "A few days ago," he wrote Nitsche, "I brought in two doctoral students . . . who are to conduct different kinds of intelligence tests with the children. I think that my daughter-in-law will also be able to resume her work on endurance tests."[140]

This daughter-in-law's name was Monika Schneider, née Jörgen; she was married to Schneider's son Wolfgang. She would obtain her doctorate in Leipzig in 1946, five weeks before her father-in-law's suicide, with a dissertation "at the University of Heidelberg Psychiatric Clinic. Director: Dr. Carl Schneider." The title of her thesis was "Metabolic Endurance Tests in Feeble-minded Children." The thesis begins by pointing out that close connections have long been known to exist between the nervous system and the internal secretory glands. In particular, it is obvious that there is a close relationship between the pituitary gland, on the one hand, and "surrounding sections of the brain" on the other. However, the connections between the internal secretory glands and the nervous system have tended to puzzle science. "Because of this, we conducted a series of experiments with children who were generally idiotic but physically healthy; we performed endocrinological function tests on them. . . . As an endurance test, we chose Volhard's water experiment, and the glucose, insulin, and adrenaline endurance tests."[141] Thirty mentally retarded children between the ages of three and thirteen were subjected to these endurance tests. The children were carefully diagnosed, and their intellectual development in relation to their age scrutinized. In order to obtain precise results in the drinking experiment, children in the research department were placed on a "uniform diet of food, fluids, and salt":

> Depending on their age, three- to thirteen-year-old children were given 300–1,000 ccm weak tea at room temperature. They were given the tea on an empty stomach, after the bladder was emptied. Drinking naturally varied in duration, but never exceeded 20 minutes. Before drinking began, we ran urine tests on the "empty stomach urine," for which the bladder was emptied completely. To achieve the greatest possible experimental consistency, we had the children empty their bladders every half hour for the duration of the experiment. We determined individual quantities using the usual glass cylinders, their specific weight with aerometers, their sodium chloride and total chlorine content. The experiment lasted four hours.

Since these brain-damaged children did not always drink voluntarily, "some of the fluid had to be force fed."[142] In her account, Schneider described this as a "circumstance making the experiment more difficult"; it also made it impossible for her to judge and evaluate the water values for six children. However, quantities excreted, temporal progress, and changes in blood values could be evaluated. This meant that Schneider drew blood continually during the four hours of the experiment.

Schneider cited abundant references in scientific literature to other doctors' discoveries regarding changes in the body's water balance. She noted that urinary inhibitions had been observed "following insulin injections"[143] and "in connection with an absence of male gonads." The relationship between water balance and the functioning of the pituitary gland had been discovered in 1883 by two doctors, "when they noted the appearance of a strong urinary flow following extirpation of the organ."[144] Schneider's dissertation described a second series of experiments conducted to study carbohydrate metabolism. Here, too, 30 children were examined; here, too, their blood sugar levels were determined. She discussed research on siblings: "Observations of our series of siblings showed that of the five pairs, three had a normal curve. . . . Unfortunately, the observations of these five sibling pairs are hardly sufficient to draw broader conclusions."[145]

"In a third series of experiments, we investigated the behavior of our children's blood sugar curves after the introduction of insulin." After 12 hours without eating, all children received injections of five units of insulin "Novo," following which blood was drawn every 20 minutes for examination.[146] Four of the 30 "cases" showed clear symptoms of hypoglycemia; they perspired and became dazed. According to Monika Schneider, "This behavior is noteworthy." The handicapped children "exhibited a stronger insulin effect" than healthy children of the same age. "In the five sibling pairs in the insulin endurance test, very similar reactions were observed. . . . This is a striking finding."[147]

This was not the case with adrenaline injections. Schneider "ascertained that the five pairs generally had very different blood sugar values." She had drawn blood from her victims—who were in perfect physical health—after 3, 8, 18, 38, 68, and 128 minutes, prepared blood smears, and checked pulse rate and blood pressure.

In the summary, she recorded the inconclusive results of her research. "It may prove the intimate, varied relationships between the nervous system and the inner secretory glands." However, the results could only be generalized once "more evidence in this area" had been collected.[148] This latter sentence is a legacy of her father-in-law, Carl Schneider, who had stated, "Complete results cannot be presented until at least 300 idiots have been systematically examined."[149]

A letter from the elder Schneider's assistant, Julius Deussen, to the director of the child extermination center at Eichberg indicates the way in which this research on internal secretions continued even after the clinical experiments: "On behalf of Professor Schneider, I would like to inquire about the condition of Ditmar K., whose parents recently transferred him to your research department from the Kork asylum. . . . Should an autopsy be performed on the child, Professor Schneider would consider it important not only that a general autopsy be done, but also that sections of the entire internal glandular system be sent here for examination along with the brain."[150]

This provided the anatomical verification of the clinical experiments described in Monika Schneider's dissertation. The Heidelberg research department turned the planned death of a child into nothing more than an intermediate step on the road to scientific knowledge. Sections of the internal glandular systems of murdered children verified and supplemented the findings reached by Monika Schneider in experiments on children while they were alive. Although the children were undoubtedly killed, it is unclear whether this anatomical evaluation was brought to a successful conclusion. On 2 September 1944, Schneider complained to his friend Nitsche: "Difficulties in processing and collecting materials" had arisen "in completely unexpected quarters." The children had been transferred to Eichberg "at our request," but after their deaths they were either not dissected at all or dissected incorrectly. "I have to assume that only half the idiots we examined here are fully available to the study."[151]

In this Heidelberg research series, doctors and doctoral candidates experimented with children who, as Monika Schneider wrote, were all physically healthy; they were put to death so as to be "fully available to the study."

The Hallervorden Collection

Like the simultaneously therapeutic and murderous psychiatrists, the pediatricians of the Reich Committee combined structural reforms in the health care system with aggressive research practices that circumvented what would otherwise have meant decades of troublesome procedure.

As far as we know today, the following child extermination departments cooperated with universities and research institutions:

Berlin-Wittenau worked with the Pathology Department of the Rudolf Virchow Hospital under Berthold Ostertag,[152] as well as with the university Pediatrics Clinic of the Charité Hospital under Georg Bessau;[153] *Leipzig-Dösen* worked with the Kaiser Wilhelm Institute for Brain Research in Berlin-Buch and with the University Pediatrics Clinic in Leipzig;[154] the extermination department in *Munich-Haar* worked with the university Pediatrics Clinic under Alfred Wiskott in Munich[155] and, like *Ansbach* and *Kaufbeuren,* with the German Institute for Psychiatric Research.[156] This Kaiser Wilhelm Institute in Munich had its own anatomical institute in Haar, led by Hans Schleusing and a Dr. Barbara Schmidt. Particularly close ties existed between the Vienna chair in pediatrics (held by Franz Hamburger) and the Reich Committee department *Am Steinhof* there; the University Pediatrics Clinic and the Psychiatric Clinic in Heidelberg cooperated in research with the *Eichberg, Kalmenhof,* and *Wiesloch institutions;* the *Eichberg Institution* also had ties to I. G. Farben's pharmaceutical research departments in Höchst;[157] the Professor von Weizsäcker Neurological Research Institute in Breslau regularly obtained children's brains from the extermination center at *Loben* (Lubliniec) in Upper Silesia.[158]

Collaboration between the Kaiser Wilhelm Institute for Brain Research in Berlin-Buch and the Brandenburg-Görden Asylum was arranged with care by the participants. In 1937, Heinze's pathologist and head physician, Julius Hallervorden, was appointed chief of the Department of Brain Histopathology in Buch. However, until 1945 he continued anatomical activities at Brandenburg-Görden, which functioned as a branch of the Kaiser Wilhelm Institute for Brain Research. In 1939, under Heinze, Görden became the "Reich Training Asylum" for juvenile euthanasia, a site where many hundreds of children were killed. In 1939, the Kaiser Wilhelm Society also gave Heinze the unusual honor of appointing him a trustee of its Institute for Brain Research. Max de Crinis joined this board at the same time as Heinze. It is likely that a child extermination department was set up at the Kaiser Wilhelm Institute for Brain Research itself. On 21 November 1942, Ernst Wentzler reported to the Führer's Office, "Dr. Soeken informed me yesterday that she is willing in principle to collaborate with the Reich Committee, and will visit me tomorrow for a detailed informational discussion."[159]

Gertrud Soeken directed a clinic at the Institute for Brain Research. In 1953 the director, Hugo Spatz, described her activities there as follows: "Finally, the institute had its own hospital (led by G. Soeken) for the treatment and study of patients with disturbances in involuntary motor functions."[160]

Reich Committee advisers were granted special privileges in conducting their research. "I would be grateful," Hefelmann wrote to Wentzler in November 1942, "if you and the other two advisers would note the cases in which Leipzig or Görden are interested on the recommendation forms. Transfers will follow accordingly."[161] This new practice was preceded by a letter from Wentzler, in which he applied for 12,000 reichsmarks for research; as he put it, once the actual work of forming the Reich Committee had largely been completed and "the actual task of this organization . . . smoothly and silently fulfilled, great new scientific goals will emerge along with the work already completed."[162] In October 1942, Wentzler reported on a "discussion among the consultants that had taken place on the fifteenth of the month in Leipzig."

. . . 2. Treatment of children with various pharmacological substances has had some unsatisfactory results. It was therefore suggested that a toxicologist be consulted. Dr. Weimann's name was mentioned. If this is approved, I request that you have Dr. Weimann contact Dr. Heinze and then Dr. Catel directly.

3. According to the consultants, assignment of pathologists to evaluate Reich Committee material has not yet been accomplished satisfactorily. In particular, it was considered desirable that Dr. Friedrich, a pathologist who works with Professor Hallervorden and is stationed at Berlin-Buch as a military doctor, be released or granted time off in order to process accumulated Reich Committee material in his hometown of Leipzig. This would have to be discussed beforehand with Professor Hallervorden, and he would have to be supplied a replacement if at all possible. In western Germany, the pathologist situation is very unfavorable on the wards (according to Dr. Heinze). It is therefore requested or suggested that the pathologist Rauch also be able to work on material from other west German institutions.

4. The assignment of scientific tasks arising from Reich Committee work was discussed, to the effect that Dr. Heinze will deal with cases of idiocy where no corresponding organic findings can be made.

In addition, he is particularly interested in the issue of Mongolism.

Professor Catel will be concerned primarily with illnesses of the main ganglia (hereditary degenerative processes) and development of fissures of the head and spinal column (split gum, cleft palate, spina bifida, meningocele, myolocele, etc.). I am informing you of this so that this perspective can be considered when assignments are made.

5. At my suggestion, Professor Catel will pursue an idea of Dr. Hefelmann's by beginning research, within the framework of the Reich Committee, on the transmission and treatment of polio. However, he needs another staff member for this, and after discussions with Dr. Kühnke, who will be doing duty on the home front for some time, I suggested him. I will eventually need the help of the office there for this. I would also very much appreciate a decision on the question of poliomyelitis research. To complete the picture, I would like to take this opportunity to point out that the Reich Committee children are serving science in two other areas: they make it possible to test the scarlet fever vaccine (Dr. Heinze) and are available for the extraordinarily important area of immunization against tuberculosis (Bessau-Hefter).

6. The consultants suggest convening an approximately three-day-long meeting of Reich Committee doctors in the first half of April 1943. This would have the character of an information and training course, and could best be held in Leipzig.

7. In addition to the above-mentioned research by committee members or their assistants, there is an acute financial issue relating to research projects in progress outside of the Reich Committee (Professor Lothar Löffler—social perspectives on genetic questions with the aid of material in our index, and Professor Ostertag—genetic research on intrauterine damage to children, utilizing autopsies at the Hefter Hospital). I have already raised these questions in a personal discussion with the Reich Leader [Bouhler] on the fifteenth of this month, and consideration has been given to mobilizing the funds necessary for research purposes through the Ministry of the Interior (Dr. Linden). On this occasion, I would like to note that this issue must still be settled.[163]

This program is nothing more than the tip of the iceberg, made visible through documents. Leading German physicians, as well as their assistants and doctoral students, were all involved in these experiments on human beings. Berthold Ostertag requested an additional assistant.[164] Heinze, Catel, Schneider, and Hallervorden advised on doctoral dissertations and postgraduate work in the context of this research; some of these projects were successfully completed and submitted to German universities, even after the war had ended and some of the dissertation advisers had committed suicide.[165]

Weimann, the toxicologist mentioned in point 2 of the previous document, was Waldemar Weimann, a specialist in forensic medicine from Berlin. In clear contravention of his professional duties, he would develop an inordinately inconspicuous, painless, and unprovable killing procedure. Weimann's *Atlas der gerichtlichen Medizin* (Atlas of forensic medicine), coauthored with his (East) Berlin colleague Otto Prokop, was published in 1963 by the East German publisher VEB Volk und Gesundheit. Weimann turned up again two years later in *Quick* magazine, a mass-circulation West German publication, as coauthor of the series "Diagnosis: Murder? Memoirs of a Forensic Physician."[166]

In 1942, the pathologist Georg Friedrich was sent from Berlin-Buch to Leipzig-Dösen on assignment from the Reich Committee to dissect brains. He wrote to his military commander that "Herr Brack has agreed to release me from my oath of secrecy in regard to you, honorable Herr Chief Staff Physician. . . . Herr Brack would like to meet you at some point."[167] The participants must have been aware of the basis upon which they conducted their research, and for whom. After this discussion, Fritz Kühnke, who was expected to conduct research on children with polio, in fact received his military orders to Leipzig, very close to Catel's children's

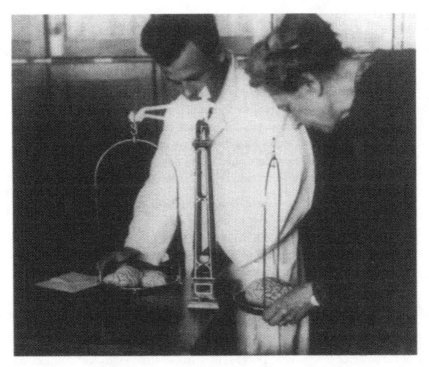

Brain research at Berlin-Buch, before the start of the euthanasia program.

hospital. In an interview with the author, Kühnke said he could not understand this transfer at the time. However, he explained that a personal circumstance put an end to his work at the Reich Committee: In 1942, this Reich Committee doctor's first daughter was born with a spinal fissure. The Kühnkes had the child examined in Leipzig by Doctors Hempel and Catel of the Reich Committee, and were told only that "you will not be happy as long as this child is alive." The girl later died of natural causes, without being placed on a "pediatrics ward."[168]

The activities of the Kaiser Wilhelm Institute for Brain Research have up to now been the easiest to describe in regard to euthanasia.

In July 1945, Julius Hallervorden showed his impressive collection of brains to an American medical officer, Leo Alexander—a Jew who had emigrated from Frankfurt in 1933, and had himself studied with Oskar Vogt at the Kaiser Wilhelm Institute in Berlin-Buch in 1928. Because of its scientific importance, the collection had been stored in 1944 on the Führer's orders at Dillenburg, in the state of Hesse. According to Alexander, the interrogation revealed the following:

Dr. Hallervorden himself initiated this collaboration. As he put it: "I heard that they were going to do that, and so I went up to them and told them 'Look here now, boys, if you are going to kill all these people, at least take the brains out so that the material could be utilized.' They asked me: 'How many can you examine?' and so I told them an unlimited number—'the more the better.' . . . There was wonderful material among these brains, beautiful mental defectives, malformations, and early infantile disease. I accepted these brains, of course. Where they came from and how they came to me was really none of my business." Dr. Hallervorden went on to say, "This thing was a beautiful mess."[169]

This description of the conversation was later vehemently disputed by Hallervorden, but it is entirely in keeping with the documents.

The Hallervorden Collection was kept and used at the Max Planck Institute for Brain Research in Frankfurt until 1990, when the samples were buried in a Munich cemetery. The accompanying documents have been placed in the archives of the Max Planck Society in Berlin for use in historical research. The collection provides clear indications of the identities of organizational collaborators behind the Third Reich's institutional murders, as well as those who simply knew about them. Although the files of the collection were later purged, they still testify to the clear connection between research and murder.

The file "Sektionen [Autopsies] 1941, 1–60" contains reports on a large number of murdered children from the Brandenburg-Görden Asylum, all of whom died on 28 October 1940. The age of the children is given in parentheses: Annelise R. (14), Werner Z. (17), Günther D. (11), Heinz R. (11), Heinz P. (10), Heinz P. (8), Hubert F. (9), Irmgard D. (16), Willy V. (13), Günther S. (12), Ursula K. (16), Wolfgang F. (10), Dora Z. (16), Elisabeth J. (15), Marie K. (?), Werner P. (13), Willy S. (16), Margarete K. (13), Henry H. (17), Erika H. (10), Berta H. (10), Herbert S. (18), Willy B. (16), Horst F. (9), Renate W. (17), Hellmuth L. (11), Vera B. (14), Werner B. (15), Günther N. (7), Siegfried G. (9), Rolf P. (12), Hildegard E. (17), Emmy K. (17).[170]

As the reports indicate, these 33 children and adolescents were not "empty husks" or "mentally dead"—terms later employed in court by their murderers. They were children who, in some cases, attended the special school in Brandenburg-Görden, and were often from difficult social backgrounds. They were obviously killed for scientific reasons. At the time, Hallervorden was researching the causes of "congenital imbecility" and the difference between "traumatic" and "genuine hereditary epilepsy," to use the terminology of the period. Added to this was the main focus of research by the director of the Brandenburg-Görden Asylum, Prof. Hans Heinze—"the abnormal character." In all three studies, anatomical examinations of brains were used to determine and describe any regular, scientifically verifiable changes in the brain that would correspond to these deviations from the norm.

A statement by one of the extermination doctors, Heinrich Bunke, before an interrogating judge in Frankfurt am Main on 16 April 1962 supplies the background of the scientific massacre of children on 28 October 1940. Beginning in August 1940, Bunke worked in the Brandenburg extermination center, housed in a prison, and was transferred to its successor institution at Bernburg at the end of October 1940.

> Children between the ages of approximately 8 and 12, perhaps 14, were also gassed in Brandenburg. The children were transferred to us from Görden by Prof. Heinze—either directly or through an intermediate institution—for the express purpose of killing them. During the period that I worked at Brandenburg, this involved about 100 children. Medical histories and documents with the consultants' decisions were sent along with the patients. You could tell what intermediate institution the children came from by the advisory opinions in the files. The medical records themselves indicated the course of illness and the original institutions from which the children came. In general, however, there was no time to study the files. In the children's cases, precise examinations and summaries of medical histories were attached to the files. They were the only cases that can be said to have been examined as one would have expected in all cases. I mean that in these cases, a non-psychiatrist could also have understood the reasons for the consultants' decisions. In all other cases, the decision was clear, but not the reasoning, aside from a general psychiatric diagnosis. Some of the bodies were dissected by Prof. Hallervorden of Berlin (histologist at the Kaiser Wilhelm Institute) and taken along for scientific evaluation. I assume this was based on an agreement with Professor Heinze. I do not know if Prof. Heinze himself also took part in killings at Görden. In any case, the above-mentioned children came from his asylum. I believe there was a total of two transports. Prof. Heinze himself was at Brandenburg at the time.[171]

According to his testimony, Bunke had gotten to know Hallervorden better on this occasion. In mid-May 1941, he spent four to six weeks in training at Berlin-Buch, after which he removed brains from patients gassed at Bernburg that he assumed "would be of interest in Buch." During this short training period he lived in the home of the director of brain research for the Kaiser Wilhelm Institute, Hugo Spatz.

The files on dissections carried out in 1940 and 1941 contain many similar descriptions of brain removals that point to the extermination centers at Brandenburg and Bernburg. The very short report forms were almost all typed on the same typewriter, with a "Be Nr." on the upper left-hand corner and a "Z Nr." on the upper right-hand corner. The Be and Z numbers are definite evidence that the killings took place in the context of the euthanasia operation. The Z number was the central number in the Berlin index; it designated the patient questionnaires that the asylums sent to the Reich Association of Mental Hospitals. The Be number designated the current number of murders. The date of death is generally unspecified. Dissection followed very shortly after death, within one to four hours. These short descriptions were dictated by Bunke at the extermination center and transported to Berlin-Buch along with the brains and pertinent medical records.

The first of these reports is reprinted here as an example:

Be Nr. 23 828   Z Nr. 55 150

Name: K., Arthur   Born: 11 June 1912 in Berlin
                      Dissection after 2 hours

Diagnosis: Imbecility
Height: 1.52 meters
Body Type: Thin
Bone Type: Fine
Circumference of Head: 55 cm.
Lengthwise Diameter: 17.5 cm.
Widthwise Diameter: 14 cm.
Brain Weight:
Dissection: Brain
Macroscopic Findings:
Strikingly small, soft brain. Soft tissues normal. The left hemisphere is better developed than the right. In the area of the right parietal brain, there are changes in convolutions reminiscent of microgyry. Nothing remarkable at the base or the cerebellum. During removal, the right pedunculus tore off, and the left was torn.
Brief patient report:
A family report could not be obtained. The patient was placed in institutional care in 1929. Is described as a completely impassive idiot who

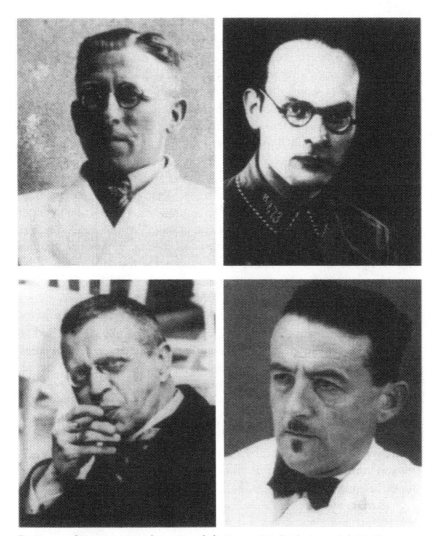

German euthanasia researchers: (*top left*) Georg Friedrich; (*top right*) Julius Deussen; (*bottom left*) Julius Hallervorden; (*bottom right*) Hugo Spatz.

reacted to neither threats nor loud noises. No verbal expression was heard from him; he only uttered animal noises from time to time. Spastic paralysis on the left side. Strong rigor in the musculature of the left arm. Slight rigor of the left leg.

Tendon reflexes are pronounced on both sides. The patient apparently survived polio, after which the symptoms of left-side paralysis appeared.[172]

There is no doubt that the files from the Hallervorden Collection on these victims are based on their murders, and that Hallervorden himself was present when the brains were removed. In 1944, he wrote Nitsche "with best regards" (rather than "Heil Hitler!"), as was typical for the kind of scientist he was: "I have received a total of 697 brains, including those which I myself removed in Brandenburg. This includes the ones from Dösen. Many of them have already been examined, but it is remains to be seen whether I will make more exact histological examinations on all of them."[173]

Among the cases Hallervorden collected in Görden is the fate of the three K. brothers. Alfred K. died at the age of seven on 6 February 1942 of a "feverish influenza infection"; 12 days later, his three-year-old brother Günther died of "bronchial pneumonia." At that time, the third brother, Herbert, had not yet been born. He died on 25 April 1944 at the age of 15 months of "pneumonia localized in the lower right lung." All three brothers suffered from the same, apparently hereditary illness. This illness involves the decay of medulla fiber from nerve cells, and, over a period of years, leads to a child's death; it is possible that the oldest brother K. died a natural death. His autopsy showed that the illness had been quite far advanced. The report on the examination of the four years' younger brother stated that "the loss of medulla is not yet very far advanced." Because this finding was somewhat similar to the one on the older brother, it provided no important leads on the course of the illness. "Much more informative are the slides from the youngest brother, Herbert K. A Spielmayer incision through the stem ganglia clearly reveals the medulla, though diminished."[174] As of 1985, the files on these three brothers were not collecting dust in basement archives. They showed signs of recent scientific use.

As late as 1974, the Max Planck Society, represented by Professor Adolf Butenandt, succeeded in getting the courts to prohibit a Munich journalist from asserting that institutes connected with the Kaiser Wilhelm Society had carried out brain research in the context of euthanasia. The society called this statement "slanderous."[175]

An Aberrant View

Much of what is known about the Nazi period has been uncovered not by historians but by police commissioners and prosecutors. They were the ones to obtain arrest warrants and subject suspects to days of interrogation. The results of the 90,000 judicial inquiries in the Federal Republic alone (not to be confused with the much less common, insubstantial verdicts) are a first-rate source—as well as, in many cases, the only one. But the prosecutors' interest is limited. They are concerned with finding individual proof of violent crimes. Thus, they did not know how to handle someone like Ludwig Trieb; they did not accept the planning files he almost forced on them. At first, they did not even look for Herbert Becker, head of the T-4 Planning Department. For two decades, they did not recognize the research department in Heidelberg as the scene of a crime. And when those they questioned began talking, unasked, about their research programs and describing their ideas on therapy and planning, judicial authorities considered their revelations as mere attempts at self-justification. No questions, no reproaches. The judiciary persistently ignored these criminals' reformist ambitions, though they lay at the very heart of their outrages.

Judicial authorities not only ignored certain files, calling them "irrelevant to criminal law"; they also excluded them, thereby limiting opportunities for later research. This began on a large scale at the Nuremberg Trials. The fate of the Nitsche files often cited in this chapter is typical. At the end of the 1940s, they were removed from a larger group of files by American prosecutors for a trial they were planning against Allers. In 1960, a prosecutor from Frankfurt named Warlo copied some of these, the so-called Heidelberg documents, at U.S. headquarters in Heidelberg. He also separated some documents from the rest. It is in this form that they are preserved as item R 96 in the Federal Archives at Koblenz— twice reduced for the purposes of criminal prosecution. In tracing the process back, it is apparent that every cut eliminated documents that could have thrown light on motives not covered by the criminal code. At some point, prosecutors excluded as unimportant almost all the planning files, the 1943 letters on equipping hospitals and nursing homes with electroshock equipment, and the 1941 "psychiatric research program." The Nitsche files can, however, be partially reconstructed. The planning files are in the military archives in Freiburg,* and the documents considered for the planned Allers trial are far more extensive as they were filmed (though sometimes only selectively) than they were as the photocopied "Heidelberg documents."

The judiciary pushed the bloody side of the Nazi regime into the foreground, thus obscuring the structures and goals at the root of the mass

---

* Since this essay was first published, these files have once again been joined to the other Nitsche files, and are therefore located in Koblenz.

murders. The crimes became individual aberrations. But Paul Nitsche was not the shady character who haunts the standard literature. He did not practice euthanasia as an incomprehensible excess in an otherwise average physician's life; he did so as a consequence of a lifelong struggle for better conditions in psychiatric institutions. The distorted image obtained from legal documents is preferred in the literature; it may be a necessary part of the process of coming to terms with Nazism. The cost, however, is the historical truth. Paradoxically, this image diminishes the real horror of the National Socialist state. The more murderous and repugnant the documents are, the easier it is for the reader to distance himself or herself from this system. However, the way in which the state actually functioned and the nature of its goals beyond the bloodbath become that much less comprehensible.

The lawyers who prosecuted Nazi criminals were forced to begin with 1933 and end with 1945. Historical research cannot do this, for the criminals continued to act both before and after these dates. Though forced after 1945 to sublimate the murderous side of their frantic desire for change, they held to their research hypotheses and reformist ambitions—research and progress, based on destruction.

Notes

1. Written testimony of D. Allers, 2 January 1949, ZStL, Testimony collection "Euthanasie." The testimony in this extensive, although incomplete, collection is arranged alphabetically and chronologically.

2. Paul Nitsche, "Städtische Heil- und Pflegeanstalt zu Dresden," in *Deutsche Heil- und Pflegeanstalten für Psychischkranke in Wort und Bild,* vol. 1, ed. J. Bresler (Halle, 1912), pp. 248–55.

3. Carl Schneider, *Behandlung und Verhütung der Geisteskrankheiten* (Berlin, 1939), p. 45 ff.

4. Testimony of H. Hefelmann, 3 July 1961, cited here and below from StA Ansbach, 1 Js 1147/62, Beiakten "Aussagen Hefelmann."

5. See Hans-Ludwig Siemen, *Das Grauen ist vorprogrammiert: Psychiatrie zwischen Faschismus und Atomkrieg* (Giessen, 1982), p. 32f. Siemen lists sources.

6. Paul Nitsche, "Allgemeine Therapie und Prophylaxe der Geisteskranken," in *Handbuch der Geisteskrankheiten,* vol. 4, ed. Oswald Bumke (Berlin, 1929), pp. 1–131.

7. Ibid., p. 32.

8. Ibid., p. 35.

9. Ibid., p. 55f.

10. Ibid., p. 99ff.

11. Hans Roemer, Gustav Kolb, and Valentin Faltlhauser, eds., *Die offene Fürsorge in der Psychiatrie und ihren Grenzgebieten* (Berlin, 1927), p. 228.

12. Nitsche, *Allgemeine Therapie*, p. 103.

13. Hermann Simon, *Aktivere Krankenbehandlung in der Irrenanstalt* (Berlin, 1929). A critical appraisal of this concept can be found in Christine Teller, "Die 'aktivere Heilbehandlung' der 20er und 30er Jahre: z.B. Hermann Simon und Carl Schneider," in *Fortschritte der Psychiatrie im Umgang mit Menschen*, ed. Klaus Dörner (Rehburg-Loccum, 1984), pp. 77–87.

14. Simon, *Aktivere Krankenbehandlung in der Irrenanstalt*, p. 84.

15. BA-MA, H 20, 463 (Report by Becker on planning in Westphalia, 27 May 1942).

16. Nitsche, *Allgemeine Therapie*, p. 103ff.

17. Testimony of Paul Nitsche, 11 March 1948, ZStL, Testimony collection "Euthanasie."

18. Nitsche, *Städtische Heil- und Pflegeanstalt zu Dresden*, p. 253f.

19. See Götz Aly and Karl Heinz Roth, *Die restlose Erfassung: Volkszählen, Identifizieren, Aussondern im Nationalsozialismus* (Berlin, 1984), p. 94f. Sources are listed there.

20. On the origin and text of the euthanasia law, see Karl Heinz Roth and Götz Aly, "Das Gesetz über die 'Sterbehilfe bei unheilbar Kranken': Protokolle der Diskussion über die Legalisierung der nationalsozialistischen Anstaltsmorde in den Jahren 1938–1941," in *Erfassung zur Vernichtung: Von der Sozialhygiene zum "Gesetz über Sterbehilfe,"* ed. K. H. Roth, pp. 101–79 (Berlin, 1984). At the time this piece was written, we were not yet aware of the connection between the euthanasia law and the 1941 law on the Reich Commissioner.

21. Ibid., p. 176f.

22. Ibid., p. 154.

23. Ibid., p. 132f.

24. Written testimony of D. Allers, 2 January 1949, ZStL, Testimony collection "Euthanasie."

25. *RGBl* (1941, I): 653.

26. *RMBliV* (1941): 1999.

27. Testimony of A. Oels, 24 April 1961, ZStL, Testimony collection "Euthanasie."

28. Testimony of D. Allers, 21 April 1950, ZStL, Testimony collection "Euthanasie."

29. Testimony of A. Wödl, 1 March 1946, LG (District Court) Wien Vg 2b Vr 2365/45.

30. Testimony of H. J. Becker, 9 October 1961, ZStL, Testimony collection "Euthanasie."

31. "Planungsbericht über Bayern vom 17.10.1942" (Planning report on Bavaria) (by Robert Müller), BA-MA, H 20, 465.

32. "Planungsbericht über Danzig-West Preussen vom 9.2.1943" (Planning report on Danzig–West Prussia) (by Robert Müller), BA-MA, H 20, 465.

33. "Planungsbericht über Pommern vom 11.12.1942" (Planning report on Pomerania) (by Robert Müller), BA-MA, H 20, 465.

34. See three letters from H. Becker to Nitsche (18 December 1943; 9 January 1944; 19 January 1944), BA-MA, H 20, 465.

35. Conversation of 19 November 1941, NAW, T 1021, Roll 12, no. 127863f.

36. Testimony of Ludwig Trieb, 3 April 1962, ZStL, Testimony collection "Euthanasie."

37. Heidelberger Dokumente (Heidelberg documents; HD), no. 127924f.

38. See Götz Aly, Chap. 2 in this book, pp. 66–68ff.

39. "Bethel-Bericht vom Wirtschaftsleiter Trieb," p. 18, NAW T 1021, Roll 1, Nos. 126898–928.

40. Testimony of L. Trieb, 5 February 1963, ZStL, Testimony collection "Euthanasie."

41. See Aly, Chap. 2, p. 91ff.

42. NAW, T 1021, Roll 12, nos. 127711–13.

43. NAW, T 1021, Roll 10, nos. 126498–502.

44. NAW, T 1021, Roll 12, nos. 128079–80.

45. Testimony of L. Trieb, 16 December 1965, ZStL, Testimony collection "Euthanasie."

46. The change in numerical guidelines and point in time can be precisely reconstructed from the numerous planning reports: BA-MA, H 20, 463, 465.

47. "Richtlinien des Reichsbeauftragten zur Planungsfrage," ca. November 1941, NAW, T 1021, Roll 10, nos. 126559–61.

48. "Bericht über 'Freigemachte Betten für andere Zwecke nach dem Stande vom 10. Januar 1942'" (Planning report on beds made available for other purposes, as of 10 January 1942), NAW, T 1021, Roll 11, nos. 12635–851.

49. Letter from Becker to Nitsche, BA-MA, H 20, 463.

50. "Planungsbericht über Sachsen" (Planning report on Saxony), BA-MA, H 20, 463.

51. "Planungsbericht über Bremen vom 28.4.1942" (Planning report on Bremen) (by H. Becker), BA-MA, H 20, 463.

52. "Planungsbericht über Hamburg vom 28.4.1942" (Planning report on Hamburg) (by H. Becker), BA-MA, H 20, 463.

53. BA-MA, H 20, 465.

54. Planning report, "Reise Sachsen" (Saxony trip), November 1942. (The numerous individual reports were written by Gerhard Wischer and Gustav Schneider). NAW, T 1021, Roll 11, nos. 125170–282. A final report on this trip, dated 18 February 1943 (by G. Wischer), with very informative interpretive comments on the question of resistance against and approval of euthanasia, can be found in the Staatsarchiv Dresden, Ministerium des Inneren (Dresden State Archives, Ministry of the Interior), no. 16849.

55. See Aly, Chap. 2, p. 76ff.

56. "Abschlussbericht über die Planung in Baden (Juli 1942)" (Final report on planning in Baden), BA-MA, H 20, 465.

57. Testimony of H. J. Becker, 13 June 1960, ZStL, Testimony collection "Euthanasie."

58. Testimony of H. J. Becker, 12 May 1966, ZStL, Testimony collection "Euthanasie."

59. Letter from Rüdin, 17 July 1941, NAW, T 1021, Roll 12, no. 128174.

60. Testimony of H. J. Becker, 15 February 1963, ZStL, Testimony collection "Euthanasie."

61. Testimony of H. J. Becker, 12 May 1966, ZStL, Testimony collection "Euthanasie."

62. Letter from H. J. Becker, 12 July 1944, to the State Asylum at Hadamar, Archiv des Psychiatrischen Krankenhauses Hadamar (Archives of the Hadamar Psychiatric Hospital), File no. 55a, "Zentralverrechnungsstelle."

63. Testimony of D. Allers, 21 April 1950, ZStL, Testimony collection "Euthanasie."

64. *RGBl* (1939, I): 2002ff.

65. "Vorschlag zur Vereinfachung auf dem Gebiet der Heil- und Pflegeanstalten vom 19.1.1944" (Proposals for simplification in the area of asylums), NAW, T 1021, Roll 12, nos. 126409–17.

66. "Gedankensammlung zur Geisteskrankenfürsorge vom 17.1.1944" (Thoughts on care of the mentally ill from 17 January 1944), BA, R 18, 3160.

67. BA, R 18, 3160.

68. Ibid.

69. Ibid.

70. See n. 62.

71. Letter from H. Becker to Nitsche, 9 January 1944, BA-MA, H 20, 465.

72. "Bericht über die Planungsbesichtigung der Anstalt für Epileptische Bethel vom 24.6.1942" (Report on a planning trip to the asylum for epileptics at Bethel from 24 June 1942) (by H. Becker), NAW, T 1021, Roll 11, nos. 126867–97.

73. See also Matthias Hamann, "Die Morde an polnischen und sowjetischen Zwangsarbeitern in deutschen Anstalten," in *Beiträge zur nationalsozialistischen Gesundheits- und Sozialpolitik,* vol. 1, *Aussonderung und Tod: Die klinische Hinrichtung der Unbrauchbaren,* p. 151.

74. Letter from H. Heinze to Nitsche, 20 January 1944, BA-MA, H 20, 465.

75. On the history of the Reich Committee, see Ernst Klee, *"Euthanasie" im NS-Staat: Die "Vernichtung lebensunwerten Lebens"* (Frankfurt, 1983), pp. 77–81, 379–400; Götz Aly, "Der Mord an behinderten Kindern zwischen 1939 und 1945," in *Heilen und Vernichten im Mustergau Hamburg,* ed. A. Ebbinghaus, H. Kaupen-Haas, and K. H. Roth (Hamburg, 1984), pp. 147–55; Götz Aly, "Die wissenschaftliche Abstraktion des Menschen," *Wege zum Menschen* 36 (1984): 272–86.

76. The association was officially registered in Berlin-Mitte on 16 February 1942, under the registration number 23742. Along with Conti, Wentzler, and Brack, the co-founders included Dr. Strohschneider, Heinz Voges (as business manager), Dr. Stark, Dr. Ramm, and Dr. Röhrs. The association's registration files are in the Landesarchiv Berlin (Berlin State Archives), Rep. 42, Acc. 2147, no. 28067.

77. Ernst Wentzler, "Das künftige 'Deutsche Kinderkrankenhaus,'" *Die Ärztin* 19 (1943): 199. The essay, which was preceded by a piece in the publication *Gesundheitsführung,* and which appeared in summary form in other professional journals, reported extensively on the founding of the association and its goals.

78. Ibid.

79. Ibid., p. 200.

80. Ibid.

81. Ibid., p. 201.

82. The association and the 200,000-RM debt to the state of Rhineland-Palatinate were annulled in 1953 as a result of the order's suit for reparations. See n. 76.

83. "Anklageschrift gegen Richard von Hegener" (Indictment of Richard von Hegener), StA Schwerin, 9 September 1949, BA, Nachlass Rheindorf, 50.

84. Evidence on treatment of retarded children in Department B of the children's ward of the Psychiatric Asylum in Lubliniec, by Kazimiera Marxen and Hipolit Latynski, quoted in StA Dortmund, Ermittlungsverfahren gegen Ernst Buchalik und Elisabeth Hecker wegen Kindertötungen in Loben, 45 Js 8/65.

85. NAW, T 1021, roll 12, Nos. 127677–80.

86. The files on the examinations, which have apparently survived, have still not been evaluated in Brandenburg-Görden. Copies of certain files were given to the Frank-

234 ■ Götz Aly

furt am Main State Archives by Friedrich Karl Kaul. Approximately 10 other files can be found among the documents connected with the case against the local asylum; they went from Görden to Ansbach when adolescents, some of whom died after 8 May, were transferred there at the end of the war. StA Ansbach, 1 Js 1147/62.

87. StA Ansbach, 1 Js 1147/62, Beiakten Krankengeschichten (Patient reports).

88. See Aly, Chap. 2, p. 81ff.

89. BAK, 96 I/9, NAW, T1021, Roll 12, no. 126420.

90. See the Bundestag's 1975 psychiatric commission report, *Bericht über die Lage der Psychiatrie in der Bundesrepublik Deutschland: Zur psychiatrischen und psychotherapeutischen/psychosomatischen Versorgung der Bevölkerung (Psychiatrie-Enquête)*, p. 62.

91. NAW, T 1021, Roll 12, no. 126428.

92. Carl Schneider, "Die moderne Behandlung der Geistesstörungen," *Gesundheitsführung* (1943): 192.

93. Archiv der Universität Heidelberg (Heidelberg University Archives), personal file of C. Schneider.

94. NAW, T 1021, Roll 12, nos. 127870–85.

95. See n. 93.

96. Aly, Chap. 2, p. 54ff.

97. Testimony of H. Hefelmann, 1 September 1960; see n. 4.

98. Anton von Braunmühl, *Insulinschock und Heilkrampf in der Psychiatrie* (Stuttgart, 1947).

99. Von Braunmühl received American investigating officer Leo Alexander in a very friendly manner and gave him some secret documents belonging to his superior, Pfannmüller, but was not himself investigated. Nuremberg Documents, L 169. Electroshock treatment would later become one of Alexander's preferred topics for publication.

100. A letter dated May 1942 from Pfannmüller to Nitsche mentions this report: BA-MA, H 20, 463.

101. Extensive documents in ibid.

102. Hauptarchiv der von Bodelschwinghschen Anstalten Bethel (Main archives of the Bodelschwingh Asylums at Bethel), 1/C71.

103. NAW, T 1021, Roll 12, nos. 127870–85.

104. List of advisers, NAW T 1021, Roll 12, no. 127891.

105. "Psychiatrischer Forschungsplan" (Psychiatric research plan), NAW, T 1021, Roll 10, no. 126472.

106. The reference to this is in a file note by Nitsche, 18 September 1941, NAW, T 1021, Roll 12, no. 127060.

107. NAW, T 1021, Roll 12, no. 128218.

108. A. Dohmen, "Anleitung zu physikalischen Untersuchungen an Hirn und Schädel bei der Leiche," *Zeitschrift für die gesamte Neurologie und Psychiatrie* 172 (1941): 667–86.

109. "Schlussbemerkungen, wissenschaftliche, wirtschaftliche, und soziale Bedeutung und Zukunft der psychiatrischen Therapien," NAW, T 1021, Roll 12, nos. 127585–91.

110. Ibid.

111. Ibid.

112. Ibid.

113. Ibid.

114. Ibid.

115. This would be the equivalent of 300 million marks today. Schneider's research plan, 12 March 1942, NAW, T 1021, Roll 12, nos. 127696–701.

116. Ibid.

117. Ibid.

118. "Vermerk über eine Reise nach Heidelberg" (Notes on a trip to Heidelberg) (by D. Allers), 4 November 1942, NAW, T 1021, Roll 12, nos. 127436–38.

119. See n. 115.

120. See n. 115.

121. Letter from Schneider to Brack, 10 December 1941, NAW T 1021, Roll 12, no. 128196.

122. See n. 115.

123. See n. 118.

124. Letter from Allers to Schneider, 17 June 1942, NAW, T 1021, Roll 12, no. 128172.

125. See n. 115.

126. See n. 115.

127. Letter from Schneider to Nitsche, 18 January 1943, NAW, T 1021, Roll 12, no. 127960.

128. Letter from Schneider to Nitsche, 19 December 1942, NAW, T 1021, Roll 12, no. 127457.

129. NAW, T 1021, Roll 12, nos. 128066–67.

130. File notes by Nitsche, "Betr.: Forschung," 18 September 1941 and 20 September 1941, NAW, T 1021, Roll 12, nos. 127149–50.

131. Ibid.

132. Ibid.

133. See n. 115.

134. Note from Schneider to Nitsche, "betrf. Zuführung von Idioten aus Anstalten in die Heidelberger Klinik im Rahmen des Forschungsauftrags," 19 June 1943, NAW, T 1021, Roll 12, no. 128038.

135. Letter from Nitsche to Schneider, 15 March 1943, NAW, T 1021, Roll 12.

136. See n. 115.

137. See n. 115.

138. Letter from Schneider to Nitsche, 28 August 1944, NAW, T 1021, Roll 12, nos. 127912–13.

139. Letter from Schneider to Nitsche, 18 July 1944, NAW, T 1021, Roll 12, nos. 127933–34.

140. Letter from Schneider to Nitsche, 1 February 1943, NAW, T 1021, Roll 12, nos. 127960–61.

141. Monika Schneider, "Stoffwechselbelastungsproben bei schwachsinnigen Kindern" (Med. diss., Leipzig, 1946), p. 1.

142. Ibid., p. 7.

143. Ibid., p. 13.

144. Ibid.

145. Ibid., p. 23.

146. Ibid., p. 26.

147. Ibid., p. 29.

148. Ibid., p. 41.

149. See n. 115.

150. Quoted from Klee, *Euthanasie*, p. 399f.

151. Letter from Schneider to Nitsche, 2 September 1944, NAW, T 1021, Roll 12, nos. 127903–4.

152. Letter from Wentzler to Blankenburg, 17 October 1942, BAP, Kanzlei des Führers (Führer's Office), no. 242.

153. Ibid.

154. Ibid.

155. Conversation by the author with Fritz Kühnke, a doctor formerly involved in euthanasia, 15 January 1985. According to Kühnke, Alfred Wiskott was among the strongest supporters of euthanasia, but did not want to have it done in his hospital. However, he cooperated with the Reich Committee, hired Kühnke as a scientific assistant, and permitted him simultaneously to carry out his activities in the extermination department in Haar. In this way, the Munich children's hospital was respectably and inconspicuously connected with the euthanasia program and ensured that its research needs were met. Wiskott wrote a popular textbook on pediatrics with Walter Keller. Keller was forced to leave the university in Giessen in 1945 despite strong opposition; as an exposed Nazi, he could not be kept on.

156. The author's research at the Max Planck Institute for Psychiatry in Munich turned up hundreds of examples of this.

157. See Klee, *Euthanasie,* p. 400.

158. Medical files of the institution, supplementary files (Beiakten) in the proceedings against Buchalik and Hecker, StA Dortmund, 45 Js/65.

159. See n. 152.

160. Hugo Spatz, "Max-Planck-Institut für Hirnforschung," *Münchener Medizinische Wochenschrift* (1953), Jubilee Edition.

161. Letter from Hefelmann to Wentzler, 17 November 1942; BAP, Kanzlei des Führers, no. 242.

162. "Antrag auf Bereitstellung eines Betrages vom RM 12 000 für wissenschaftliche Forschungszwecke im Rahmen der Reichsausschussarbeiten," from Wentzler, 20 November 1942; BAP, Kanzlei des Führers, no. 242.

163. See n. 152.

164. See n. 162.

165. For example: Josefine Bassek, "Beitrag zur Röntgentherapie des chronischen Hydrocephalus," dissertation research at Leipzig University Clinic (December 1945); Karl Heinz Pospiech, "Encephalographische und anatomische Befunde bei angeborenem Balkenmangel und bei Erweiterung des Cavum septi pellucidi," dissertation research at Görden State Asylum, near Brandenburg on the Havel (Berlin, January 1942); Arnold Asmussen, "Ein charakterologischer Beitrag zum Adoptionsproblem," dissertation research at Brandenburg State Asylum at Görden (Kiel, September 1943); Werner-Joachim Eicke, "Gefässveränderungen bei Meningitis und ihre Bedeutung für die Pathogenese frühkindlicher Hirnschäden," postdoctoral thesis in the Department of Histopathology (director: Prof. J. Hallervorden) of the Kaiser Wilhelm Institute for Brain Research (director: Prof. H. Spatz) (Berlin, 1944).

166. Waldemar Weimann, with Gerhard Jaeckel, *Diagnose Mord: Die Memoiren eines Gerichtsmediziners* (Bayreuth, 1965).

167. BA-MA, H 20, Personalunterlagen des Heerespathologen (Personal files of the army pathologist).

168. See n. 155.

169. Nuremberg Documents L 170, "Neuropathology and Neurophysiology, Including Electro-encephalography in Wartime Germany" [in English]. Benno Müller-

Hill provides important information on the context of this research in *Murderous Science: Elimination by Scientific Selection of Jews, Gypsies, and Others in Germany 1933–1945*, trans. George Fraser (Oxford, 1988).

170. The author was able to look at the following autopsy files: 1936, 1937, 1–90; 1939, 1–70, 71–111; 1940, 1–60, 61–110, 111–170; 1941, 1–60, 61–119, 120–185, 186–282; 1942, 1–60, 61–102; 1943, 76–130; 1944, 1–83. Furthermore, 30 case histories of euthanasia victims that are apparently considered particularly interesting are indexed under the title "Hallervorden Collection."

171. Testimony of Heinrich Bunke, cited here from StA Hamburg, 147 Js 58/67, supplementary files (Beiakte) Vernehmungen Bru-El.

172. See n. 170.

173. Letter from Hallervorden to Nitsche, 9 March 1944, NAW, T 1021, Roll 12, no. 127898.

174. Hallervorden Collection, index.

175. Bayer. Oberlandesgericht München (Bavarian Superior Court, Munich), Urteil gegen (judgment against) H. Brendel, AZ: 30 o 106/73 LG Mü.I.

CHAPTER FIVE

Selected Letters of Doctor Friedrich Mennecke

Introduced and Annotated by Peter Chroust

Introduction

Little light has ever been shed on the paradoxical ability of doctors to take part in human extermination projects without significant moral scruples—be they projects involving human experimentation, euthanasia, or torture. The dialectic of healing, research, and extermination continues to be denied, as medicine is separated into "good" and "helpful," on the one hand, and "destructive" and therefore "unscientific," on the other. Yet, a number of reconstructed biographies prove that the main supporters of human extermination under National Socialism were not murderous beasts, but in fact well-adjusted, progressive, well-qualified doctors.

The correspondence of the "euthanasia doctor" Friedrich Mennecke, of Eichberg in the Rheingau, helps us to reconstruct the social and biographical conditions behind medical crime.[1] This issue was largely ignored in postwar trials, starting with the Nuremberg doctors' trial of 1946–47 and ending with the 1986 euthanasia trial against Heinrich Bunke and Aquilin Ullrich before the Frankfurt State Court (probably the last of its kind). Friedrich Mennecke's letters to his wife, colleagues, and relatives were written during the period in which he worked as a euthanasia doctor, and thus do not contain the slightest degree of conscious or unconscious editing after the fact. The extracts published until now have been limited, in typical fashion, to particularly drastic citations that allow readers easily to distance themselves from the writer. But the more one becomes aware of the human and scientific "normality" of even a medical offender such as Friedrich Mennecke, the more apparent become the links between a mentality of progressive-minded extermination and the average German physician's life. The fact that these letters also reveal details of his private life is not merely voyeurism disguised as scholarship. Hermann Langbein explained the legitimacy and necessity of publication of the Mennecke letters three decades ago:

> The effusive emotion with which Dr. Mennecke greets his wife in his daily letters, and the talkativeness with which he tells her of even the most unimportant details of daily life, remain the couple's exclusive business only as long as Dr. Mennecke is not traveling from concentration camp to concentration camp selecting people for the gas chambers. Once this becomes the case, however, the public has the right to read along as Dr. Mennecke rejoices over a good night's sleep before hurrying off to his workplace—the concentration camp.[2]

The majority of the Mennecke letters available so far are preserved in the Main State Archives of Hesse in Wiesbaden;* a smaller number are still on file with the general prosecutor in Frankfurt-Main but will also be given to the Main State Archives. We thank the employees of these institutions, especially Dr. Helfer, Dr. Eichler (both in Wiesbaden), and Chief Prosecutor S. Schmidt (Frankfurt-Main), for their support.

Friedrich Mennecke's Biography

Friedrich Wilhelm Heinrich Mennecke was born on 6 October 1904 in Gross-Freden, in the district of Alfeld-Leine (near Hanover). His only brother, Karl, was four years old at the time. Both grew up under difficult material conditions. Their father, Karl Mennecke, worked as a stonecutter and mason; their mother, Lina, cared for the children and household. Af-

---

* The complete edition of the Mennecke letters is as follows: Friedrich Mennecke, *Innenansichten eines medizinischen Täters im Nationalsozialismus. Eine Edition seiner Briefe, 1935–1947*, 2 vols. (Hamburg: Hamburger Institut für Sozialforschung, 1987; 2d ed., 1988). Most of the letters can be found in volumes 15–19 of the *Eichberg Trials* (archive no. 461 32442); however, certain documents can also be found in the actual files of the trial (vols. 2–4).

The first work to describe the various phases and functions of the Eichberg asylum was written for a high school students' contest on German history and later published: Armin Kreis et al., *Der Eichberg — Opfer und Täter: "Lebensunwertes" Leben in einer hessischen psychiatrischen Anstalt, 1935–1945* (Geisenheim, 1983). In 1988, the tutor of the students' working group, Horst Dickel, published a document collection on Eichberg: *"Die sind doch alle unheilbar": Zwangssterilisation und Tötung der "Minderwertigen" im Rheingau, 1934–1945*, vol. 77 (Wiesbaden: Hessisches Institut für Bildungsplanung und Schulentwicklung, 1988).

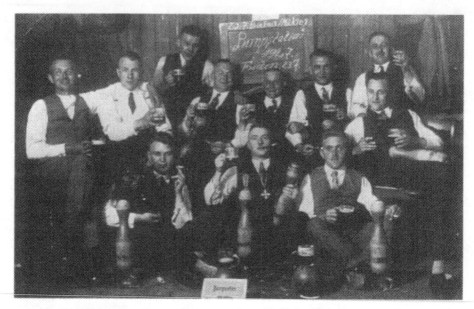

Mennecke's bowling club, 1927; Mennecke is fourth from the left, second row.

ter attending a three-year primary school, Friedrich Mennecke transferred to the *Gymnasium* in nearby Alfeld, and in 1920 to a *Gymnasium* in Einbeck. From 1920 until receiving his diploma in 1923, he and his brother lived in their grandmother's home, with their mother's unmarried sister. The elder Mennecke, an active Social Democrat, had gone off to fight in the First World War at age 42; like thousands of other veterans,[3] he returned in 1917 a shell-shocked cripple. Mennecke's father withdrew into himself as a result of his disability, and died in 1923 at not quite 51 years of age. It was probably within this constellation that Mennecke's wish to make a profession of a "healing" science was formed. This is made more likely by the fact that Friedrich Mennecke experienced not only material want, illness, and resignation within his own family, but also the economic and social crises of the period; his graduation from school and his father's death coincided with the peak of the inflation. Thus, Mennecke had to wait four years to begin his studies. An uncle—probably his mother's brother—supported the family after the father's death, but as a middle-level judicial official he was able to finance studies for only one of the two sons.

After receiving his diploma in 1923, Friedrich Mennecke first took up a commercial apprenticeship in the Deutsche Spiegelglas AG (German

Mirror Glass Company) in his hometown of Freden. After only a year of apprenticeship, he was temporarily made head of the entire export department at the firm's headquarters in Hanover. Returning to the branch in Freden, he worked as an export salesman. In a later résumé, Mennecke stated, "On 1 January 1927, the Freden factory, which had been economically undermined by Jewish members of the board of directors, was sold to a concern supported by French and Belgian capital. I was taken on by the new firm, but remained only until 15 October 1927."[4]

In another letter, also written later, Mennecke translated his office activities into political resistance: "I became a salesman, and in the firm in which I worked . . . I experienced Jewish corruption and egoism on the part of the directors of this German commercial firm in the truest sense of the word—sometimes even through personal experience. Even at that time my political views turned firmly against such dealings, and I longed for the moment when I could escape the economic power of my Jewish director and take up my studies."[5]

After his older brother had completed the legal exams to become a civil servant, Friedrich Mennecke was able to begin studying medicine in Göttingen in the winter semester of 1927–28.[6] In the summer semester of 1929 he transferred to Marburg-Lahn for two semesters, returning to Göttingen in 1930. There he passed the state medical exam on his second attempt and received a doctorate on 11 May 1934, with a grade of Good, for a thesis in pathology that he had already completed under Professor Georg Gruber two years previously ("Haemosiderin Nodes on the Epicard"). A particular medical attitude is already perceptible in this academic paper—incidentally, the only one Mennecke published. The dissertation describes only findings made on organs, without linking them in any way to the patient histories that accompanied them. It goes without saying that no dialogue between doctor and patient is possible with pathological preparations—only medicine as monologue. This distancing mechanism would appear again in Mennecke's later work as a consultant to the National Socialist euthanasia program, when he selected hundreds of people each day from psychiatric facilities and concentration camps.

Mennecke's Scientific and Political Career

Mennecke joined the Nazi party (28 March 1932) and the SS (1 May 1932) even before Hitler's seizure of power, during his studies in Göttingen. There, although just a student, he took charge of investigating SS applicants. He is not known to have been more than a simple party member before 1933, even though Mennecke later liked to call himself an "old fighter." The fact that he voluntarily joined the Nazi party in the final phase of the Weimar Republic, however, as did thousands of other students, is significant.[7]

Mennecke's social background and financial problems were typical of students of his time. Like him, tens of thousands of (primarily) sons of lower civil servants, white-collar workers, and small independent businessmen entered the universities during the Weimar Republic. These students experienced the catastrophic effects of the inflation of the early twenties and the Great Depression at the end of the same decade, which were intensified by insufficient mechanisms to aid students (government grants, dormitories, student cafeterias, etc.) and permanent academic unemployment; yet apparently it was not so much these difficulties that led these students to join fascist organizations. The National Socialist Student Union (Nationalsozialistische Deutscher Studentenbund; NSDStB), in particular, saw itself as the only political university association that could articulate and channel the deep crisis of meaning emerging at the universities, which extended beyond the increasing chasm between property and education. Thus, problems such as the social responsibility of science (which they termed "*völkisch* science"); the ivory-tower mentality of German professors; the separation of intellectual and physical labor, of work and the private sphere; and the demand for student participation in determining academic content were taken up mainly by National Socialist students. The issue of a "functional transformation of academic education" (Habermas) was probably decisive in making fascism attractive, more so than class-based political demands. The transformation of German universities from centers of education and contemplation into facilities for training natural scientists and teachers apparently was perceived as more of an issue than rampant undernourishment and threatened unemployment.[8]

Added to this was the fact that the sons of railroad officials, small farmers, and white-collar workers could hardly identify with the antiquated lifestyles of the fraternities and dueling societies. By propagating a reconciliation between workers and students, the SA, the NSDStB, and the Nazi party seemed to offer a "modern," realistic alternative. Their program foresaw an expanded politicization of scholarship through politicization of daily life, with new lifestyles and types of work. Living and working as a "political academic"—a scholar equally active in study and in the fraternity clubhouse, in the academic sphere and in the military training camp—would provide an escape from the ritualized lifestyles of the fraternities and the new isolation at these early "universities for the masses."

Mennecke's later efforts as a "political doctor" seeking to "redeem" society from unproductive or disruptive influences through medical means follow naturally from a social and biographical background defined in this way.

Immediately following his first state medical exam, Mennecke completed his internship at the Göttingen University Surgical Clinic, in the Department of Internal Medicine at the Peine City Hospital, at the Göttingen State Mental Hospital (with Professor Ewald, later one of the few German doctors who would openly oppose the Nazi euthanasia program), and in the Gynecological Department of the Frankfurt-Main University Clinic. Given the main focus of training during his internship, he might have been expected to specialize in internal medicine or psychiatry (four months each). Probably because of the continuing scarcity of jobs for doctors even after 1933, following a number of unsuccessful applications[9] Mennecke on 1 July 1935 began studying for a specialization in the Department of Surgical Gynecology of the Bad Homburg (Taunus) District Hospital. Because conditions there apparently did not suit him, he transferred after only two months to an internship at the Eichberg State Mental Hospital in the Rheingau. In another two years, Mennecke had advanced to chief physician; on 30 January 1939, he became director of the hospital. On 4 June 1937, during this extremely successful phase of his professional career, Mennecke married medical technician Eva W., eight years his junior.

As a political doctor and scientist, Mennecke enjoyed as-yet unheard of opportunities after 1933 to combine research and therapy with political practice. For the first time, a practical fusion of health care and social utopias became possible; a "healthy" world without the handicapped, the infirm, and the poor seemed attainable, to be achieved by young, active, idealistic doctors who had themselves come of age in "unhealthy" times.

For a young, ambitious, politically minded doctor like Friedrich Mennecke, advancement was all but inevitable. Thus, promotions followed rapidly: 1 February 1937, adjutant to the SS regional chief physician for the Rhine-Westmark region in Wiesbaden; 2 February 1937, SS master sergeant; 26 May 1937, SS second lieutenant; August 1937, district representative of the Racial Politics Office of the Nazi party for the districts of Rheingau and St. Goarshausen; 1 April 1939, local group leader of the Nazi party in Erbach-Eichberg; 20 April 1939, first lieutenant; October 1940, captain.

Mennecke was appointed troop physician at the beginning of the Second World War—behind the lines, however, in the Westwall zone between the Moselle and Saar rivers, although at the time he headed his letters "in the field." But his military service was terminated in January 1940 by a "special order" from the Adjutant Desk of the Führer's Office.[10] This "special assignment" was employment in the euthanasia program, begun in German psychiatric hospitals in the autumn of 1939. Mennecke's work mainly involved selection tours to psychiatric facilities (for example, Bethel, Lohr on the Main, Bedburg-Hau in the Rhineland, and Hall in the Tyrol), and later, more and more often, to concentration camps such as Dachau, Buchenwald, Ravensbrück, and Auschwitz. There he was responsible for selecting for extermination rebellious prisoners and those no longer able to work, particularly within the framework of Operation 14 f 13. At least 2,500 prisoners fell victim to Mennecke's "advisory activities."

Mennecke could not himself carry out the second planned focus of his special assignment: heading a so-called pediatrics department ("Kinderfachabteilung"), that is, a clinic in which children would be killed, in his hospital at Eichberg. Because of his frequent absences on selection tours, and also because of conflicts of principle with the expert in charge of hospitals in Hesse, Fritz Bernotat, he had to transfer direction of the "pediatrics department," established at the beginning of 1941, to his deputy, Dr. Walter Schmidt.

Also unable to make it past the early stages was the "modernization" of the Eichberg Hospital that Mennecke actively planned. This meant introduction of "active therapy,"[11] such as the new shock treatment, especially electroshock, supplemented by work therapy, also a relatively new method.[12] Mennecke hoped to introduce the newest types of diagnostic and therapeutic treatment, in order to be able to separate patients who were curable in the short term from therapy-resistant cases or those "unworthy" of therapy. The victims of this psychiatric triage—at the Eichberg Hospital, they were mainly children—were authorized for "therapeutic extermination" through overdoses of medication. After they were murdered, their brains were used for research on the physiological and morphological symptoms of certain mental illnesses, or conditions and behavioral patterns that were seen as such.

The scientific analysis of euthanasia victims occurred in cooperation with the Heidelberg University Neurological and Psychiatric Clinic, headed by Professor Carl Schneider. The structuring of this "division of labor," as well as the modernization of Eichberg, was slowed by the above-mentioned hospital expert, Bernotat. While Mennecke represented the dialectic of intensive cure and specific extermination, Bernotat demanded indiscriminate killing of "useless eaters" in order to gain hospital beds and reduce costs. Through an old war buddy of Hitler's, the *Gauleiter* of Hesse, Jakob Sprenger, Bernotat's influence reached as far as the Führer's Office. As a result, in 1943 Mennecke was assigned "probation at the front" as a troop physician, first on the French Channel coast, then on the eastern front.

As Red Army troops approached and an order home on "special assignment" failed to materialize, Mennecke wrote his wife:

> If it continues this way much longer, I will consider going to the hospital with a "heart ailment" and traveling "home to the Reich" on a hosp. train. I'm not chickening out, but I don't want to destroy myself either.[13]

Mennecke, who otherwise cynically treated so-called actors so they could return to the front as soon as possible, actually did become ill— right on the deadline he had set of "10 or 15 August" (1943).[14] The illness of choice, however, was not a heart ailment, but goiter.

Even after his recovery in various hospitals back home, however, Mennecke was not allowed to return to the Eichberg Hospital he had headed. Instead, he was transferred—again as a military doctor—to a hospital in Bühl (Baden).

Mennecke continued to work with the Berlin euthanasia authorities, once again taking part in conferences of the T-4 advisers. With the help of Professor Heyde's successor, chief consultant Professor Nitsche, Mennecke attempted a number of times to assume direction of another psychiatric facility. Temporarily under discussion were the Meseritz-Obrawalde (Pomerania) euthanasia facilities or Bernburg-Saale and the Plagwitz hospitals (Silesia) or Graz. After only a few months as a neurologist, however, Mennecke switched roles yet again. During a routine x-ray examination, a (most probably old) tuberculosis was discovered in his lungs. Not until March 1945 could he once again work in a hospital as a neurologist, but after a short time he again became ill with tuberculosis. Mennecke experienced the end of National Socialist rule as a patient. In autumn 1945 he moved to Northeim, not far from his mother's home. Shortly thereafter, his wife, Eva, who now lived near her—unmolested—husband, was arrested. Because no assistance in her husband's "consulting" work could be proven against her, she was quickly released.

The two lived together inconspicuously until the spring of 1946. Not until Mennecke tried to begin working as a doctor in a refugee camp—

the former youth concentration camp Moringen—at the beginning of April was he arrested.

The Trial

The so-called Eichberg trial in the Frankfurt-Main State Court against Mennecke, Walter Schmidt, his deputy and head of the "pediatrics department," and two nurses, one female orderly, and two male orderlies ended in a death sentence for Mennecke. The court found him guilty of the murder of at least 2,500 people through his work as "consultant" in psychiatric facilities and concentration camps and as head of a facility and its attached "pediatrics department." The letters found (probably with his wife) after his arrest served as evidence, although only a third of the original 8,000 pages had survived.

The life sentence against Dr. Schmidt was commuted in 1953 as a result of continuing public pressure. Two of the accused nurses and orderlies received prison sentences of between four and eight years; three were acquitted.

The court justified handing down different sentences for Mennecke and Schmidt by arguing that Mennecke acted out of base motives such as careerism and profit-seeking. In Dr. Schmidt's case, on the other hand, the court discerned a therapeutic idealism and activism, which it considered "mitigating circumstances."

Mennecke escaped his punishment—which would not have been carried out in any case, as appeals and new trials in similar cases later proved—on 28 January 1947 in the Butzbach prison near Frankfurt am Main. Two causes of death are possible: one is the acute tuberculosis from which he had been suffering for over two years, combined with his generally bad physical and mental state. The second was suggested in a newspaper article on 1 February 1947: "Dr. Mennecke dead: Dr. Friedrich Mennecke, condemned to death at the Eichberg trial, was brought to Butzbach state prison several days ago. Mennecke died suddenly yesterday evening, two days after a visit from his wife. The prison administration would not comment on the cause of death." [15]

The Letters

The extraordinarily extensive, at times almost simultaneous, description of daily life in his letters cannot be explained as a normal need for communication on Mennecke's part. The conspicuous precision of the letters (which his wife matched), the significance of times, exact dates, places, titles, details like exact amounts of money, etc., most likely fulfilled a broader function. Such a framework of figures, titles, and details provides orientation in disturbed times. Particularly given Mennecke's biography, characterized by difficult material conditions, a delayed career, and socioeconomic crises, one can understand such a need for stability and a binding orientation pattern. This deep insecurity, reinforced by rapid social ascent from a working-class family, extended to behavioral insecurity in daily life. Thus, shortly after his arrival at a sanatorium in which his tuberculosis was to be treated, Mennecke, long since the director of an institution, adviser on euthanasia, and protégé of influential scientists like Nitsche and Carl Schneider, wrote:

> This afternoon for the first time I will go—in uniform—to eat in the dining room. . . . It's like this: breakfast is eaten around eight downstairs in the dining room in "free dress"—that is, a track suit or the like. A second breakfast is brought to your room. We have lunch and dinner in the dining room at 12:30 and 6:30—after a gong—either in uniform or a civilian suit; in any case, dressed up. Afternoon coffee may be taken anytime downstairs in the dining room. So that's the new routine nowadays! Monday and Thursday we go to the movies—in addition to the half-hour walk that we take during the afternoon hours from 4–6 o'clock (that is, not exactly half an hour!) . . .
>
> We sit at single tables. I have been asked to sit at the colonel's table, with an elderly major and a planner. . . . The diners here are quite colorful; most of the gentlemen wear *civilian clothing*. Soon I'll only be wearing civilian clothes myself. Here one wears the Nazi insignia on civilian suits. *So please send me my party and SS insignia,* preferably packed well in a strong envelope, by registered mail. . . . For a while I will continue to show up in uniform, but starting around Sunday only in civilian clothes.[16]

His obsession with detail extended even to the reason for writing itself:

> So this "very last letter" is going to be written after all—for various reasons:
>
> 1. I feel a need to describe to you the course of my very last solo day in Heidelberg today,
> 2. the chronological chain of my report on my Heidelberg "student" days should not end without the links being completed,

3. this is now letter no. 15, the "last one" in five weeks, which means I have written you three letters a week, and

4. I still have to say good night to you.[17]

The reason for this unusual precision was not only the most extensive possible communication with his wife. On the first document that has survived, a 1927 photograph of Mennecke's bowling club, he noted, "Keep for the chronicle of my life!" In later letters, he wrote, "He who writes, lives!"[18] or "They [the letters] should bear witness for a long time to these greatest of all times!"[19] In the face of a life and letters that he considered more or less a higher duty, the importance of his wife as a correspondent fades. She often seems little more than a projection screen for her husband's "essential reports to history," or at least to a hoped-for reader of a future generation.

In addition to social orientation and fulfillment of what he seemed to see as a historic mission, Mennecke's letters served other purposes. They achieved a linguistic symbiosis when Mennecke was forced to live separately from his wife—whether because of "advisory" trips or "probation at the front." Their mutual infantilization ("Mommy," "Pa") could not conceal the patriarchal structure of the relationship, which is expressed when Mennecke calls his wife a "Mommy-*child*," while she calls him "Master."

The dichotomy characteristic of such a symbiosis[20]—an idealized, conflict-free interior and a threatening, aggressive exterior—is also present in Friedrich Mennecke. Thus, one searches in vain—aside from one exception in an early letter before their wedding—for differences of opinion between the partners. There is not even a hint of such conflict. But Mennecke's relationship with his wife is marked by yet another dichotomy. On the one hand, he describes his wife as "Mommy," "Mommy-child," "little guy," or "Eva-comrade"; on the other, he describes "Jew-wenches" in the East or his "Bolshevik" sister-in-law: "I think she boozes and whores a lot!!"[21]

This points to the crucial factor separating "Mommy-child" and "Bolshevik whore." Linguistic desexualization of one's own, as well as of politically or socially acceptable women, contrasts with the sexualization of women who behave autonomously or even simply differently. This also explains the "diagnoses" of mainly female concentration camp inmates, which basically reproduced again and again the association "sexuality—Communism." The barely concealed connection between deterioration of

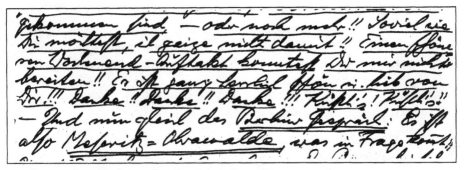

Excerpt from the letter of 23 June 1944.

a "coerced sexual morality" (W. Reich) and deterioration of the power relations in which Mennecke had established himself with great effort had to be repelled through aggressive devaluation, even to the point of killing these representatives of "subversion" and rebellion. The dichotomy between the desexualized "Mommy-child-comrade," on the one hand, and the "Bolshevik whore," on the other, also reflects a separation of aggressions. Employing a projective defense that was already familiar from the *Freikorps* literature [22] and anti-Soviet propaganda of the early twenties, Mennecke, too, wished to protect his "Mommy-child" from the "cruelty of the Soviets . . . with rape and slaughter of women": [23]

> Caution is always advisable! Never walk alone in the dark, and if possible not in daylight, in empty places! This is especially important for you now, dearest Evelyn!! I often think with concern of your walk up to the Eichberg from the railroad station in the dark!! . . . It would be the most horrible thing if I had to go through something like this with you! [24]

The enemy without was, so to speak, everywhere:

> And if the world were full of devils, "the two of us" are together, come hell or high water—even if the whole world conspires against and attacks us!! [25]

Their conflict-free symbiosis was the opposite pole:

> *I am soooooo happy, dearest Evalein,* to possess *you completely,* and to be able to rely on you in everything—and to know that you think and feel exactly as I do—that "the two of us" can be truly wrapped up in each other!! [26]

Separation phenomena, idealization, and devaluation can be found not only in Mennecke's symbiotic relationship and not only in regard to women. He constructed his entire social environment around such defense mechanisms—at least to the extent that it appears in his letters. Thus, Mennecke wrote admiringly of the "many books in the study"[27] at Professor Zucker's (a colleague of Professor Carl Schneider's in Heidelberg), or of his trip to the eastern front:

> The commander sat in my compartment. . . . My good map with the country borders and railways is very much in demand. They all like to orient themselves by it; the commander was just here.[28]

Or on his position as physician to the troops:

> Today the true focus of our entire unit was here *with me!!* This is not presumption on my part, but *reality,* for whatever information had to be passed on went through my telephone!! It is rare, after all, that the entire strategic service is focused on the office of *Dept. IVb,* but I have achieved this here in this department!! Actually it is not a big deal, when I consider that I could be the father of all these influential information officers. They are all attracted to me and enjoy being here.[29]

On the other hand, Mennecke described the concentration camp inmates he selected simply as "Pat" (patient)[30] or "antisocial . . . to the highest degree."[31] The victims were literally objectified as "portions" and registration forms:

> First there were some 40 forms still to complete on the first portion of Aryans, which my other two colleagues had already worked on yesterday.[32]

Mennecke, who himself planned to be sent home because of a "heart ailment," defamed subordinate soldiers as "wash-outs"[33] when they collapsed during a cholera inoculation.

Entire peoples were denigrated if they were considered Bolsheviks:

> You can tell by looking at the Russian people that they are born and raised right in the dirt, so they don't know any better. These people are really only silhouettes in human form that Jewish Bolshevism had an easy time molding in its image. No other people would be better suited to be misused for an idea as absurd and crazy as Bolshevism. This is not a master race, but the most primitive, stubborn, and shabby heap of humanity that we have in Europe. A single human life means as little here as in any lower order of animals.[34]

His thorough refusal to feel empathy for the victims and patients who did not behave acceptably brings forth sentences like this one:

> So, Mommy, Pa has now thrown together a recommendation that he is pleased with. The man will probably be condemned to death.[35]

or:

> Then we drank another *bottle of Eisenthaler* and conversed quite flowingly and pleasantly about the *problem of the antisocials,* with me exclusively the giving (pontificating) side. It was very, very pleasant . . . ![36]

Nevertheless, Mennecke was not entirely the unfeeling medical technocrat that these quotes make him seem. The astonishing thing about his written language, in fact, is precisely the often completely unexpected juxtaposition of extreme objectification and almost melting sentimentality. The separation phenomenon sketched above is accompanied by a contrast between "external" and "internal" language. While Mennecke acted deliberately martial in front of colleagues, superiors, and subordinates (see Doc. 7), to his wife he at least hinted at feelings of fear or helplessness. Thus emerged Mennecke's typical language, a combination of military private and petit bourgeois, local party leader and doctor. Finally, it is remarkable which functions Mennecke's letters did *not* serve. In the approximately 2,500 pages that have survived, one searches in vain for feelings of guilt about his participation in the Nazi euthanasia program. Friedrich Mennecke had so firmly internalized the "historic mission" of a cost-reducing modernization of German psychiatry that he did not even begin to experience ethical doubts.

Selected Letters *

Doc. 1

Letter no. 8   Weimar, 25 November 1941
                                        (Hotel Elephant) (8:58 P.M.)

My dearest, best little Mommy!

I have been waiting almost an hour to speak to you; I have not yet made it "urgent," but if it doesn't come through soon I will register it as

---

* The letters by Mennecke that have so far been located can be divided into the following phases: (1) search for a position as intern (1935); (2) resident physician at Eichberg-Rheingau (1935–39); (3) consultant to Operation 14 f 13, which selected for

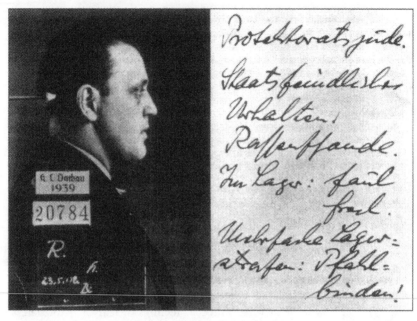

A diagnosis by Mennecke, which amounted to a selection for death. This is an example from Dachau. The diagnosis, translated, reads: "Jew from the Protectorate. Antistate behavior, miscegenation. In the camp: lazy, impudent. Many punishments in camp: tied to the post!"

"urgent." I am sitting here in my room, No. 235 (third floor), listening to music on the radio, with freshly bathed feet and a delicious dinner (little delicacies: bouillon, Hamburg herring salad, Swiss cheese). Now Barnabas is playing his lively tunes—are you listening too? I hope I'll be able to send them to you soon over the telephone, when I get you on the line.

extermination disruptive prisoners and inmates of psychiatric facilities and concentration camps who were unable to work (1940–42: see Doc. 1); (4) classes with Prof. Carl Schneider at the University Neurological and Psychiatric Clinic in Heidelberg (1942: see Docs. 2, 3, and 5) (5) army doctor on the French Channel coast near Dunkirk (1943); (6) army doctor on the Eastern front near Charkov (1943, see Docs. 6–10); (7) patient being treated for goiter in various hospitals (1943–44); (8) army doctor in the Bühl-Baden and Bruchsal hospitals (1944: see Doc. 11); (9) tuberculosis patient at hospital in St. Blasien, Schwarzwald (1944); (10) tuberculosis patient at hospital in Rockenau-Odenwald (1944–45).

From the few available letters written by Mennecke's wife, Eva, I have selected one from the period when Mennecke was observing the work done at Professor Carl Schneider's clinic, because this letter refers to a letter of Mennecke's that is also presented here (see Doc. 4). Sections in italics are underlined in the original.

Earlier I had two evening drinks with Schmalenbach and Müller* in a little restaurant. At 7:00 P.M. we ate dinner here in our hotel restaurant, and now each has returned to his own room. At 7:00 tomorrow morning we will wake up, have coffee at about 8:00, and be driven out in Schmalenbach's car, which will then drive off to Dresden. On Thursday and Friday there is a meeting in Pirna connected with the Operation† at which the future is to be discussed, and in which Schmalenbach is to take part as the medical adjutant to Herr Brack (Jennerwein).‡ No consultants will be there. Now I want to read until I hear your voice, my love! Come soon—in person!! Youyou.

9:25 P.M.: Hey!! I can still hear you say: Ahoy!!ǁ And eight days from today I will have you here, my love!! I'm looking forward to it very very much!! But it's hard that the post takes so long. Well, at least the telephone is reliable, it is a *beneficent institution!!*

Now I'm going to read a bit longer, and at 10 o'clock I will lie down. The conversation cost four marks. Are you already turning in, or will you also stay up until ten? Kissy, kissy—many many loving ones, youyou!!!!

10:30: So, little mouse, now I've finished the brochure "The Wartime Goals of the World Plutocracy." Like any German who reads this brochure, I am shaken by what we will face if we lose this war. But it will not be lost, it is already won! Now I'm going to go again . . . and then get into this snug bed that does honor to this hotel, which is distinguished as a "model enterprise"; it is modeled exactly on the Deutscher Hof hotel in Nuremberg. Now sleep well, my little heart, pleasant dreams, and get enough sleep!!

Loving good-night kisses from Pa!!

Wednesday, 26 November 1941, 7 A.M.: Brring—brring—brring: seven o'clock!! Wake up! A hearty good morning, Mommy!!! Kissy! Still snoozing, eh? Now up, shave! Ahoy!!!

7:30: I'm through, even with sh . . . ; now off to start another day. This evening I'll write again. Kissies!! Ahoy!!!

* Kurt Schmalenbach, resident physician at Sonnenstein-Pirna near Dresden, and Robert Müller, resident physician at Königslutter near Braunschweig, were consultant colleagues of Mennecke's in the euthanasia program.
† The reference is to euthanasia.
‡ Viktor Brack directed Main Office II of the Führer's Office; this main office formed the top administration of the euthanasia program, within which Brack used the cover name "Jennerwein."
ǁ This nautical term was occasionally in vogue in Germany as a greeting.

7:50 P.M.: Home again, my little mouse!! My first day at work in Buchenwald is over. We went out early this morning at 8:30. First I introduced myself to the most important leaders. The deputy camp commander is SS Captain Florstedt, the camp doctor SS First Lieutenant Dr. Hofen.* First there were some 40 forms still to complete on the first portion of Aryans, which my other two colleagues had already worked on yesterday. Of these 40, I worked on around 15. When this whole portion had been completed, Schmalenbach left for Dresden; he won't return until we have finished working here. Afterwards came the "examination" of the pat.; that is, appearance of the individual and comparison with the entries in the files. We were not finished with this until noon, for our two colleagues only worked theoretically yesterday; so I "reexamined" those that Schmalenbach (and myself, this morning) had prepared, and Müller did his own. At noon we took a break and ate in the officers' mess (first class! Soup, boiled beef, red cabbage, boiled potatoes, apple compote—for 1.50 marks!), *no* ration coupons. While being introduced to all the SS leaders, I recognized the second lieutenant who was adjutant in the Hinzert[†] camp in December 1940. He recognized me immediately, too, and also inquired after your health.[‡]

At 1:30 P.M. we began the examinations again, but Ribbentrop's speech began and we stopped to listen to it. He said a lot of good things, did you hear the speech? After that we did examinations until around 4:00; I did 105 pats., Müller 78 pats., so that in the end our first installment of 183 forms was completed. The second portion followed, a total of 1,200 Jews, none of whom are even examined; it is enough to take the reason for arrest (often very comprehensive!) from the file and enter it on the form. Thus it is purely theoretical work, which will certainly occupy our time until Monday, maybe even longer. For this second portion (Jews), we did the following today: 17 for me, 15 for Müller. At exactly 5:00 P.M. we "threw in the towel" and went to dinner: a cold plate of salami (nine large slices), butter, bread, and a helping of coffee! Cost: .80 marks without coupons!! At 5:30 we were driven back to Weimar by a crim. [criminal] investigator, an SS master sergeant (Leclair), who lives in Weimar but takes his car here every day. He picks us up at the hotel every morning at 8:00 and brings us back at 5:30; in exchange we give him our gasoline coupons. He already has 10 liters that Schmalenbach

* Dr. Hoven is meant.
† A concentration camp near Hermeskeil in Hunsrück.
‡ Paragraph indentions are added for the reader's convenience.

had left over, and we'll get another 5 liters from Berlin; the distance is 10 kilometers. The man (Leclair) drives very carefully and responsibly. In the city, I checked at the post office to see if the cigarettes from Emil Schmidt* had come; they aren't here yet. Then we sat for an hour in the café of the Weimar Hall, where Müller is going to see the comedy "Wednesday Evening Music" tonight. I haven't gone yet, because it seems to me this comedy is nothing special. If it is good, I can still see it anytime—or with you next Wednesday. So after 7:00 I wandered slowly back to the Hotel Elephant from the Weimar Hall.

Yesterday afternoon I sent the gray suit in to be pressed; it came back just before, but one rear seam had split again. So I just had the chambermaid sew it up, provisionally, for one mark—*I really missed my Mommy!!* Now everything is all right again; I have put on the gray suit and will have the blue one pressed tomorrow morning. I just listened to the address by Rear Admiral Lützow, then the news, and now the evening concert (8:40 P.M.), which you are probably also listening to. I want to sit in the hall downstairs for a while (I live on the third floor) and read to music on the radio. Maybe the orchestra will be playing as well. The next few days will be like today—with exactly the same program and the same work. After the Jews, some 300 Aryans come next as the third portion to be "examined." Thus, we will have work to do here until around the end of next week. Then on Saturday, 6 December, we will go home, on 7 December the people from Frankfurt† can come, on 9 December there is the concert in the hall, and on 13 December (Saturday) we'll leave again for Berlin, from where we will continue on to Fürstenberg‡ on 14 December, because work begins there again on 15 December. We'll be through with Ravensbrück by 20 December, and then we'll go to your parents for Christmas. Whether Gr. Rosen‖ near Jauer will follow has not yet been decided in the affirmative; we can almost certainly expect it for the beginning of January. That is the program for "this year," so we won't be able to take part in the Christmas celebration at the Senior Section [of the SS] in Mainz. That won't do us any harm!

I'll mail this letter now, so you will quickly find out how our program is structured. Müller is going home from Sat. afternoon to Mon. afternoon, Königslutter near Braunschweig. I'm going to wander around

* The cook at the Eichberg asylum in Rheingau headed by Mennecke.
† The reference is to Mennecke's brother, Karl, and his wife, Beli.
‡ Near the Ravensbrück concentration camp.
‖ Gross-Rosen, concentration camp near Breslau.

Weimar; too bad you won't be here yet!!! Tomorrow I expect your (third) letter. *So, my dearest Mommy, once again you get soooooo many loving kisses, and I hug you very, very tightly in joyful expectation of your coming, you leetle mouse, from your faithful Pa.*

Doc. 2

Letter no. 9

Heidelberg, 30 June 1942
Hotel Reichspost
Annex, Rm. 57

My dearest and best little Mommy!

It is *Tues. evening, 10:45 P.M.;* this new letter—already in my night-shirt—must still be started. I just devoured a delicious "Mommy roll" with "Mommy butter" and "Mommy sausage." It tasted very much like peace. Before that, I took my usual foot bath—and now I'll be turning in very soon. You'll probably be doing the same thing soon, or already have. At 8:00 I mailed the other letter, then took a little walk on the Neckar-staden, and at 9:00 sat in the Reichpost restaurant for the length of two beers. There I looked around for awhile, then read the paper and listened to the ten o'clock news. At ten it became quite crowded, because the Sere-nade concert was over. So I made for home. At the train station I inquired about my Sunday train: *3:04 P.M. from Heidelberg, 4:59 arrival in Mainz.* There is no connection from there to the passenger train from Wiesbaden at 5:25 P.M. that arrives in Eltville at 5:46. To catch the pass. train in Wiesbdn. I would have to take the streetcar, but I don't know how often it runs or whether I would be sure to catch the pass. train at 5:25; I don't think so. Therefore it would probably be best if you (Massing* and you) would *pick me up at the main train station in Mainz with the Kadetti at 4:59 P.M..* We can talk about it more on the telephone; I'll call on Friday evening at the latest, around 8:00. You'll probably be at home—if not, you can call me earlier at the clinic† (tel. 4851—the switchboard for *all* clinics, so you still have to ask for the psychiatric clinic!); the best time is during meals, that is, between 12:30 and 1:00 or between 6:30 and 7:00. However, if you do not *call the clinic, then I will call* on Friday evening at 8:00 at the latest.

---

* Driver for the Eichberg Asylum in Rheingau.

† University Psychiatric and Neurological Clinic in Heidelberg, in which Mennecke studied for several weeks with the scientific protagonist of the Nazi euthanasia program, Prof. Carl Schneider. Prof. Schneider killed himself on 10–11 December 1946 while in pretrial detention, by slitting his wrists and hanging himself.

So, heart's Mommy, now get in bed quickly and have another wonderful sleep—peacefully and undisturbed! Go on now!!

Loving Daddy-Kissies! Ahoy!

Good night!!

Wed., 1 July 1942, 7:30 A.M.: A hearty good morning, Mommy!! I slept sooooo well once again and now I'm ready to go. The sun is streaming in through all the cracks; it's really summer at last! Now, off to start another day and to work! Kissies!! Ahoy!!!

1:15 P.M.: Wow! Is it ever hot! July can really do a better job than June! Is my Mommy sweating too? I only went the distance from the clinic to here and had to take off my thick wool socks and rinse my feet, and then take off my pants, shirt, and underpants. Nobody can see me here, the door is closed and no one can look in the window—so only my Mommy sees me, and she doesn't mind her naked Pa! Your letter hasn't come yet, it won't turn up until tomorrow; instead a registered letter came, a new package* from Berlin. It's like this all the time; they always make sure Pa has something to do. God knows, he's not here to laze about; but in exchange Berlin should be sending something too—I mean money! I will write to Nitsche† and ask him to cover the cost of your one-week course, since if they want to do things here to promote clinical research methods, diagnosis of spinal fluid cells is part of that, and this in turn requires technical laboratory work. I want to be sure to write the letter to Nitsche this afternoon. I don't have much time outside of the work on the ward, but I'll manage it. From three to five o'clock P.M. today, we have more lectures by Schneider. There was a great deal of work again this morning: visits, shocks,‡ occipital aspiration,‖ blood tests, reexaminations, taking patient reports from relatives, etc. The scholars could not agree this morning on *one* very interesting case: Schneider said schizophrenia, Zucker# said "delirium." Then Zucker aspirated the case himself; he was very interested in it, and of course, so was I. For breakfast there was the

---

* Of euthanasia registration forms.

† Professor Paul Hermann Nitsche, director of the Sonnenstein-Pirna killing facility near Dresden, main consultant on euthanasia of adults, successor to Professor Heyde (after 1945, Heyde used the cover name Sawade) after December 1941. He was executed on 25 March 1948.

‡ Electroshocks.

‖ For diagnosing inflammations of the central nervous system.

Professor Theodor Zucker, deputy to Professor Carl Schneider and euthanasia consultant.

usual quantity of butter, bread, two rolls, and one (triangular) cheese. I took along a little cheese and two rolls for this evening, as it was too much for me. For lunch there was an excellent bouillon with homemade noodles, three Heine's Halberstadt sausages (one of them will be eaten tonight), mangold root and potatoes, and a green salad. So, dear heart, I will end this letter now, so you'll hear as soon as possible that you have to pick me up in Mainz. We hold to the agreement above: I will call you on *Fri.* evening if you don't call me before that at the clinic. I'm only bringing the small suitcase with me. Now I will finish working on the Berlin package that I've started; tomorrow and the day after I will do the one that arrived today. *In three days I'm leaving for Mommy's — hurray! I already fly to you in my thoughts and am right beside you!* Are you at the Henkels'* today? Please, always greet our friends the Henkels and Friedrichs† from me. *I hug you very tightly, my good little Mommy, and kiss you over and over again!!*

Ardently!
Your faithful Fritz-Pa

Doc. 3

Letter no. 10   Heidelberg, 1 July 1942
                                                 Hotel Reichspost, Annex

My dearest, best little Mommy!

It is *Wed. evening, 10:25;* I want to start the last letter this week to tell you how the afternoon went. Shortly before 3:00 I mailed letter no. 9‡ in the box at the main post office, and quickly read today's Wehrmacht report containing the German *summer offensive on the central and southern sections of the eastern front.* Let's hope they'll be followed by special reports of successes! At 3:10 I was at the forensic lecture at the clinic, where Professor Schneider introduced a 21-year-old epileptic who murdered his wife, who was a lesbian, in April by throwing her into the Neckar. The man suffers from epilepsy (probably traumatic), but he shows no signs of dementia and was therefore declared completely sane— and thus condemned to death! That was also my feeling about this rec-

---

* Dr. Otto Henkel, retired director of the Hadamar facility and former chief physician of the Eichberg Hospital.

† Dr. Hans Friedrich, physician to the top SS "Rhine" section (SS-Oberabschnitt), independent dermatologist in Wiesbaden.

‡ Doc. 2.

ommendation. Then, between lectures, I had a meeting with Professor Schneider in his office:

(1) Dr. Schmidt* is going to come here during the semester break, even if there are no lectures. Prof. Sch[neider] explained this more or less as follows: With me it's different than with Dr. Schmidt, since I am older and director and chief at Eichberg; therefore I cannot and must not do the therapeutic and examination work of a physician myself, but should only direct—just as he does here. Therefore he had insisted that I come as quickly as possible, so that I would be able to attend this semester and the lectures. My responsibility—in contrast to Dr. Schmidt's—is to gain insight, especially here, into his *completely new concept of psychiatry,* so that, thus armed, I can shape the Eichberg facility with regard to the Operation according to his model. He pointed out that he purposely, *thinking of me, presented his new theories* in his lectures whenever it seemed appropriate—always keeping in mind the problem of the Operation. He thought I probably had noticed this; he had sensed it in our frequent discussions of these problems. He didn't want to be only a teacher of students; with his knowledge, based on a National Socialist world-view, he addressed above all those destined to take part in the Operation. Thus I was *the first one* to learn his completely new ideas in context, and his goal was to pass on these ideas to all "leading" members of the Operation. Unfortunately, there was not enough time and opportunity for all those involved. In this context, he then said that Dr. Schmidt (and possibly "the new doctor"), along with his (Schneider's) assistant, would have to learn the method through practical work on the wards, which he (Dr. Schmidt) could then apply practically at Eichberg. Thus, Dr. Schmidt did not need the coherent scientific and ideological training that he (Schneider) could and wanted to give *me.* So, even if he himself and Professor Zucker will not be here while Dr. Schmidt is attending classes, as they will be on vacation in August and September, still Dr. Schmidt's participation here is desirable. Thus, he advised me to send Dr. Schmidt here approximately 14 days after my return to Eichberg, rather than waiting for the winter semester, especially since our new department is to be set up as soon as possible. This version from Professor Schneider means a lot to me; it basically corresponds with the opinion I had already formed myself on these issues. It also clearly defines my own position. He also said he had already discussed all this with Professor Nitsche.

* Mennecke's deputy at the Eichberg Hospital, head of the "pediatrics department" (*Kinderfachabteilung*), that is, the child-killing facility.

(2) He is completely agreeable to *your* training on the technical aspects of collecting data on spinal fluid cells; he very much advocates my plan, and advised me to approach Professor Nitsche officially on the question of expenses, which is actually not his responsibility, since he charges no fees for our training, and any assumption of costs from Berlin can only be an advantage to our pocketbooks. I have already drafted a letter to Nitsche, which I will type and send tomorrow. (3) I asked him to send Dr. Schmieder* to Eichberg after I return, so that I can discuss with him on the spot how to set up our photo work for the Reich Committee cases.† I already told you that there are many important scientific aspects to consider. Prof. Sch[neider] agreed that Dr. Schmieder will come, and we spoke about future Reich Committee work. This discussion today was once again very, very important to me! Apparently it was also important to him, for we even missed the punctual beginning of the following "psychology lectures" by almost 10 minutes. The latter, in turn, was extraordinarily impressive! Especially for those who—like me—see behind all these things the enormous question of eu., the psychology lectures are uniquely enjoyable. . . .

1:15: Hey there!! Hey there!! A letter from my Mommy with 30 marks in cash has arrived! Hearty Pa-thank-you-kissies for it, my good Pommy-Mommy. Now I want to go through the course catalog. But that's news, that H.‡ will no longer be an E.‖ facility and is being set up as a state mental hospital once again. But I can imagine the reasons for this measure: temporarily to save the expenses the E. facility ran up despite the pause in activity, and also probably its unfavorable location, which was often mentioned. We will have to wait and see what happens next. The "dissolution" of the Public Foundation# was probably an expedient measure, as at the moment minor financial work can be taken care of in other ways. The name was only camouflage anyway, and it was actually only a

---

* Dr. Friedrich Schmieder, intern to Professor Schneider; mainly responsible for scientific photography of euthanasia victims.
† The Reich Committee for the Scientific Processing of Serious Genetic Diseases (Reichsausschuß zur wissenschaftlichen Erfassung von erb- und anlagebedingten schweren Leiden) was the organization that camouflaged the euthanasia of children.
‡ Hadamar.
‖ Euthanasia.
The Public Foundation for Asylum Maintenance (Gemeinnützige Stiftung für Anstaltspflege) was particularly responsible for personnel and financial matters in the euthanasia program.

small department in the entire Operation. Things will continue for us as before, except we may receive more patients at Eichberg. Well, that wouldn't be such a terrible thing, but it mustn't detract from our ability to set up the new department. In this regard I have to be careful with Berno,* or he will bungle everything for me with his eagerness to accept patients. At a suitable opportunity, I will ask Professor Nitsche in detail about the state of affairs. . . .

I didn't hear about the fall of Sevastopol until this morning. It's fabulous! Now we're attacking heavily again on all fronts—hopefully for the last time! This morning, in addition to my work I also wrote to Nitsche; I am enclosing both copies. I already spoke early today with the financial counselor about your taking meals in the officers' mess. So the week after next you will be able to take part in everything here. But we will still take some "easy" days for ourselves—summer vacation!! Otherwise, nothing special happened this morning. Of the gentlemen from the reserve hospital, staff physician Dr. Schmidt of Klingenmünster and Dr. Gutterer, the physician's assistant, who is assistant here in peacetime, will have to leave tomorrow. They have to report to Bad Kreuznach, and will very probably be sent to the eastern front for the offensive. I hardly think Dr. Dieke will be furloughed. Let's wait and see what he writes. I wonder if they might even take me again. But I don't really think so, for who would do everything at Eichberg then? In any case, they are again making enormous efforts to end the war. Probably they have already assembled the forces needed for the offensive. We must anxiously await what the future holds! It is now 2:05 P.M. and I want to start on the photocopies† in the new package. There is always something to be done; Pa has no time for napping! I always sleep very well at night, so during the day I am bright enough to work straight through. It is not advisable to move around much in this humid heat, especially since the ball of my toe is pricking again; it has to go back to Mommy for treatment! *Now I hug you very, very tightly, my Goody, hug, caress, and kiss you lovingly and fervently, like I did eight or nine years ago! The day after tomorrow I will be ready to come to you!! Ahoy!!! Most fervent kisses, my good Mo . . . y, from*

Your
Faithful dear Pa.

---

* State administrator (Landesrat) Fritz Bernotat, responsible for the asylums in Hesse.
† Euthanasia registration forms.

Doc. 4

Wife's letter   Eichberg, 1 July 1942

My best and dearest Daddy!

With great happiness and pride over the special report* read out an hour ago, I begin this letter, which my beloved husband will read when he returns home. Did you also hear the announcement of the fall of Sevastopol? They have finally succeeded; the battle was long and hard, but the strongest bulwark in the south has fallen, and things will move along briskly now. This war will end someday after all!! Now a bit about my day: Your sweet letter came with the mail, and I'll hug and kiss you for it as soon as I have you here. For now, a thousand thanks. In addition, there was: one letter from the parents, one letter from Nalaba† with 1,019.56 marks' credit, and one letter from the civil servants' home. The cherries took two days to arrive home; some of them were rotten, but Mommy still canned 12 jars. Daddy is going to Salzbrunn at the end of July after all; he got a room, and the school board granted him vacation. Everything else you can read for yourself.

It was very decent of Gareis to deliver 50 bottles of wine; however, they are not cheap. I just wrote the remittance for 228.50 marks, which will go out tomorrow. Maybe the wine will be here by Sunday.

The cherries for the Friedrichs did not arrive today, which is all right with me. I hope now I can go to Wiesbaden tomorrow. Otherwise, the morning passed in housework, fixing up the room to let, etc. . . . Today, Fräulein Fay helped me; after eating, I first organized my work basket, then darned until 5:00 P.M. Then Herr Wirges‡ called and asked if our air-raid shelter was in order, as an inspection commission was coming from St. Goarshausen. I checked everything, and refilled the water and sand on the staircase, so now everything is in order. However, they did not inspect it; they were only more or less at Herr Wirges'. I saw them standing down at the hothouse for a long time. From 5:30–6:00 I picked a small basket of strawberries, which I have just prepared for the Frankfurt people‖ so I can send them from Eltville tomorrow. In the meantime, a storm had been brewing since 5:00, and the whole sky was gray on gray; gradually it began to rain, while I sat on the balcony again and darned. The storm wasn't bad; it came and went and gradually cooled down. After 8:00 I ate dinner,

---

* On the radio.

† Nassauische Landesbank (Nassau State Bank).

‡ Head gardener at the Eichberg Asylum.

‖ Mennecke's brother, Karl, and his wife, Beli.

and then typed eight registration forms. Things are progressing slowly—but it will end eventually. *All* of them have to be finished by the time you get back from Heidelberg. Yes, yes, I'm not bored, as so many like to claim. I could use an assistant. If I didn't sleep so well at night, I could continue working, but the eyes also need their rest. So—into the hay! In three days I'm going to be with the master, hurray!! How quickly that day will come! Good night—kissies, Mo!

Thursday, 10:35 P.M.: I just closed the machine; now a few lines to the master. The day after tomorrow I won't have to write any more; Pa will be sitting by me. Are you looking forward to it as I am? Today went as planned. The cherries did not come, so I could go to Wiesbaden. There's always something with the fruit; almost every day there is a new announcement in the newspaper. Now all gardens and allotments have to hand over their fruit and vegetables, and you cannot sell anything within your own district. In that case, the Friedrichs would not be able to get any more cherries through us. I wanted to send a basket of strawberries to Frankfurt by express, but now they won't accept that either. If the Frankfurt people want anything from now on, they'll have to get it themselves. I would like to send everything else to Kiedrich, as there may be heavy penalties. I took one basket of strawberries and a bouquet of lilies along for Frau Henkel; Massing* took the other, which was actually intended for Frankfurt, to his mother, as she doesn't have any more.

I got up at 7:00 A.M., did some housework, and then picked another basket of strawberries. We left at a quarter to ten; Massing was supposed to deliver the strawberries and flowers to the Henkels so they would be fresh, but then Frau Henkel came down and invited me to lunch. I tried to talk her out of it as best I could, but nothing helped; she did not stop talking. I could not get an appointment at the beauty parlor right away; there was nothing free until 5:00, so I went to do some shopping. Herr Massing picked up your suit from the tailor's. At noon I sat in Café Opel and wrote you a card, then read the paper at length. At 1:00 I went to the Henkels'. He did not come home from the office until 1:30, and then we ate: soup, cutlets and peas and boiled potatoes, and sugared strawberries. It was excellent, better than a restaurant, and used up only 50g's worth of meat coupons. He left right afterwards; I had to lie down on the couch and rest while she set the table for coffee. I got up at 3:00. At 3:30 another friend, who incidentally suffers from severe multiple sclerosis, came for

---

* Driver for the Eichberg asylum.

coffee. She can hardly walk, walks with a stick, and sways back and forth badly. The time passed quickly in conversation, and at 5:00 I called Massing again. First he drove me to the beauty parlor, while he and Fritzchen* sat in Café Opel, where I picked them up. We got back here at exactly 7:00. I ate dinner right away and darned socks on the balcony until nine, as it is a warm summer evening. It was almost a shame to sit inside, but I have to finish the forms; I've done 43 so far.

A letter from the *Gauleiter* came in the mail regarding Party member Bidert,† files from the state court of Limburg reg. Hella B., and of course your sweet letter, which I already thanked you for. Kisses for it once again!!

Now I am going to go to bed alone for the second to last time; you must also stop writing and get some sleep. Very, very, very hot Mo-kisses, my "old man," and have a good, undisturbed night without bombs!!

Friday, 10:45 P.M.: I just stopped typing for the day; 60 forms are finished. How is the punch? I hope you won't have a bad hangover after all that sweet stuff, because I want a fresh, lively Pa, okay? I already told you almost everything about my day on the phone; overall I had a lazy day. Yesterday evening I could tell already what was going to happen; this morning everything was all right until 10:00, but then I had to lie down after all. The attacks were quite strong; the pain was so strange this time, more sharp than cutting. At 2:00 P.M. I got up again, as I couldn't really sleep. I quickly made myself something to eat, fed the chickens, and sat on the balcony darning socks until 5:00. Then I went to the store and into the garden. Everything is growing well because of the rain last night and the warm weather today. Tomorrow morning I have a lot to do in the garden: picking strawberries, raspberries, currants, and sugar peas. I want to bring the raspberries down to Käthe right away. At 6:00 P.M. I began typing, but stopped for dinner and the telephone call. The cherries for the Friedrichs are still not here; now they want to can them themselves after all, since there have hardly been any police checks, as they simply don't have enough officers. Well, I don't mind, in that case we'll just pick them up in Erbach; we haven't yet decided when. Tomorrow the Friedrichs are going to spend the whole day on a bicycle trip; they will call again tomorrow after 8:00 P.M. They received sad news today: their brother-in-law, her sister's husband, died suddenly in Berlin of an infectious disease. That was

* Massing's son.
† District head of Eltville-Eberbach (Rheingau).

my day today, Daddy. In the mail there was only your sweet letter,* which made me very happy and for which I kiss you warmly, until tomorrow!! I'm only afraid it will be hard for me to leave because of the garden; the next few weeks will bring a rich harvest, but not everything will be done. Today the truck took the empty wine bottles to Eltville. Now I'm going beddy-bye, hopefully without any disturbances. I'll tell you everything else in person, darling! I'm sooooo looking forward to seeing you!! Come to your dear, dear Mo!!

Good night!!

Doc. 5

Letter no. 15 (the very last)   Heidelberg, 11 July 1942
                                                        Blumenstr. 8
                                    (Psychiatric-Neurological Polyclinic)

My dearest and best Mommy!

So this "very last" letter is going to be written after all—for various reasons:

(1) I feel a need to describe to you the course of my very last solo day in Heidelberg today,

(2) the chronological chain of my report on my Heidelberg "student" days should not end without the links being completed,

(3) this is now letter no. 15, the "last one" in five weeks, which means I have written you three letters a week, and

(4) I still have to say good night to you.

It is now 1:00—midnight has gone by—you are already slumbering peacefully—and I have just had the most pleasant of Heidelberg evenings, aside from those with you. I have just come from visiting Frau and Professor Zucker; I spent three and a half hours at their home, with (a) a bottle of 1940 Kiedrich Gräfenberg and (b) a bottle of Haute Sauterne, along with cookies, pretzel sticks, and "war" cake. The nicest part, though, was the pleasant, flowing conversation with these two dear, good people. They have an attractive apartment, with many books in the study, where we sat. Facing the rear, they have a small balcony right under the old walls of the Heidelberg Castle, and facing the front they look out on the plane trees of Karl Square; otherwise, it is an old apartment building. First we conversed about garden fruits. Professor Zucker raved about how many raspberries he saw in Kiedrich—and Frau Zucker complained that she had re-

* Doc. 2.

ceived only her allotment of one and a half pounds. I suggested she call and ask you to bring a few more pounds for her tomorrow—either our own or other people's. At 9:30 we requested an urgent telephone call to you, but by 11:00 it had not yet come through. Frau Zucker then canceled the call, because she did not want to get you out of bed. It might have been possible for you to bring a few more pounds. Then we talked about traveling, especially by ship; they had a number of stories to tell. Finally the conversation turned to the future of psychiatry, not forgetting neurology, of course. In short, it was a very pleasant evening.

Unfortunately, to Frau Zucker's great regret, we couldn't sit out on the balcony, as the very, very heavy storm between seven and eight was still rumbling. It rained terribly, as it had in the afternoon. Just as I was speaking to you from the Reichspost Hotel (around 7:30), thunder crashed and lightening flashed and the rain beat like waves against the window. I got away from the clinic at seven, just in time, and was able to buy a bouquet (carnations) before the storm really hit. At work, from four to five there was another phenomenal lecture on medical psychology; afterwards, we (Professor Schneider, Chief Medical Officer Dr. Holzer, Dr. Rauch,* and I) took a look at the seven brains that had come from Eichberg today. I heard a lot of nice, gratifying things. In fact, Professor Schneider today told me a number of "edifying" things. As I stood in the hotel entrance after the telephone conversation with you and the rain wouldn't end, one of our night nurses came by on the way to work. I asked her to send down my coat, hat, and flashlight, as I did not want to ruin my shoes and suit in the rain. Soon after, a young nurse in training brought me my things, and I took the Number One to the Corn Market and Number 6 Karlstrasse.

Now rain has gotten in the way again, but since it was a storm, maybe tomorrow and the day after the weather will be good after all; *let's hope!! The second bed was set up here in my room today, but they don't fit together, so each is in its own corner. But that's not so important; the room is not bad.*

So now your Pa is going to bed alone in Heidelberg for the last time!! In fifteen hours Mommy will be here!! Hurray!! Good night, my dear!! Heartfelt sleep-kissies!! Sweet dreams!! Good night!!

7:33 A.M.: A warm good morning kissy, Mommy—Phooey!!! It really is a jinx: every time you come to Heidelberg, the good weather has

* Dr. Hans-Joachim Rauch, who interned with Prof. Schneider. He was the subject of an investigation that began in 1985.

just ended. It's really raining again!! Well, maybe things will improve! Now to work!! Once again, have a good trip!! Kissies! Ahoy!!

1:30 P.M.: It's the weekend! Another weekend with Mommy, who is still not here. Did you already leave Wiesbaden—or are you still eating? How often I looked at the sky this morning to see if it would take pity, but it won't! At the moment it's raining again, and as I was on my way here, it thundered. So we will just have to accept that you will never see Heidelberg in the sunshine, since that's how it's been so far. Let's hope things get better next week! Now I must give a precise description of a cardiazol shock I did for an epileptic in *status epilepticus* a while ago. This case is going to be published in a paper; so Professor Schneider asked me earlier, downstairs in front of the building, to give him an exact description of the shocks. That is, written down while fresh in my memory! Besides that, I did 10 more electroshocks today. Today was my last day as a temporary replacement; starting Monday I will be a free man, and will work with you in the basement now and then. This morning the hundred-liter gas card from Berlin came in the mail. And in addition, I now own a half-size pipe!!!

Kissies—Ahoy!!

The end!! Over—finished! Done!! Pa!! July 12, 1942

Doc. 6

Letter no. 41 Czschenstochau,* 20 April 1943
Tuesday, 12:15 A.M.

Dearest, sweetest Eva-Mommy!

I am writing and sending you this letter, after having sent so many "last letters before going into action," not because I'm a "mama's boy" without toughness and soldierly discipline, but simply because my feelings and thoughts of you require it; and I have another opportunity after all, without grossly offending against my soldierly duties, to let you know my thoughts and experiences. You see that I remain consistent; for I wrote you in the many "last letters" that I would take any opportunity to send you news of myself. If this is the opportunity to send you the same number of letters as I did a year and a half ago from Warsaw, and "the two of us" did a year ago from Cracow, with G.G.† stamps that I have acquired, it

---

* The Polish name is Czestochowa. The Germans renamed cities in occupied Poland.
† The Generalgouvernement (occupied Poland).

does not reflect the tone of a "mama's boy" who cannot leave his mother; it is simply the exploitation of all opportunities to write, as long as they are quicker than military mail.

This evening's situation practically *forces* me to inform you of it quickly; I hope you won't be angry with me, especially since I'm only paying you back in kind, as I know quite well that you are still writing me regularly about your daily life. Anyway, I want to tell you the following: I am writing by the light of my service flashlight, while our express train is being switched so it can begin the second act of the great journey.* That is, it changes direction here; until now "forward" was always "forward," but from here on in it will be the other way around: "in back" will become "in front." Not because Czschenstochau is a dead end station (it is a continuous station), but because we are going in another direction—that is, due east (until now, we were going north); so it is backing up. But the passenger cars have to remain in front and the M.G. cars in back for air defense. A fair amount of switching is necessary to reverse the sequence of the cars. I want to use the time while they are switching to describe what happened this evening.

When we arrived in Czschenstochau at around 6:00 P.M., I gave the engineer from Kreuzberg, with whom we had all conversed whenever we stopped on the way, letter no. 40, so he could mail it in Kreuzberg. At the time I did not think I would be able to mail anything in the G.G. with G.G. stamps, especially since they told us to send as much private mail as possible before crossing the Reich border! At first I had put a question mark ("?") on the back of the envelope of letter no. 40, because I didn't know what direction we would be proceeding in. But when I could tell, soon after, I had the engineer give me back the letter, crossed out the "?", and wrote in "2." Now, at 12:50 A.M., our express train is finally leaving—we are starting Part Two of the great journey (G.G.). Our second-class car is no longer the first one after the locomotive; it is now the fifth car. When letter no. 40 was finally sent off successfully, I went to the second-class waiting room with Lieutenant Colonel Koller and Lieutenant Zobel, as we had heard that we would not be continuing on to Kielce until 12:08. First we drank just one glass of beer. In the station vestibule, I bought five postcards that already had G.G. stamps glued to them. It is impossible to continue writing, as the train is jerking too much!! I'll con-

---

* Mennecke and his medical corps had been transferred from the Channel coast at Dunkirk.

tinue my report tomorrow. Now just one more thing: a fond good night!!
Sleep well, without bombs!! Sweet dreams!! Good night, dearest Mo!!

Kissies!! Ahoy!!
Good night!!

6:50 A.M., Tuesday, 20 April 1943, Kielce: Good morning, dearest
Mommy!! We went only a relatively short distance during the night, but I
slept through it. *7:01* news: Göring's appeal! Otherwise, nothing special.
The first impression of the day was the begging, starving Polish children
who descended in hordes from the nearby city upon our train, which had
stopped somewhat outside the city; with miserable faces, they begged:
"Bread, please!" They've already learned how to say that. I threw two
slices to them. As I said, the night was good again; I slept well and feel
very good and cheerful. Aside from a slight tautness at the site of the injection, I have had no reactions. In any case, my general health is very good,
as always. So, little heart, now I will continue the report from yesterday
evening: I could not get any loose stamps at the newspaper stand in the
station at Czschenstochau, and therefore took the five postcards with
stamps already glued on. Then I went back to my compartment and had
a thorough wash, shave, change of socks, etc. When I had freshened up,
we all sat together in the section of the first- and second-class waiting
room reserved "for Germans only," and ate: one glass of good cognac for
five marks, one piece of marinated fish (cod) as an appetizer for three
marks, one cold roast meat patty (no food coupons necessary) (as big as
one's palm) for five marks. We ate bread with it and drank one glass of
beer. I paid *only* eighteen marks for this dinner!! It's absurd, but not unusual in our situation. Afterwards, on the train, we listened to the Nazi
party's birthday celebration* and Goebbels' address. The commander sat
in my compartment. I wrote you a card, which I mailed at the Czschenstochau station in the box labeled "German Post Office East."

  After Goebbels' speech I talked for a long time with Captain Mäu-
rich about National Socialism. I got to know him a little better, and know
how to deal with him psychologically. He is not a BMW automobile representative in civilian life after all; he is primarily chief of staff of the senior
Dresden NSKK† group, an old Nazi often sent to Nazi celebrations in
Berlin on special occasions. He also worked in Berlin for two years on the
staff of the deceased corps leader Hänlein, and has even been invited to

---

* For Hitler's birthday.

† National Socialist Automobile Club (Nationalsozialistisches Kraftfahrkorps).

small gatherings with Goebbels. Thus he was interested in my connections to the Führer's Office, etc. In any case, there is a good basis for the mutual feeling between the two of us. During our conversation, we emptied a bottle of red wine from the quartermaster's for 2.50 marks (one cognac = five marks!). Around 11:00 we walked around Czschenstochau a bit, in order to see some of it ("parole" from the transport train!). Czschensto-chau has some 250,000 inhabitants and is a very clean, well-built city; in appearance it is not far behind Cracow. We walked along a big, wide avenue that led to the Marii Pamny, the church with the famous Black Madonna; it was Pilsudski Street. We didn't go all the way to the Marii Pamny, as we wanted to be back at the train on time. At the Railway Station Hotel (German-run), we had another glass of beer for 80 pfennigs. There I could also buy loose stamps that I can, fortunately, use for this letter! . . .

9:15 A.M., Skarzysko: Finished with my morning toilette, as usual. There was water to wash with. Breakfast just now was good. This is a larger station in a small country town, and we have been here for half an hour. A "transport-supervision officer," an old captain, has come aboard; he is to accompany and supply our transport in the G.G., as well as supervising any other provisioning. He is seated for the present in a compartment with Lieutenant Colonel Koller and Lieutenant Zobel. He just spoke with the commander. I hope they do not put him in my compartment to keep me "company"; I would rather be alone with you, my little heart!! I assume we will reach the Russian border this evening, so the captain will no longer be with us tonight. But until then I don't want to be disturbed in my chat with you. Let's hope for the best! I don't know yet where I can and will mail this letter; before nightfall, in any case, since during the night at the latest we will cross the Russian border. . . .

I am going to put on my new boots now and go for a walk along the train. *Kissies! Ahoy!*

10:10: All aboard! We're on our way. The second battery of one of our infantry regiments (the same division) just rolled up on the siding in a transport train. I just talked for a while with the troop physician (staff physician). We also had a detailed conversation with the transport-supervision officer. Our route through the G.G. is now perfectly clear. From here we will travel by way of Radom—Deblin—Lublin—Chelm. We will cross the Russian border at Dorpkusk (border station) tomorrow morning at 3 A.M.. We're off, and I am still alone. Lunch break will be in Deblin. *Kissies!! Ahoy!!*

11:30 A.M.: We have reached Radom. The train passed through the station, and we have stopped somewhat outside the station. This also seems to be a very nice city; like all significant locations in the G.G., it is strongly influenced by Germany, with German firms, German offices, and the German Wehrmacht. Particularly today, with flags fluttering everywhere for the Führer's birthday, one can see so well how extensively German saturation has progressed. There is building going on everywhere, on the railroad, country roads, in the cities. On the other hand, the flat landscape is typically Polish. The villages we have traveled through generally consist of miserable straw-thatched peasants' huts; the people are ragged, barefoot, dirty, hungry. One often sees women doing difficult work on construction sites; they are Jewish wenches or expelled enemies of the state, of the concentration camp type! Here, over Radom, there is a great deal of aerial activity; there must be a training airbase in the neighborhood. The infantry transport is following us again on the siding as we begin moving again. Now we are going to *Deblin*. Our train is 550 meters long; I could calculate it from the kilometer markers. Now I'll look out the window again!! *Kissies!! Ahoy!!*

1:10 P.M.: We just passed through Bakowice and are approaching our afternoon destination, the junction of *Deblin*. There we will cross the Vistula—the great curve of the Vistula! My good map with the country borders and railways is very much in demand. They all like to orient themselves by it; the commander was just here. *Kissies! Ahoy!!*

1:57 P.M.: Deblin: I just ate my afternoon meal (two and a half mess-tin covers full of goulash with noodles) in the middle of a desert of sand many kilometers wide. We have stopped on a stretch with many tracks next to each other. The sand is thin and warm, and in places has blown over the tracks. *The news* is on: you have had no bombardments—that's the most important thing to me! This place is about one kilometer on the far side (east) of the Vistula on a great railway bridge. . . .

The infantry just rolled up again, the transports meet—on all the lines! Now we are moving again, continuing in a southeasterly direction toward *Lublin. Kissies!! Ahoy!!*

3:05: It's raining! The first rain of our trip! The sky has been cloudy all over since the afternoon and there's a full moon today. Spring is still a long way off here; one hardly sees any green, but it's not winter anymore either. The crops are not bad in places, but on the average agriculture is mediocre. Kissies!! Ahoy!!

4:50: Lublin is in sight; in a few minutes we will be there. I will see to it that I send off this letter here. So tonight we will be crossing the border to Russia, toward Kiev—probably then *Poltava?*

> *Fondest greetings and kisses, dearest Mommy, until the first letter by military mail from Russia! Stay well and cheerful! Your faithful, good Fritz-Daddy-Pa*

Doc. 7

Chief Physician of the Reserves
Dr. Mennecke
02296*   In the East, 3 May 1943
Dear Colleagues!

I purposely waited before sending you news of myself. I wanted to be at the scene of the fighting first, in order to describe the impressions I have received so far during this assignment at the front.

When I left you on 18 January, I was first deployed in my area of specialization as the departmental physician of the Neurology Department of Res. Hospital I in Metz. At the same time, our comrade Dr. Sehr was transferred from Metz to Kiedrich. I headed the Neurology Department in Metz until 3 March, and had a great deal to do during this period. My patients were mainly soldiers with bullet wounds to the nerves or neurologically-organically disturbed soldiers; purely psychiatric cases appeared to only a very small extent. A few court-martial cases requiring recommendations also arose. As assistants in my department, I had two older medical orderlies who had been hospital orderlies in civilian life, from Merzig (Gierden, who worked in Weilmünster for a time) and Alzey (Raddey). Except for the military context, the work in Metz differed little from the activity of the neurological ward of a mental hospital. From a purely professional standpoint, the work was very interesting, particularly since in a hospital one sees nowhere near as many organic cases; but the entire time I hoped for another assignment that would bring me closer to the actual scene of combat.

Thus, on 20 February I was transferred to a field infantry division, but could not leave my position in Metz until 3 March, as a replacement could not be found until then. My successor in Metz was Staff Doctor Fuchs of Mannheim, who until then had worked in the reserve hospital of the Heidelberg Psychiatric Clinic, where he had been chief physician. I

---

* Mennecke's military mail number.

reached my division on the Channel coast on 14 March, by way of Medical Replacement Dept. 12, Bad Kreuznach and the transit office in Darmstadt. The division was still being organized and was to be deployed to the East after being restaffed. As in 1939–40, I was again assigned as troop physician, which gave me general medical responsibilities; that had been my personal wish for this assignment. During the time I spent at the front on the Channel coast, I had the opportunity to observe the destruction wrought by the Battle of Dunkirk in June 1940. Dunkirk itself is in bad shape. I stood on the 60-meter-high lighthouse that extends farthest into the sea; from it, one faces westward toward the British coast, and can view the extensive wreckage left by the battle along the European coast. In terms of combat, during this period there were only disturbances from the air, which were no more difficult for us to bear than the attacks that threaten you night after night. Attempts to land on our section of the Channel would not have been very good for the British; there was no need for defense, but it may become necessary in the future. During my final days on the Channel coast, I learned that Hans Lang was in my neighborhood, but I had no time to meet with him.

It is now 1:50 P.M., and I and my comrades have just heard the D.A.F.'s Reich appeal and Dr. Ley's* address, which you probably also listened to, together in the hall. I feel that I am with you in spirit, joining you in the vow: Never again a 9 November 1918! He who fights Judas saves our people and our Reich! Yes, Dr. Ley's words were stirring enough to make us constantly aware of the necessity of our victory for the preservation of German life and German thought! Now I will report further: On 16 April, we began the "great military journey to the East" in railway transports. We went through Belgium, crossed the Reich border at Aachen, then crossed Westphalia and the province of Hanover by way of Düsseldorf; in Kreiensen we were only a few kilometers from my home; then we passed through Magdeburg—Dessau—Silesia, Liegnitz—Breslau—Kreuzburg on the S.; we took two days and two nights to cross our beautiful Fatherland. Then we traveled through the Generalgouvernement by way of Czschenstochau—Radom—Lublin. After crossing the Russian border we crossed the wide area of the Reich Commissariat of the Ukraine, richly endowed with natural resources. When one has seen these fields of the most fertile soil, one realizes that if there were a just social

---

* Dr. Robert Ley, head of the German Labor Front (Deutsche Arbeitsfront). He escaped the Nuremberg war crimes trials by killing himself on 25 October 1945.

distribution, these resources would provide all of Europe with enough to eat. As far as the eye can see, there is nothing but fresh sowings, thousands of acres of kilometer-wide connected fields! There lies the task for the next generation of German farmers. All generations to come will find work there; one can only begin to imagine its extent when one has seen the land itself! It is worth fighting for this country, and keeping the uncivilized hordes of the steppe once and for all away from this fertile land. Kiev and Poltava are attractive cities; they will become a hub of trade one day.

After six days and six nights' train ride we were unloaded, and our motorized overland march began. We rode through the ruins of Charkov that came about during the last battles in March; they are worse than the ruins of Mainz. Then we crossed the battlefield on which, in mid-March, the SS Division Greater Germany [Grossdeutschland] put an end to the Soviets. This enormous tank field still shows all the fresh marks of the disastrous battle of annihilation against the advancing hordes of the steppe. There I became acquainted for the first time with the paradisical "roads" in this enormous country. Indeed, you find here, in its purest form, a dilapidation and degeneration of streets and houses that in Germany one would not believe possible. You can tell by looking at the Russian people that they are born and raised right in the dirt, so they don't know any better. These people are really only silhouettes in human form that Jewish Bolshevism had an easy time molding in its image. No other people would be better suited to be misused for an idea as absurd and crazy as Bolshevism. This is not a master race, but the most primitive, stubborn, and shabby heap of humanity that we have in Europe. A single human life means as little here as in any lower order of animals. This is the only way to assess the deployment of these hordes—and unfortunately it must be judged a serious, obstinate host fighting under the lash of the Politruks.* For the last fourteen days we have been in position at the front and are waiting to see what will happen. The upper reaches of the river† that is often mentioned in Wehrmacht reports will not cause us any great difficulties. At the moment, the front is relatively calm here; nevertheless, there are daily losses on both sides. Just today, on the first really rainy day at the edge of the worldwide steppe, the battle is proving difficult and arduous. This small amount of rain was enough to make the "roads" impassable; trucks slide in the slippery, sticky mud, their tires cannot get a

* Political officers of the Red Army.
† The Donets.

grip [here a word is unreadable], they can only drive with snow chains. I am quartered with several comrades in a typical Russian peasant's hut, which holds all the charm of these tidy people. Our night camp consists of a plug of straw in a strip of canvas and wool blankets for cover; for obvious reasons, we cannot undress—the old soldiers among you are familiar enough with this!

We will do our duty here at the front at all times for Führer, Volk, and Reich—and if necessary, give our lives doing it. You people back home have no less great and important tasks to fulfill. And thus our entire nation, men, women, and children, stands together in a single front like a wall to repel the onslaught of our enemies and end this war happily through total victory. When this happens is not important, but it is necessary that it happen—for the sake of our lives! [here a sentence is only partly readable, as the margin of the letter is damaged. Most likely: "Katün (Katyn)* threatens us all!"]

I hope to see you all, healthy and cheerful, at our beautiful Eichberg, and send you all my warmest regards! Heil Hitler!

Your Fritz Mennecke

Doc. 8

02296   Russia, 19 June 1943
Dear Mother!

You have heard nothing from me since 3 June, and so today I am sending you some news of myself. I am still well, and hope the same is true of you. Nothing has changed for me yet. It is not yet certain when I can expect things to change. I have been a soldier for five months now, and I do not know how much longer it will last. Heinfried Laue† recently tried to call me, but the connection was bad. We could only make ourselves understood through a middle man. He is also well. He will come on vacation again around the middle of August. Well, best wishes and my warmest regards!

Your Friedrich

---

* In April 1943, mass graves were discovered at Katyn containing the corpses of 4,250 Polish officers. According to experts, they had been shot before the German attack on the Soviet Union.

† A cousin of Mennecke's.

Doc. 9

02296   Russia, 19 June 1943
Dear Parents!*

It is time that I send you some news of myself. But the old rule—he who does not write is doing fine—applies here. For I am indeed well, and there have been no changes. Five months of my assignment have already passed. How much longer it will last, I don't know; but it could come quite quickly. I am waiting patiently and calmly. I have to thank you warmly for the kind packages numbers seven and eight, and I hereby do so. They arrived on 14 June, and the cigarettes and cigarillos have already been smoked. We receive six cigarettes a day, which is not very many. I hope your health is improved.

Best regards and kisses!
Your Fritz

Doc. 10

Letter no. 70
02296   Russia, 19 June 1943
                                                          (Saturday)

Florian† is here!!! 21 June 1943
My dearest Mommy!

May this new letter no. 70, *the weekend letter at the beginning of summer,* begin like this! It is 4:00 P.M., and I am sitting behind the house again in the sun at the garden table—in my birthday suit, letting the pleasant, mild, windy summer air stroke me—it does sooooo much good! Pöllen just set up our radio outside, so out here our "Gustav" intones its beautiful Saturday afternoon concert, the "Colorful Afternoon." Ulla Burmeister (soprano) is just now singing "Homeland," the first performance of the afternoon. The program, with announcements etc., is again taking place at the broadcast studio, full of privates. After I sent my letter no. 69, together with those for Professor Nitsche, your parents, and my mother, I read the paper. . . .

After lunch (beef, boiled potatoes, peas), I lay down on the bed to read, but my eyes soon closed. But first I put on my track suit just in case, so as not to catch cold lying there in my birthday suit. And then I fell

---

* The reference is to his in-laws.
† Mennecke's orderly.

asleep and took *the* weekend nap *between letters!* As ordered, Pöllen woke me for the Wehrmacht report, which I listened to half asleep, but took in enough to know that no *terror flights had taken place in the Reich—thank God!* Right after that, Daddy slept blissfully on—until 4:00, when I began to write. Now my upper body is smeared with vaseline and is broiling in the sun. I have the sun on my back, and it burns, but the wind stirs it pleasantly! . . .

My whole "IVb family" is gathered around the radio here on this lovely spot; while I chat with you, Brochner is reading, Pöllen is sunning himself lazily, and so are my three patients. All three cases are surgical ones; one cut off half his big toe with a sharp spade while digging (work detail in the company). I sewed on the dangling front half (no bone damage) with a few stitches of silk. The second has a cell tissue inflammation on his foot, near the joint; the third has a pulled tendon in the left forearm. All three are sitting around us in their bandages—a typical military hospital, *"front hospital"!* On the radio, Hans Moser and Theo Lingen are being imitated diligently—fabulously lovely! There are also some nice pieces of music. And what are you doing now, little heart? You've already finished work. Do you have Sunday duty again tomorrow, after your four days' vacation over Pentecost? Now they've interrupted the "Colorful Afternoon" to announce the *5:00 news:* active sinkings in the straits of Sicily, 17 shot down during terror attacks on Italy. Our fighter pilots attack the port of Astrachan on the Caspian Sea! Twenty-two thousand tons lost to the Russians—altogether forty-five thousand tons. American losses to the Japanese by Guadalcanal—*Bose** in Japan! *Vavel* Vice-King in India— Military dictatorship! Wehrmacht report again—no attacks! 5:08—and the program continues with the "Pizzicato Waltz" by George Boulanger— and now the "Street Singers of the Anti-Tank Unit" (a quartet) is singing a Hawaiian song, "Yearning for Hawaii," with guitar accompaniment. My pipe tastes sooooo good. Cigarettes are gradually becoming scarce; I hope Räder-Grossmann† sends some more. But I can also make cigarettes *myself,* as I still have plenty of tobacco. . . .

Now they are telling a funny story on the radio: a telephone connection is made with Germany, and they ask for various switching stations— "salad bowl," "fruit salad," "pancake," etc. (nice code names). Now the first lieutenant in charge in the East has finally gotten through to the home

* Subhas Chandra Bose, president of the Indian National Congress, was allied with Nazi Germany against Great Britain and fought with the Japanese in Burma.

† Hans Räder-Grossman, administrative official in the Bernburg-Saale killing facility.

of the major (who is home on vacation); the maid picks up the phone. The major is not home; he should call his regiment at the front when he gets back—through "old cow," "strawberry sauce," "foot cloth," etc. Funny misunderstandings with the maid—everyone laughs!! And now a saxophone solo, "Capricious Waltz." I am still sitting facing the wall of the house with my back to the sun—and roasting. These two hours from four to six (on Saturday) are always pleasant. I hope it isn't too boring when I describe the program as well as I can. But this is also my *"war diary"*!! My letters in general are supposed to be reports of my experiences. And now, wrapping up the "Colorful Afternoon," the Soldiers' Choir: "Soldier's Heart." Then we go "into the water"; Pöllen is preparing everything. A pity these two hours are over, they went by so quickly! Did anything come in the mail? I don't think so. See you later! Kissies!! *Ahoy!!*

7:25 P.M.: Two announcements: *"Clean little pig!"* and *"so full!!"* Oh, what bliss the bath was! Washing and soaping off the roasted-in grease on my skin was so lovely! And now I have such a wonderful warm—but not too warm—feeling on my skin under the clean clothes. Then came dinner: three pieces of bread and butter with pork sausage and one helping of semolina pudding!! Oh, was it good!! Florian gets his portion tomorrow evening; hopefully it will keep until then.* Orderly Private First Class Herling just reported back from the NCO training program. He passed the test; now he can become an NCO, and in autumn he will start college. No mail came, not even the paper. This evening we will have a round of skat. Incidentally, my supply of cigarettes is looking better; Fabian (department paymaster and quartermaster) just brought me, at my request, nine packs of Salem cigarettes with twelve cigarettes each. So things always work out well; I'm never really short. Now *Hans Fritzsche*[†] is speaking, time to listen! *Kissies! Ahoy!!*

0:30. That was a long round of skat; I came out of it plus-minus 0, but still stood at +.46. I won almost every game—the way it always goes! It was quiet again the whole evening, like yesterday; no "runway whores" appeared—unless they come later. Very far away we can hear flak—far to

* They have to be eaten up, since Florian is not here yet. [Mennecke's note.]

† Hans Fritzsche was head of the German Press section of Goebbels' Propaganda Ministry starting in 1938; from 1942 on, he was head of the Radio Section, responsible for "political propaganda broadcasts by the Greater German radio." He was known for his regular "political newspaper and radio review," which is probably what Mennecke means. Fritzsche was indicted at the Nuremberg war crimes trials for his propaganda work, but later acquitted (see Ansgar Diller, *Rundfunkpolitik im Dritten Reich*, Munich, 1980, pp. 107, 350, 354, 362, 443f.).

the north. I hope it stays quiet there, too. Now sleep well into Sunday, my heart's child!! Be spared bombs, and have a good rest!! Tomorrow will bring Florian, and with him *"Mommy" once again!!! Good, good night!! Sleep well!! Kissies!! Good night!!*

Sunday, 20 June 1943, 8:30: A fond good morning on this lovely Sunday, my dear Mommy, and lots of loving, hearty welcoming kissies!! A weekend night of six and a half hours of the deepest, most wholesome slumbers, and I hope very much that you, my darling, also had such a nice, quiet night!! If you are on duty, you are once again working at your laboratory bench; but if you are off duty, I hope you're still lying in bed— whether in Wiesbaden or at Eichberg! (How are things with your p.?* I suppose it's over for now? There was nothing in your letters about it yet.) Here the weather today is like every day recently: *hot!* The sun is already blazing, and it's best to stay in the shade. I have been "undressed" since I got up! The air burns your skin, even if it isn't always sunny. Today, Sunday, I am entirely taken up with *waiting for Florian!* . . .

Now I have some work to do. More later! *Kissies ahoy!!*

11:45: Lieutenant Colonel Knüpfer and Radiomaster Colonel Heinecke just left for their quarters. At 10:30 they came for a Sunday morning visit, which turned into a game of skat that we just interrupted for lunch. They will come back after they've eaten—and then we'll keep playing here in our room! That is, today it's different than otherwise on Sundays; I'm not *their* guest, *they are mine.* I don't want to go away today *because Florian is coming! I want to be home when he arrives!* We will have our *good Sunday coffee and cake* served here! Last night there was a *big raid* here, looking for male and female Ukrainian workers. It was a decree by *Gauleiter* Sauckel.† Right now, the population is greatly agitated, as they remember the deportations to Siberia they experienced for many years; they do not yet realize that it will be very different in Germany than in Siberia! After they have been in Germany for a while, they will know better. Women between 20 and 25 without children were collected, as well as young fellows between 18 and 22; there are no older men here anymore, except ancient grandfathers!

---

* Period.

† Fritz Sauckel, *Gauleiter* of Thuringia. Starting in 1942, he was also General Plenipotentiary for Labor Mobilization, and therefore responsible for the deportation of forced laborers to Germany. Sauckel was condemned to death at the Nuremberg trials and executed.

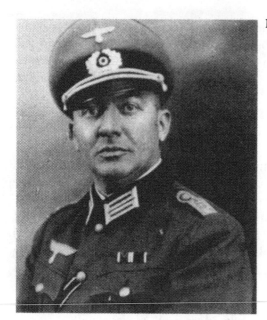

Friedrich Mennecke, 1943.

There is said to be a lot of lamentation among the people; four girls from our neighborhood were apparently taken as well. Our "Matka" is too old for a work detail in Germany. Just today—independently of the operation last night—the family in the neighboring house (my local sickroom) was thrown out by the local commander on my initiative. There was a woman of around 35 with three children; the family has been taken into another house. You cannot imagine what dirt and filth this "tidy" family's former dwelling held!!! I got a mild shock when I saw the room in which these people had lived! I simply could no longer be responsible for treating my inpatients in the same house. I am now having this filthy room (smaller than the local sickroom that has already been fixed up) newly whitewashed—walls, ceiling, and floor; I will leave the room empty for a few days and then set up two new beds there. So much for this Sunday's "happenings." . . .

6:30 P.M.: Florian is still not here and can hardly come tomorrow, since the vacationers who came back today have already arrived . . . so I have to wait—but he'll come tomorrow!! We have been playing skat here very professionally since 4:00: Knüpfer, Köpf, Heinecke, and I, with Zobel kibitzing. First we drank good "coffee" (beans) and ate cake, then began to play skat. There was one bottle of Steinhäger from the Second Company. Now the gentlemen have left for a while to check up on their

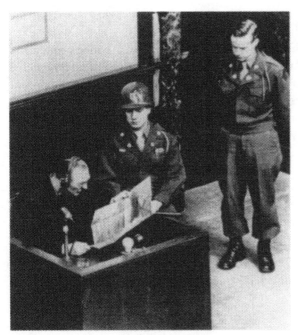

Friedrich Mennecke, 1946, testifying at the Nuremberg doctors' trials.

companies—soon they will be back for dinner, which we will follow with more skat. I am sitting outside again in my track suit and bare upper body in the evening sun, and again feel the mild wind pleasantly caress me. *My thoughts always turn to you as soon as I am alone, my heart! What are you doing now?* Unfortunately, I don't know where you are today. Enjoy your dinner!! *Kissies!! Ahoy!!* The mail just came (7:00): *one "Reich"* * *from you*, otherwise nothing!

11:30: Sunday is over, and *Florian* has not come!! My guests just left. We had a very nice skat evening—we officers here in our room, my orderlies in the neighboring house doing the same thing! It was quite a harmonious evening on both sides, and I was top winner in *our* skat with +3.25 marks!![†] But it disturbs me *that Florian did not come today!!* What can it mean? Will he come tomorrow, at least? Today the true focus of our entire unit was here *with me!!* This is not presumption on my part, but *reality,* for whatever information had to be passed on went through my telephone!! It is rare, after all, that the entire strategic service is focused on the office of *Dept. IVb,* but I have achieved this here in this depart-

---

* *The Reich,* a weekly paper published by Goebbels.

† See the note! [Mennecke's note.]

ment!! Actually it is not a big deal, when I consider that I could be the father of all these influential information officers. They are all attracted to me and enjoy being here. Of course, I anticipate these young gentlemen's wishes correctly, and thus lend the office of "division physician" *the* status it deserves—without the person involved being the most important thing. . . . You understand, don't you? In this division it is relatively easy for me, as all the officers are very young men! Now I will close for today— although I am still listening to nice melodies from the *Ostland* station in Minsk, while Brochner and Pöllen are still in neighboring houses, also spending a quiet Sunday evening at the front. Now I am going to sleep. I am very sorry *Florian didn't show up today;* he has to come tomorrow! *I will not send this letter until Florian is here.* It is 12:02 A.M.; the late news is on, but they are bringing nothing new. I wish you, good Mommy, a pleasant, peaceful "bolona,"* like what we have here (because nothing has happened here yet)—sleep well and sweet dreams!! *Good, good night!!*

Kissies!! Good Night!! . . .

21 June 1943
1:15 P.M.: Florian is here!!!
Oh, the packet from Mommy!!

2:45: Oh, dear Mommy, the last hour and a half were irretrievably beautiful—so beautiful that I can hardly describe my feelings accurately and completely!! Darling, oh, if you could only have been here, you would have seen how I ran to Florian as he climbed from the truck that brought him!! And you could have heard yourself how nicely and frankly he told me about you; how he said, "Herr Chief Physician, after seeing your wife and speaking with her, I understand why you two have to write to each other so often." He is full of praise for you, and he is so trusting and innocently confidential that, in the last half hour that he sat here alone with me, he told me so much about his girl and said his girl was *like you,* that he is also very fond of her and can't leave her; and as he said it, the tears flowed from this big strong boy's eyes!! He takes us as an example, and God knows "the two of us" are not a bad example, Florian is right about that!! Now I will describe to you in context the scene of *Florian's arrival;* but one thing first: In the Wehrmacht report today, they said that *southwestern Germany* was bombed and there were *losses among the ci-vilian population!! Oh good, darling Eva-Mommy, I hope you are alive*

* *bombenlose Nacht,* bombless night.

and unhurt??? Pommily, what would I do if something happened to you? Oh, I don't even want to think about it!!! They didn't mention Wiesbaden, they didn't mention any city, and that is not very reassuring!! Nevertheless, with a firm heart and trusting completely in our "two of us Providence," I will simply assume you are alive and well!!! I hope I am not mistaken about this.

I had just lain down on my bed and begun to read "The Love of Lieutenant Warenstein" when Matka came in and said, with a great effort to make herself understood, that the "shoemaker" from the neighboring house (a private who left *with* Florian) was back; she mentioned the name of a place and indicated that Florian also came from there. I got up immediately—and as I was listening to the shoemaker, whom I had brought to me, say that he had last seen Florian three days ago in Warsaw, I saw a truck stop outside the window and vacationers get out. Among them I immediately recognized *Florian*—and ran outside, mother-naked as I was, *grabbed my Florian and got him!!* Yes, one is happy as a child when a *"personal tie from home"* arrives!! In he came with his packets—four altogether!!! Right away I had your *Mommy-packet* in my hands!! Oh, Mommy, was that a wonderful moment!! *Florian looked totally dirty and dusty — he had been through terrible nights!!* Brochner and Pöllen and I—first we stood around Florian for several minutes and stared at him! Yes, that's what happened!!! Then I immediately set to work on your packet; I tried to loosen the strings, but it took too long, so I cut it open!! *Then came the contents!! I immediately had Pöllen uncork a bottle of "Mirapommapriko" and pour out four glasses of schnapps!! Our own cellars!!! Oh, Mommy!!!* All three bottles are unscathed. Then came *the big sausage!!! Wonderfully preserved!!!* Then the *small Brägen sausage, also no problem!!!* Then the *heavy wonderful cake!!!!* Ach, now I have to drink a quick "Eichberg spirit" to your health, Mommy—*Prost!! Aaaaah!!! I smack my lips*—ta-ta-ta-ta-ta!!!!

Anyway, darling, the cake is quite enchantingly beautiful!! I have not tried it yet, but in the transparent paraffin paper it looks as if Mommy's hands had just taken it out of the electric oven!! Oh, *it will taste good!* Florian's girl (or her mother) baked a similarly shaped cake and gave it to him to take along; both are now in front of me on the table, wrapped up. I also found the four nice cigarettes and am now smoking a Mommy-four thirty!! I found the lighter, which already works. Florian also gave me the *epaulettes with stars* that he received on the last day before leaving Duisburg. And he also gave me the *candles* and *your letter!!* Ach, darling, you *really showered me!!!* Everything ended up in my hands, safe and sound and guarded faithfully by Florian. *Thank you, and a thousand, many thousand kisses for it, you good, good Mommy!!!!!!* I immediately had two bottles of spirits brought down to chill; one opened bottle—the third—proved *Eichberg's kindness* many times over in our "circle of four." It is now three-quarters empty!! But that hardly matters!!! Soon after, Brochner and Pöllen took our "Peugeot" to the H.V.Pl.* to pick up medical supplies—and *I was alone with Florian!!* We had a sincere, comradely talk—even fatherly, I must say—and downed some quick spirits in the process!! Florian described his trip to me in true "Florian style," and spoke of you—he *appreciates you as much as he does me.* With enthusiasm, he described *your great joy* when he visited you on May 1. He described you personally with the same enthusiasm: *how you already had your head scarf on, and how good you looked! Can you imagine, Mommy, what was going on inside your Pa at that moment?!!* Ach, Florian is a good guy!! (Brochner is not half as sincere!!) Florian spoke of the bitterness of the bomb nights in Duisburg, of the patience of his mother, whom he loves above all, of the determination of his father, to whom he feels very close. Florian is a man with heart!! His girl is getting a good man!! He "confessed" to me that he will probably "have to" marry his girl soon, as he believes she is expecting a child from him! But they also love each other very much!! He said this vacation brought him very close to his girl—and that he had always seen how you and I—"the two of us"—stand by one another!! Oh, Evali, don't we understand *that?!!* . . .

7:15 P.M.: Hurray!! And another letter from Mommy!! And a letter from the Elena clinic in Kassel! Let's get to it!!

7:55: There's nothing to be done but bring you here, you good Mommy, because besides the Florian package you made *me so very happy again* today!! *You get countless fervent Daddy-kisses—quick, quick, catch them!!* Today your *letter no. 56* arrived, *no. 55 in between is missing!!* It has probably been delayed and will stroll in later. But I'm that much happier now that I know everything you've been doing, up until your departure on Pentecost vacation (Saturday evening)!! This letter no. 56 of yours was postmarked 12 June 1943, so once again it took only nine days. Now first I'm going to listen to the *8:00 news!* Gangs† in the Balkans!! Three years since Compiègne!‡ And tomorrow will be two years

* *Hauptverbandsplatz,* military first aid station.
† The reference is to the partisans.
‡ The signing of the Franco-German cease-fire agreement on 22 June 1940 in Compiègne, near Paris.

since the beginning of this war in the East (Hotel Kasten, Hanover!!)! Before I begin the second reading and response to your no. 56, one more indication of frugality: our dinner (four of us, since Pöllen doesn't leave again until tomorrow) was very big today. Incidentally, this afternoon when I opened the package I *immediately* devoured a *juicy Mommy-sandwich with Brägen sausage* and drank *"Mirapommapriko"* with it! *That was the first "visible" Mommy-greeting!!* For dinner, in addition to butter and cheese from our evening provisions, we had pork sausage and ham from packages Florian received while he was away. The big sausage you sent—as well as the one from Florian's parents—are still untouched down in our bunker. But the pork sausage we devoured this evening, and especially the ham, tasted great!! *If only I could have made you a ham sandwich too!!!* . . .

It is now 9:15. Florian is already in bed, so he can sleep off the difficult journey. Brochner is writing, and Pöllen is sleeping next door in the hospital tonight so he can leave tomorrow. The head physician of the *Elena clinic in Kassel, Dr. Voeller,* is willing to grant Daddy* *"preferred admission."*† He also sent two special publications on the clinic and the special therapy. I'll look into all this more closely tomorrow and write you more about it. Now I want to end this wonderful Mommy-day soon, my good little one, and lie down myself; *it will be another good night.* If only that would be true for you too; but after the Wehrmacht report today, I'm worried about you again! I gather from the news that the attack on southwest Germany was not so bad, as only four enemy flyers were shot down. Either there weren't many of them, or our defense is not as strong there as in the Rhineland-Westfalen industrial area. At any rate, I hope quite confidently *that nothing happened to you!* Nothing *can* have happened to you—and *nothing must ever happen to you!!!* I cross my fingers tightly for you, my dearest Mommy, and wish you a real "bolona"!!! Here they are roaring overhead again, but they must be German flyers. *My most heartfelt thanks once again for all the love I received from you today!! My warmest good-night kissies!! Sleep well!! Sweet dreams!! Good, good night!!*

Tuesday, 22 June 1943, 8:45 A.M.: Good morning, dearest Mommy!! Two years of war in Russia!! Two years ago today, "the two of us" were eating breakfast at the Hotel Kasten in Hanover—and today? *I just*

---

* The reference is to Mennecke's father-in-law.

† For treatment of Parkinson's disease.

had the wildest Russian night yet, and am healthy!! My most ardent wish is that you, too, good Evalein, are just as healthy and cheerful!! When I stopped writing yesterday evening, I actually wanted to lie down soon to sleep, but that's not what happened! The "Gustavs" continued to rumble over us, so we preferred to take cover in our underground bunker. Around 10:20 the first bombs fell nearby! A few minutes later the second load, and soon after that the third! Only then did flares light up directly above us, as bright as day. By their light, on-board machine-guns clattered and raked the area heavily!! After that, no more bombs fell. Around 11:00 it became quiet, and we left our bunker. We stayed outside until around midnight, but no more "Gustavs" entered our area. So we lay down again peacefully. I fell asleep, but was *torn from sleep shortly after one A.M.* by *incredible detonations and the sound of splintering glass*—all three of us woke up immediately!! *Five heavy bombs crashed down nearby at short intervals!* Getting out of our straw beds—outside—into the bunker—was the work of seconds!! Three more bombs burst, but none hit. As in the first attack, flares then came on and threw their light, as bright as day, as far as our bunker. *And once again the on-board MGs and two-centimeter on-board cannons clattered — but nothing hit us!!* Around two it became quiet, and we crawled out again; then it remained quiet. Since today was the *shortest night,* around this time a glowing red "dawn" had pushed its way up in the east-northeast, and I thought involuntarily of *22 June 1941, two o'clock in the morning** — *Dwinger*[†]—think!! In the light of dawn we took a look around outside and saw two of the strikes, both of which were some 60 meters away. Fortunately, we can claim no dead; I know of only one injured from our unit so far, a slight wound that I'll take care of now. More later. *Kissies!! Ahoy!!*

10:00: Back again! It was only a very small, superficial skin wound from a small bomb fragment; not even enough for a "wounded" badge. But it could have been worse, because this noncommissioned officer had even more fragments in his bed that had smashed through the wall! On the runway in front of our house this morning I also found two small bomb fragments (little things) that aimed in our direction but did not quite reach us. I am keeping them. So that was the *night of the summer solstice of 1943 — exactly two years after the beginning of the global conflagration in the East!* Now I want to close this weekend letter, which took one

---

* German attack on the Soviet Union.

[†] Edwin Erich Dwinger (1898–1981), one of the most successful authors of Freikorps literature.

day longer than intended because of Florian's delayed return. I just want to copy for you what the head physician of the Elena clinic wrote:

> Queen Elena Clinic   Kassel-Harleshausen, 9 June 1943
> Chief physician: Dr. Walther Voeller
> Dear Senior Medical Officer!
> I received your letter of 18 May 1943 and am prepared to grant preferred admission to your father-in-law, Herr *Theodor W., Schacksdorf über Sorau-Lausitz,* even though your registration dates only from 22 January 1943. Of course I am willing to submit intermediate reports to you.
>
> At the same time, I thank you for your interest in our clinic and attach two special publications for your information.
>
> With collegial greetings and Heil Hitler!
>
> Yours   Voeller

I will send the original letter to Daddy, as well as the two special publications, which I will read first. One publication is for a general readership: "The Social Significance of the Italo-Bulgarian Cure Carried out at the Queen Elena Clinic in Kassel"; the other is scientific: "Pharmacology and Expanded Therapeutic Measures in the Italo-Bulgarian Cure," both by Med. and Dent. Dr. Walther Voeller. Hopefully Daddy will soon be able to [one word unreadable] to Kassel; he will probably be called up. Maybe I will write Daddy today. Now I want to read this letter over one more time. Once again it contains all kinds of things, but please, please, little Mother, don't worry about me because of last night's bombing or in the future; it may be even worse where you are!! All my warmest wishes go to hoping that nothing should happen to you and me, *because "the two of us" must remain invulnerable — for "the two of us"!! In this heartfelt hope, I hug you very, very lovingly, my dearest Mommy, thank you again for all your love — and kiss, kiss, kiss you most fervently — your healthy, cheerful, forever faithful and good Fritz-Daddy-Pa.*

This afternoon at 2:15 I am going to the next village (with Florian) for injections.

Doc. 11

Letter no. 50   (17a) Res. hospital Bruchsal, 23 June 1944
                                   Nerve damage section

My dearest Mommy!!

Fifty letters each quarter = two hundred letters a year! That's not too many! It is *Friday evening, 10:30.* I just managed to post the last letter with the 10:05 train to Heidelberg-Frankfurt—right to the mail conductor who dispatched the train. Maybe you will have it by tomorrow. No. 50 is going to be the weekend letter, and since it isn't the weekend yet, I'll only start it. I'm going to throw myself down and sleep in a moment. Are you coming too? Please!!! Off to bed!! Sleep well, my dear, undisturbed!!! *Dearest kissies!! Good night!!*

Saturday, 24 June 1944/7:15 A.M.: Good morning, my good Mommy!! Slept excellently again—with no disturbances. You too? The weather is also good again—so nothing stands in the way of a pleasant weekend. But first, a few hours of work. What will be the result of the Berlin meeting? And when are your strawberries coming? I hope I can answer both questions by this afternoon! And now—to work!!

Warmest kissies!! Ahoy!!

2:25: Weekend!!! Dearest, best Mommy, as a weekend greeting, in front of me on the table, beaming and resplendent, in glowing, delightfully smiling beauty and savor, a bowl full of sugared Mommy-strawberries!! If you were here in person, you would be totally squashed!!! Much, much more squashed than your lovely strawberry basket, from which I licked the first drops of juice when I came home at 1:30. It dripped more when I picked up the basket to unpack it immediately. Anyway, it came this morning and was already on the chair in my room with four or five drops of strawberry juice beneath it. *And not only that, but somebody had been pinching them!!* As I reimbursed him the 20-pfennig delivery fee, young Herr Beerweiler, who was standing out here in the hall, told me right away that the basket had been *opened!!* And in fact, some pig of a thief had bent up the cardboard cover on the end and *pinched one or two handfuls of strawberries* (theft of food, not robbery!!). This is most likely permitted in the fifth year of war, and one can't do anything about it!! However, the thief "generously" left me the lion's share!! I hurriedly untied the basket and saw that some of the strawberries were already pretty mushy. I immediately got a medium-sized glass bowl from downstairs and peeled off the stems. I had to throw away only a few strawberries. I devoured a good handful immediately, since they were very soft, and the good ones ended up tidily in the glass bowl—by far the larger part, the bowl is full!! Then I crumpled the paper in which the strawberries had been packed—all full of juice as it was—and placed the basket in the sun on the window sill to dry. I went right away to the delicatessen across the street and bought myself a half pound of granulated sugar. This took the 200-gram sugar ration coupon and the 25-gram jam coupon from the seven-day card. In addition, I got 60 grams of cheese spread and 50 grams of (hard) salami sausage slices. I immediately sugared the wonderful strawberries, and the sugar is just melting. *Delicious, the glass bowl looks so delicious!! I am already sooooo hungry for it!!! And now come very close to me, you dear good Mommy, and have as many Pa-kisses as the strawberries you sent — or even more!! As many as you want, I'm not stingy!! You couldn't have started my weekend more pleasantly!! It is so wonderfully lovely and sweet of you!!! Thank you!!! Thank you!!! Thank you!!! Kissies! Kissies!!*

And now the *Berlin meeting: Meseritz-Obrawalde* is the one being considered!! Around 10:30 came the call from Dr. Borm,†* and the line was very good. The directorial position in *Graz* for which I am definitely designated will not be filled *until after the end of the war.* But *Meseritz-Obrawalde is to be filled as soon as possible, and they may ask me to go there "for now."* Dr. Borm could not give me any more details on the structure of the facility or whether I am being considered for director of the planned hospital. He said it could be discussed in more detail at the conference in Vienna.‡ The K.d.F.‖ had no papers on my application, and no résumé; they had probably been destroyed in the bombing, and therefore Herr Blankenburg# had asked him to get in touch with me about sending a résumé. Blankenburg is apparently going to the provincial administration in *Stettin* shortly, and will recommend me. Well, good, that may happen, but *still* I have neither applied for Meseritz-Obrawalde in writing to any office, nor have I agreed to go there. So I can still reject the "appointment." I won't commit myself, in any case, until the question of overall director or merely department head is cleared up; and besides, we *both* will look at everything in person first!! I will stand by these principles at any possible discussions in Vienna!!

3:15: I just listened to the *Wehrmacht report* downstairs and polished off one cup of coffee and cake. *Cherbourg* is as good as lost, even if

---

* Killing facility in Pomerania.

† Dr. Kurt Borm, first a euthanasia doctor in the Sonnenstein-Pirna killing facility headed by Professor Nitsche near Dresden; starting in late summer of 1941, adjutant to his boss, who had since risen to become medical director of the Berlin euthanasia administration.

‡ Conference of a number of euthanasia consultants in Vienna 3–5 July 1944.

‖ Kanzlei des Führers, Führer's Office.

Werner Blankenburg, Viktor Brack's representative (see Doc. 1) at the Führer's Office, responsible for nonmedical euthanasia personnel.

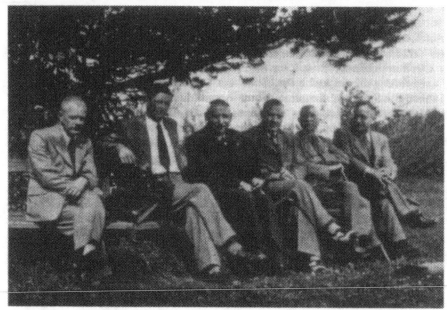

A commission of T-4 consultants on the road. *Left to right:* Erich Bauer (the driver), Dr. Lonauer, Dr. Ratka, Dr. Mennecke, Professor Nitsche, and Dr. Wischer.

our defense nests are still fighting at the enemy's rear; they will soon be snuffed out. Our lines have been *penetrated* in Italy and the central section in the East! It is heart-breaking!! Our luck in battle is gone!?! Bombs on *Bremen*. Additional long-distance bombardment from London. What will happen? Everything is coming to a head in gigantic leaps!! Will the final decision come in the next three months?

That is precisely the reason I am delaying the question of changing facilities; there is no big hurry at the moment!! I am anticipating these things *cold-bloodedly,* and will not push anything myself. I'll learn more in Vienna. In any case, I will return immediately to Bühl from Vienna; so I definitely won't go directly to Meseritz or Graz. First I want to discuss everything with you at leisure, and then we will see if we should go to Meseritz together.

Regarding the Vienna conference, Dr. Borm told me a room had been reserved for me at the *Hotel Astoria, Vienna, Sührich-Gasse* * for the two nights of 3–4 July and 4–5 July, that vacation had been requested for

* It should read "Führichgasse."

me for 2–7 July incl., and that I would be picked up at 8:00 in the morning by car on 4 July, along with the other gentlemen who will be staying at the Hotel Astoria. That was all we discussed on the telephone. Herr Allers* is in Italy at the moment, not as a soldier, but on Operation business. A special delivery letter containing the above information re: the Vienna conference is on its way to me. . . .

4:50: *Oh, dearest Mommy, if you had only been here in the last quarter hour and had seen and heard (!!!) how I feasted on the lovely strawberries, you would certainly have experienced pure Mommy-joy!! I sat before my bowl of strawberries like a little boy, looking alternately at the strawberries and your picture in front of me — and gorging myself at the same time!!* But I have not yet managed to polish them all off. I'm leaving some for this evening—and I look forward to them already, although my stomach is full for now. Strawberries are like asparagus, the kings of their species—*and I place you at their side, "you in your species!!" I can munch you as well as these sweet strawberries! Ha-ha!! I did much too little of that eight days ago, but just wait till you're here in fourteen days!!!* Now I am going downstairs to listen to the 5:00 news and read a little—and then I'm going to a concert at Professor Voss'! What a wealth of weekend joys!! Is this war? The fifth year of war??

Kissies! Ahoy!! . . .

10:50 P.M.: Beg to report: *all strawberries polished off!! Oh, did they taste good!!* I just put aside the empty glass bowl. I took a walk earlier, and at a quarter to ten took a seat downstairs in the restaurant with Chief Paymaster Breuning and Angerbauer, and had a pleasant conversation with them, accompanied by a pot of tea. At another table sat Chief Medical Officer Bopp with a large group of ladies: his wife (a doctor), two daughters (15 and 17 years old), Fräulein Klein (our T.A.)† and Fräulein Jantz (our dietitian's assistant). The same group also sat in a row in front of me at the concert. Frau Bopp is a typical female doctor, around 40 years old; they had children late. Our new secret weapon is called *V-1*, have you heard? When are the next ones going to follow, up to V-100? By the time these V-100's are deployed, the world will already have ended!!! Now I'm

---

* Dietrich Allers, manager of the euthanasia organization at 4 Tiergartenstrasse in Berlin (T-4). Following prisoner revolts in the Treblinka and Sobibor extermination camps (August and October 1943), the gassing personnel were transferred to Istria to murder Jews, partisans, and followers of Mussolini's successor, Marshal Pietro Badoglio, who was fighting on the side of the Allies. This explains Mennecke's formulation, "in Italy . . . on Operation business."

† Technical assistant.

going to sleep! A lovely "bolona" here and there!! Most fervent kisses!!
Good night!!!

It's *Sunday!!* The bells are ringing!! I'm still lying in bed, but I've
been awake for half an hour. It is *Sunday, 25 June 1944, 8:15 A.M.*. I have
undarkened and opened the windows, and through the fresh, sunny summer Sunday air I call out the most fervent *good-morning-greetings* to you
from my bed, dearest Mommy!!! Are you working already? How blissful
the night was again!! No disturbances, just a sound, deep, and refreshing
sleep from 11:45 to 7:45: seven hours! I woke up by myself and read a
couple of pages of *Bodelschwingh* until just now. But I'll get up in a
moment!! I am lying here on my left side, my left arm propped up and
the writing pad on the edge of the bed—still covered—but I'm going to
jump up right away, on the double!!! First some more sweet kissies from
Daddy's bed!!! *Up!! Ahoy!!*

9:05: Ready to go!! Freshly washed and clean, I take on the solo
Sunday! First I'll coax two boiled eggs from it for breakfast; I would rather
eat them before they go bad. Then I'll go to H. Sch. Sch.* to see whether
any mail has come—and then we shall see! Once again I broadcast *loving
kissies* to you at your laboratory bench!! *Ahoy!!* . . .

5:00: *Wehrmacht Report: Cherbourg* is as good as gone!! Ship sinkings and hits! Heavy destructive fire on *London* and its suburbs! Italy:
unchanged. In the East: heavy pressure!! *Bremen* terrorized, bombs
around *Berlin,* 59 shot down. Difficult situation in *Finland!* The *Daily
Mail* admits that the V-1 is hard on the British!! Now I will get going
again! See you this evening!!

Kissies!! Ahoy!! . . .

10:10 P.M.: The final "Brusel† Sunday" is ending, dear heart! I'm
sitting again on my camp bed by the window, and I just turned on the
light; we still have a little time before blackout. I just had my "ten o'clock
snack," two slices of bread and salami and one bread-and-cheese, along
with one glass of beer. I can't hear the news downstairs, as the radio is
broken. But nothing new will have happened. The "K.d.F.‡ program" in
the auditorium was very, very nice! It was neither an operetta nor an evening of Lehàr, but a *Lortzing opera evening.* It was put on by (1) an an-

---

* Hans Schemm School, named for the founder of the Nazi Teachers' Association, who
died in 1935.

† Mennecke meant Bruchsal.

‡ *Kraft durch Freude* ("Strength Through Joy"), a Nazi recreational organization.

nouncer of quality who only spoke in verse, (2) a chamber singer as the bass, (3) a good stage singer as the soprano, and (4) a second chamber singer as the tenor—and (5) a very good pianist. There was a "survey of Lortzing's operas" which I enjoyed in particular: Waffenschmied, Zar and Zimmermann, Undine, Wildschütz. All the concise arias from these four operas were performed to perfection. "Father, mother, sister, brother . . ." is a tenor aria after all, not a bass! I really got my money's worth. Afterwards I talked for a long time with Chief Med. Off. Bopp. In addition to general conversation about art, politics, etc., I brought him greetings from Chief Med. Off. Waltz, and we decided that I will go next Friday. Thus, I am going to break camp in the hospital here next Thursday, and travel to Bühl in a suitable train on Friday; I'll write to you on the train. In any case, by Friday evening I will be in Bühl. So I still have four days in Busel. And eight days from today, I will be back here to take the *12:40 A.M. train* to *Vienna*.

It is now 10:30 P.M. and I have to observe the blackout—too bad, the evening air is so lovely! I'm going to read this letter over again, then crawl into bed and read myself to sleep. But I want to close this letter now, and just add the morning greeting tomorrow morning. *The whole day today I was very much with you* in spirit, dearest Evali—and I still am, at this moment!! I hope you didn't have any problems at the Eichberg!! I'm so looking forward to your next letter!! Now I hug you lovingly and press you very tightly to me. I caress and kiss you good night; a "bolona," fervent and loving—and I know you're doing the same in spirit to

Your sooo good, forever dear and faithful Fritz-Daddy-Pa.

Notes

1. See Ulrich Schultz, "Soziale und biographische Bedingungen medizinischen Verbrechens," in *Medizin und Nationalsozialismus: Tabuisierte Vergangenheit — ungebrochene Tradition? (Dokumentation des Gesundheitstages Berlin 1980,* vol. 1), ed. Gerhard Baader and Ulrich Schultz (Berlin, 1980), pp. 184–201; see also Charles Roland, Henry Friedlaender, and Benno Müller-Hill, eds., "Medical Science without Compassion: Past and Present" (Proceedings of Fall Meeting, Cologne, 28–30 September 1988; photocopied and distributed 1992).

2. Hermann Langbein, " . . . *wir haben es getan": Selbstporträts in Tagebüchern und Briefen, 1939–1945* (Vienna, 1964), p. 15.

3. See Hans-Ludwig Siemen, *Das Grauen ist vorprogrammiert: Psychiatrie zwischen Faschismus und Atomkrieg* (Giessen, 1982), p. 14ff. See also Christian Pross, "Militärpsychiatrische Untersuchungen an KZ-Überlebenden und Panikpersonen im Dienste des Zivilschutzes," paper presented to Discussion Group 4 of the Sixth Con-

gress of International Physicians for the Prevention of Nuclear War (IPPNW), Cologne, 30 May 1986.

4. Doc. 6 of the complete edition.

5. Doc. 4 of the complete edition.

6. See Michael H. Kater, "Professionalization and Socialization of Physicians in Wilhelmine and Weimar Germany," *Journal of Contemporary History* 20 (1985): 677–701.

7. According to Michael H. Kater, within the Nazi "elite" of academic professions, businessmen, higher civil servants, white-collar workers, and students, in 1930–32 students represented the largest single group among party members with higher educational degrees or functions. See Michael H. Kater, *The Nazi Party: A Social Profile of Members and Leaders, 1919–1945* (Oxford, 1983), p. 250.

At German universities, the National Socialist German Students' Union (NSDStB) was even more popular than the Nazi party. Thus, by 1931 the National Socialists had already seized power in the umbrella organization, the Deutsche Studentenschaft (German Student Body). See Michael H. Kater, *Studentenschaft und Rechtsradikalismus in Deutschland, 1918–1933: Eine sozialgeschichtliche Studie zur Bildungskrise in der Weimarer Republik* (Hamburg, 1975), pp. 120, 140, 170–73; see also Konrad H. Jarausch, *Deutsche Studenten, 1800–1970* (Frankfurt am Main, 1984), p. 152ff.

8. See Kater, *Studentenschaft*, p. 43ff.

9. There are 14 letters of application in the complete edition (Docs. 3, 4, 9–19).

10. On this occasion, Mennecke's certification as a specialist in neurology and psychiatry was also "taken care of" by the top euthanasia consultant, Professor Heyde (see Doc. 63 of the complete edition).

11. See Angelika Ebbinghaus, "Kostensenkung, 'Aktive Therapie,' und Vernichtung: Konsequenzen für das Anstaltswesen," in *Heilen und Vernichten im Mustergau Hamburg,* ed. A. Ebbinghaus, H. Kaupen-Haas, and K. H. Roth (Hamburg, 1984), pp. 136–46, esp. 141–45. See also Siemen, *Das Grauen,* pp. 14–63 and 154–66, and Benno Müller-Hill, *Tödliche Wissenschaft: Die Aussonderung von Juden, Zigeunern, und Geisteskranken, 1933–1945* (Reinbek, 1984), p. 46f.

12. See Christine Teller, "Die 'aktivere Heilbehandlung' der 20er und 30er Jahre: z.B. Hermann Simon und Carl Schneider," in *Fortschritte der Psychiatrie im Umgang mit Menschen: Wert und Verwertung des Menschen im 20. Jahrhundert* (36th Gütersloh Continuing Education Week), ed. Klaus Dörner (Rehburg-Loccum, 1984), pp. 33–55.

13. Doc. 243 of the complete edition.

14. Doc. 238 of the complete edition.

15. *Frankfurter Rundschau,* 1 February 1947.

16. Doc. 330 of the complete edition.

17. Doc. 139 of the complete edition.

18. Doc. 132 of the complete edition.

19. Doc. 238 of the complete edition.

20. See Margret Mahler, *Symbiose und Individuation* (Stuttgart, 1972), p. 13ff.; Melanie Klein, *Das Seelenleben des Kleinkindes* (Hamburg, 1972).

21. Doc. 290 of the complete edition.

22. See Klaus Theweleit, *Männerphantasien,* 2 vols. (Frankfurt am Main, 1977).

23. Doc. 380 of the complete edition.

24. Doc. 386 of the complete edition.

25. Doc. 356 of the complete edition.

26. Doc. 362 of the complete edition.
27. Doc. 139 of the complete edition.
28. Doc. 186 of the complete edition.
29. Doc. 219 of the complete edition.
30. Doc. 77 of the complete edition.
31. Doc. 68 of the complete edition.
32. Doc. 87 of the complete edition.
33. Doc. 182 of the complete edition.
34. Doc. 191 of the complete edition.
35. Doc. 152 of the complete edition.
36. Doc. 313 of the complete edition.

Chapter 1 has been adapted from "Nazi Doctors, German Medicine, and Historical Truth," in *The Nazi Doctors and the Nuremberg Code: Human Rights in Human Experimentation,* edited by George J. Annas and Michael A. Grodin. Copyright © 1992 by Oxford University Press, Inc. Reprinted by permission.

Chapter 2 originally appeared in German in *Beiträge zur Nationalsozialistischen Gesundheits- und Sozialpolitik,* vol. 1, *Aussonderung und Tod* (Rotbuch Verlag Berlin, 1985). Translated, re-edited, and reprinted by permission of author and publisher.

Chapter 3 originally appeared in German in *Beiträge zur Nationalsozialistischen Gesundheits- und Sozialpolitik,* vol. 4, *Biedermann und Schreibtischtäter* (Rotbuch Verlag Berlin, 1987). Translated, re-edited, and reprinted with permission of annotator and publisher.

Chapter 4 originally appeared in German in *Beiträge zur Nationalsozialistischen Gesundheits- und Sozialpolitik,* vol. 2, *Reform und Gewissen* (Rotbuch Verlag Berlin, 1985). Translated, re-edited, and reprinted with permission of author and publisher.

Chapter 5 is a heavily edited version of an interpretation written for an edition of the Mennecke letters, published by the Hamburg Institute for Social Research. Approximately one-third of the Mennecke letters have been located so far. This chapter originally appeared in German in *Beiträge zur Nationalsozialistischen Gesundheits- und Sozialpolitik,* vol. 4, *Beidermann und Schreibtischtäter* (Rotbuch Verlag Berlin, 1987). Translated, re-edited, and reprinted with permission of the annotator and the publisher.

Library of Congress Cataloging-in-Publication Data

Aly, Götz, 1947–
     Cleansing the fatherland : Nazi medicine and racial hygiene / by Götz Aly, Peter Chroust, and Christian Pross ; translated by Belinda Cooper ; foreword by Michael H. Kater.
         p.   cm.
     Consists primarily of edited translations of articles which originally appeared in German in the journal: Beiträge zur Nationalsozialistischen Gesundheits- und Sozialpolitik.
     Includes bibliographical references.
     ISBN 0-8018-4775-3 (hc : alk. paper). — ISBN 0-8018-4824-5 (pbk. : alk. paper)
     1. Human experimentation in medicine—Germany—Moral and ethical aspects.
2. Medical policy—Germany—History—20th century. 3. Eugenics—Germany—History—20th century. 4. World War, 1939–1945—Atrocities. 5. World War, 1939–1945—Medical care. 6. National socialism—Moral and ethical aspects.
I. Chroust, Peter. II. Pross, Christian. III. Title.
     [DNLM: 1. Concentration Camps—history—Germany—collected works.
2. History of Medicine, 20th Cent.—Germany—collected works. 3. War Crimes—history—Germany—collected works. 4. Human Experimentation—history—Germany—collected works. 5. Ethics, Medical—collected works. W 50 A477c 1994a]
R853.H8A42 1994
174'.28—dc20
DNLM/DLC
for Library of Congress   93-42564

Printed in the USA
CPSIA information can be obtained
at www.ICGtesting.com
LVHW101559291123
764733LV00006B/24